Radiology of Orthopedic Implants

Sanjeev Agarwal · Gaurav Jyoti Bansal
Editors

Radiology of Orthopedic Implants

Springer

Editors
Sanjeev Agarwal
Department of Trauma and Orthopaedics
University Hospital of Wales
Cardiff
United Kingdom

Gaurav Jyoti Bansal
Cardiff and Vale University Health Board
Cardiff
United Kingdom

ISBN 978-3-030-09378-5 ISBN 978-3-319-76009-4 (eBook)
https://doi.org/10.1007/978-3-319-76009-4

Softcover re-print of the Hardcover 1st edition 2018

This Springer imprint is published by Springer Nature, under the registered company Springer International Publishing AG
The registered company address is: Gewerbestrasse 11, 6330 Cham, Switzerland

To our parents—Rekha and Dev,
Padam and Ramesh
For all what you have done

Preface

The idea for this book owes its provenance to our weekly combined orthopaedic–radiology multidisciplinary meetings. We realised that discussions around radiographs of orthopaedic implants were not accompanied with the usual adroitness of non-implant radiographs and scans.

The array of orthopaedic implants is bewildering, to orthopaedic specialists and radiologists alike, and continues to proliferate. Combining the historical implants, the range of metalwork used by orthopaedic surgeons is so extensive that it is near enough impossible to catalogue the features of all the implants ever used.

The purpose of this book is to give the reader an insight into the radiological features of implants and to pick up any signs of impending failure. In many situations, the orthopaedic specialist who is familiar with the implant may be best placed to interpret the radiological findings. However, close working between radiologists and orthopaedic surgeons is of the essence. With increasing sub-specialisation in orthopaedics, a surgeon who operates on the knee may not be entirely comfortable with interpreting spine radiographs. Hence, the contributors to this book cover the whole range of orthopaedic and radiological specialties.

We hope this book helps improve interaction and promotes a common language between orthopaedic surgeons and radiologists.

Cardiff, UK

Sanjeev Agarwal
Gaurav Jyoti Bansal

Acknowledgement

The authors are greatly indebted to the contributors of this book. Each of them is an expert in their chosen field, and despite their busy schedules, they kindly set time aside for this project.

We are very grateful to Liz Pope and Julia Squarr from Springer for their support throughout the process.

Contents

List of Contributors

Sanjeev Agarwal University Hospital of Wales, Cardiff, UK

Sashin Ahuja University Hospital of Wales, Cardiff, UK

Gaurav Jyoti Bansal Cardiff and Vale University Health Board, Cardiff, UK

Vineet Bhat University Hospital of Wales, Cardiff, UK

Juliet Clutton University Hospital of Wales, Cardiff, UK

Abdul Gaffar Dudhniwala University Hospital of Wales, Cardiff, UK

Patrick Fielding University Hospital of Wales, Cardiff, UK

Mark Forster University Hospital of Wales, Cardiff, UK

Carlos Heras-Palou Pulvertaft Hand Centre, Derby, UK

Monier Hossain Wirral University Teaching Hospital, Wirral, UK

Vetri Sudar Jayaprakasam University Hospital of Wales, Cardiff, UK

Sridhar Kamath University Hospital of Wales, Cardiff, UK

Faiz Khan University Hospital of Wales, Cardiff, UK

James Lewis University Hospital of Wales, Cardiff, UK

Kiran Lingutla University Hospital of Wales, Cardiff, UK

Ashish Mahendra Glasgow Royal Infirmary, Glasgow, UK

Timothy Matthews University Hospital of Wales, Cardiff, UK

Devdutt Neogi University Hospital of Wales, Cardiff, UK

Anthony Perera University Hospital of Wales, Cardiff, UK

Ryan Trickett University Hospital of Wales, Cardiff, UK

Tamsin Wilkinson University Hospital of Wales, Cardiff, UK

1 Introduction to Skeletal Radiology

Gaurav Jyoti Bansal and Vineet Bhat

Orthopaedic surgery has developed tremendously over the last 100 years.

Many developments in associated specialities have resulted in a significant change to the practice of orthopaedic surgery. Three of these milestones were the development of anaesthesia, asepsis and radiology. Before considering the development of orthopaedics, it is befitting to consider these three disciplines.

Development of Anaesthesia

The first impetus to surgery came from the development of anaesthesia, which initiated following the discovery of nitrous oxide by Joseph Priestley in 1772. Nitrous oxide was initially used for recreational purposes. In 1799, British chemist Humphrey Davy suggested that nitrous oxide could be used for anaesthesia, but the idea was not pursued, and nitrous oxide continued to be used as 'laughing gas'.

Horace Wells, a dentist in the Unites States, used it for dental extractions and documented its utility as a pain-relieving agent. The gas was collected in an animal bladder and administered through a wooden tube. Wells had his own tooth extraction to prove its safety.

Subsequently, a demonstration was organised in 1815 at the Massachusetts General Hospital in Boston by Horace Wells. The patient was William Morton, also a dentist. However, the gas was not administered properly and failed to produce the desired effect. Diethyl ether, commonly known as ether, had been used by Crawford Long in 1842 for general anaesthesia, but this was not publicised.

Morton continued the search for a suitable anaesthetic agent and tried using ether on himself and his assistants. In 1846, in the same operating theatre, ether was used by William Morton as an anaesthetic for removal of a tumour from the neck. An ether-soaked sponge was used, and the patient inhaled through the sponge. The procedure was witnessed by medical professionals and was successful. Anaesthesia gained rapidly in popularity.

The administration of ether often led to vomiting in patients, and an alternative—chloroform—was tried by James Simpson, an obstetrician in Edinburgh in 1847. This became popular and was widely used. In 1885, the anaesthesia machine was patented. Improvements in equipment continued to make the administration safer and reliable. Intravenous anaesthetic agents were introduced in 1874, and spinal anaesthesia started in the 1890s.

G. J. Bansal (✉)
Cardiff and Vale University Health Board, Cardiff, UK

V. Bhat
University Hospital of Wales, Cardiff, UK
e-mail: vineet.bhat@wales.nhs.uk

S. Agarwal, G. J. Bansal (eds.), *Radiology of Orthopedic Implants*,
https://doi.org/10.1007/978-3-319-76009-4_1

However, asepsis was not established at the time, and profusion of surgical procedures subsequent to anaesthetic developments still resulted in poor outcomes for many patients.

Development of Asepsis

Asepsis has its origin from the work of Robert Koch (1843–1910) who proposed four postulates establishing the connection between infecting organism and infectious disease. He worked on linking tuberculosis with *Mycobacterium tuberculosis* and was awarded the Nobel Prize for medicine in 1905. Louis Pasteur, a scientist working in France, made significant improvements to the understanding of microbes and infection. His work helped to refute the theory of spontaneous generation and replace it with the germ theory, which links microbes with infection and contamination. He also recognised the ability of carbolic acid to reduce infections.

Joseph Lister, professor of surgery at Glasgow, was influenced by Pasteur's work and started using carbolic acid dressings for wounds in 1867 [1]. He also introduced handwashing, sterilisation of instruments and spraying of carbolic acid in operation theatres, which greatly reduced infection rates. In 1869, a spray of carbolic acid and local anaesthetic was devised. Lister is considered the 'father of antiseptic surgery'.

Further advances in asepsis came with the work of Scottish Surgeon William Macewen, who used steam to clean surgical instruments. He advocated instruments made entirely of steel, which could be heated to a high temperature for decontamination. Rubber gloves were introduced in the late 1890s, prior to which surgeons used to operate with bare hands. Laminar flow was introduced in the operation theatres with the pioneering work of Sir John Charnley in Wrightington, England. With modern techniques of asepsis, maintaining normothermia in the anaesthetised patient and the use of prophylactic antibiotics, infection rate in orthopaedic surgery is lower than ever before.

Development of Radiology

Radiology owes its origin to the work of Wilhelm Roentgen, a German physicist.

Roentgen was working with cathode ray tubes in 1895 and noticed fluorescence on a barium platinocyanide plate on one side of the tube. He placed different objects between the tube and the plate. When placing his wife's hand in the path of the rays, he observed an image of the hand, showing the shadows thrown by the bones of her hand and that of a ring she was wearing. This famous image was the first 'roentgenogram' ever taken. Because the nature of these rays was then unknown, Roentgen called them 'X-rays'. Later, Max von Laue and his pupils showed that they are of the same electromagnetic nature as light but differ from it only in the higher frequency of their vibration. X-rays had been observed by many others before Roentgen, but he was the first to interpret the results and realise the importance of the discovery. Roentgen received the Nobel Prize in 1901. The uptake of radiographic imaging was dramatically quick following this discovery, and within months, many hospitals had set up X-ray machines.

The next major step in radiology was the development of cross-sectional imaging. Dr Godfrey Hounsfield, an engineer in Middlesex, England, was trying to determine the contents of a closed box using X-rays projected from different directions. Instead of using photographic plate, he developed a computer, which could record multiple images. This work led to development of a computed tomography (CT) scanner, and in 1971, a CT scanner was installed at a hospital in Wimbledon, London.

Hounsfield shared the Nobel Prize in 1979 with Alan Cormack, who was a physicist in Cape Town, South Africa, and worked out the theoretical mathematics for cross-sectional imaging. The radiodensity scale used in CT scans is named after Hounsfield (Hounsfield Unit, HU) with air being −1000 HU, water is 0 HU and dense cortical bone is +1000 HU.

Nuclear magnetic resonance (NMR) was discovered by Felix Bloch and Edward Purcell for which they shared the Nobel Prize in 1952.

Magnetic resonance (MR) creates a strong magnetic field leading to magnetisation of small biological magnets (protons) within the nucleus of the hydrogen atom within the body. In the 1970s, medical application of this technology gave rise to magnetic resonance imaging (MRI). MRI uses harmless radio waves to change the steady-state orientation of protons. Radio waves are then detected to register the body's electromagnetic transmission. Lack of ionising radiation makes MRI superior to CT scan for many clinical applications. The first image of two tubes of water was produced by Paul Lauterbur at Stony Brook University, USA, and further work by Peter Mansfield of University of Nottingham, UK, led to both scientists sharing the Nobel Prize for medicine in 2003. Lauterbur was credited for using magnetic field gradients for spatial localisation that led to rapid acquisition of 2D images and Mansfield for the mathematical formalism. The actual work that won the prize was performed 30 years earlier in Stony Brook University, where Lauterbur was a professor of chemistry.

The first whole-body MR scanner was built by a Scottish Professor John Mallard [2] and his team in 1970 at the University of Aberdeen. In August 1980, they used this machine to produce the first clinically useful image of the chest, abnormal liver and secondary cancer in bones. This machine was later used at St Bartholomew's Hospital, UK, between 1983 and 1993, leading to widespread popularity of MRI.

Ultrasound (US) is a nonionising, noninvasive technique which is now widely used in orthopaedic practice. In 1794, Lazzaro Spallanzani was the first to study ultrasound physics by deducing that bats used ultrasound to navigate by echolocation. In 1826, Jean Daniel Colladon, a physicist, used an underwater church bell to calculate speed of sound through water. He proved that sound travelled faster through water than air. In 1880, Pierre and Jacques Curie discovered the piezoelectric effect, which is a basic principle of modern ultrasound.

Karl Dussik, neurologist and psychiatrist at the University of Vienna, is generally regarded as the first physician to use ultrasound for medical diagnosis (of brain tumours) in 1942. In 1948, George Ludwig, an internist, first described the use of ultrasound to diagnose gallstones. The use of ultrasound for obstetrics and gynaecology conditions was pioneered by Ian MacDonald in 1958.

Ultrasound can be used as a primary diagnostic tool and as an adjunct to other radiological modalities. Apart from its excellent diagnostic capabilities, ultrasound can also be used for joint aspirations, drainage of abscesses/collections and targeted biopsies. Musculoskeletal ultrasound can visualise superficial/deep soft tissues and can diagnose soft tissue abscesses, fasciitis, pyomyositis, bursitis and soft tissue tumours. Following implant or prosthesis surgery, the presence of metalwork makes it difficult to interpret CT and MRI imaging due to degradation of image quality. Ultrasound is less affected and can be helpful in evaluating fluid collections or joint effusions and can be used to guide aspiration for microbiological diagnosis.

Radioisotope scanning started in 1961, when Fleming produced the first bone scintigraphic image using strontium 85, which is a gamma ray-emitting radionuclide. On the basis of these scans, he was able to diagnose metastasis and fractures. The use of technetium-99-labelled methylene diphosphate was proposed by Subramanium and McAfee in 1971. This, along with high-technology gamma cameras, has vastly improved the application and utility of bone scanning.

Increasing research is being carried out to assess the usefulness of positron emission tomography (PET) in osteomyelitis, and the results are encouraging. The accuracy of PET in the diagnosis of musculoskeletal infections was 94% compared with 81% for combined bone and white blood cell scan [3]. A recent meta-analysis found PET to be the most accurate diagnostic modality for osteomyelitis.

Orthopaedic surgery could not develop without adequate anaesthesia, asepsis and radiology, and once these aspects were developed, the profusion of orthopaedic implants has been tremendous.

Development of Orthopaedic Implants

Various substances were tried for use as orthopaedic implants. Some—like gold, silver and aluminium—were not strong enough. Others like nickel and copper caused local reactions. In the late eighteenth century, two French surgeons, Lapejode and Sicre, used brass wire for cerclage wiring of long bone fractures. This is one of the earliest attempts at internal fixation using metalwork. In 1843, Malgaigne devised a claw-shaped metal instrument, which could be used to approximate the two fragments of patellar fractures.

One of the earliest pioneers of internal fixation was Albin Lambotte (1866–1955) from Belgium. He devised internal and external fixation methods and carefully kept records of his operations. He coined the term 'osteosynthesis' and is considered the 'father of modern fixation methods of the bone'.

Sir William Arbuthnot Lane, working at Guy's Hospital, London, devised methods to internally fix displaced fractures using wires and screws. He published his results in his book entitled *The Operative Treatment of Fractures* in 1905. He used aseptic techniques and specified dressings to reduce infection rate. He also used long steel plates fixed with screws for fracture fixation. Stainless steel had not been discovered, and Lane's implants were made of ordinary steel, which was prone to corrosion.

In 1912, William Sherman devised self-tapping fully threaded vanadium machine screws. He laid down exact dimensions for screw design, which were largely similar to the screws used in metal and wood industry. He also designed a plate for use with screws, which remained in use for nearly 50 years.

The development of orthopaedic implants was closely linked to improvements in metallurgy. Stainless steel with 12.8% chromium and 0.24% carbon was first made by Harry Brearley in 1913. In 1926, stainless steel was used for orthopaedic implants for the first time. In 1936, Venables and Stuck introduced cobalt-chrome alloy. Martin Kirschner, a German surgeon, devised steel wires for fixation, which remain in use even today.

Gerhard Kuntscher, working in Hamburg, Germany, developed the intramedullary nail. He used a hollow nail with a clover leaf cross section to achieve fixation in the medullary canal. His work was presented in 1940, but the Second World War delayed general knowledge and acceptance of his work. Prior to development of the nail, standard treatment of femoral shaft fractures involved traction and cast. A faster recovery was made possible with the use of nail and avoidance of casts.

Robert Danis, a Belgian surgeon, made design changes to the Sherman screws to adapt it for use in orthopaedics in 1940s. He also developed the compression plate and laid down the principles of internal fixation—accurate reduction, rigid fixation, early mobilisation and healing without callus formation—also known as healing by primary intention. One of his students—Maurice Muller—took his concepts and, along with his colleagues, formed the AO (*Arbeitsgemeinschaft fur Osteosynthesefragen*) group in Switzerland in 1958. The AO group was instrumental in advancing orthopaedic trauma management. Over the years, the AO group has continued to innovate and expand the armamentarium.

The development of hip replacements by John Charnley and knee replacement implants by Insall and Walker made these procedures reliable and immensely popular. The profusion of implants over the last three decades has been truly exponential, and the range of tools available to the orthopaedic surgeons today would have been unimaginable few decades back.

References

1. Lister J. On the antiseptic principle in the practice of surgery. Lancet. 1867;90:353–6.
2. Mallard J, Hutchison JM, Edelstein W, Ling R, Foster M. Imaging by nuclear magnetic resonance and its biomedical implications. J Biomed Eng. 1979;1(3):153–60.
3. De Winter F, Vogelaers D, Gennel F, Dierckx R. Promising role of 18-F-fluoro-D-deoxyglucose positron emission tomography in clinical infectious diseases. Eur J Clin Microbiol Infect Dis. 2002;21(4):247–57.

Hip Implants

2

Sridhar Kamath, Sanjeev Agarwal,
and Ashish Mahendra

Hip replacements became popular in the 1960s following pioneering work by Sir John Charnley at Wrightington, England. Over the last 50 years, there has been a profusion of various types of hip implants alongside the number of operations performed worldwide.

The radiological assessment of hip replacements is based on anteroposterior (AP) view of the pelvis and lateral view of the hip joint.

The parameters to note are:

1. AP pelvis radiograph:
   - Acetabular abduction angle
   - Distance of the acetabular component from the medial wall
   - Degree of covering/uncovering of the acetabulum
   - Cementation of the acetabular component
   - Femoral stem placement in the canal
   - Cementation of the femoral component and any radiolucencies in the cement mantle
   - Level of femoral neck cut
   - Leg length discrepancy
   - Periprosthetic fracture
   - Restoration of offset of the femur
2. Lateral view of the hip:
   - Acetabular version angle
   - Femoral stem placement in the canal—quality of cementation
   - Any impinging osteophytes along the anterior acetabular margin
   - Periprosthetic fracture
3. On long-term follow-up radiographs, note:
   - Evidence of loosening of the femoral/acetabular component
   - Wear of the acetabular liner—as evidenced by eccentric migration of the femoral head
   - Periprosthetic fracture
   - Stress shielding
   - Remodelling of the bone around the implant

The acetabular version is an important determinant of the stability of the hip. The version is the angle between the face of the acetabular component and the coronal plane of the patient. Most studies indicate the desired version is between 5 and 30°. Hip replacements done through a posterior approach are more reliant on adequate version to maintain stability.

The anteversion of the acetabular component gives the opening (equator) of the cup an elliptical appearance on the AP radiograph (Fig. 2.1). If the equator appears as a straight line, it implies that it is parallel to the radiographic beam and is in neutral alignment (Fig. 2.2).

S. Kamath (✉) · S. Agarwal
University Hospital of Wales, Cardiff, UK
e-mail: sridhar.kamath@wales.nhs.uk

A. Mahendra
Glasgow Royal Infirmary, Glasgow, UK

S. Agarwal, G. J. Bansal (eds.), *Radiology of Orthopedic Implants*,
https://doi.org/10.1007/978-3-319-76009-4_2

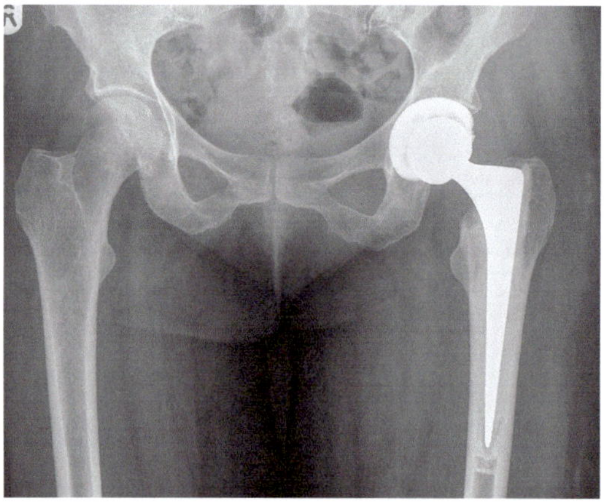

Fig. 2.1 Left total hip replacement with a cementless acetabular component and cemented femoral component. The equator of the acetabular component has an elliptical outline, as is desirable. The acetabular component has a polyethylene liner, and no screws were used for fixation of the acetabular shell into the pelvis

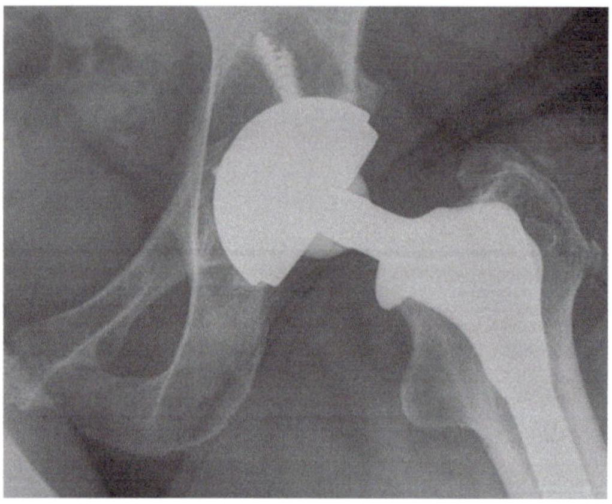

Fig. 2.2 The equator of the acetabular component has a nearly straight projection. This implies that the equator of the component is parallel to the beam and is in neutral version. Anterior or posterior tilt of the pelvis would also influence the projection of the acetabular component

A lateral radiograph is essential to accurately assess anteversion, as a retroverted acetabular component may appear similar to anteverted radiograph on the AP radiograph (Fig. 2.3a–c). The positioning technique for shoot-through lateral radiograph of the hip is demonstrated in Fig. 2.4. In this view, the angle between the equator of the acetabular component and a line drawn vertically represents the acetabular version. Methods to measure anteversion are described later in this chapter.

Hemiarthroplasty of the Hip

Hemiarthroplasty of the hip is replacement of the femoral head with a metal prosthesis. It is commonly done for displaced intracapsular fractures of the femoral neck in the elderly.

The mode of fixation of the implant to the femur depends on whether the implant is designed for use with or without cement. Examples of uncemented hemiarthroplasty are the Austin Moore and the Furlong Hemiarthroplasty (JRI Orthopaedics, Sheffield, UK). Cemented hemiarthroplasty includes Thompson's prosthesis.

In addition, hemiarthroplasty can be unipolar or bipolar. A unipolar prosthesis is made of a single block of metal without an inbuilt articulation—like the Austin Moore and the Thompson's prosthesis. These were widely used in the past few decades but have now largely been replaced with modern designs which allow better cementation/fixation and offer a wider range of stem sizes and offsets.

The Austin Moore prosthesis (Fig. 2.5) was designed by Austin T. Moore in early 1950s. It is inserted without cement, and the surface does not have any special coating to encourage bone ingrowth or ongrowth. It has two large fenestrations in the stem which theoretically allow the bone to grow through for stability, and a hole proximally which is to aid removal of prosthesis if required. The prosthesis has a collar which rests on the cut surface of the femoral neck and the calcar. Although widely used in the past, the use of this prosthesis is now largely historical as it provides inadequate fixation in the femur.

The Thompson prosthesis was introduced by Frederick Thompson at St. Luke's Hospital, New York, in the early 1950s. This is generally cemented (Fig. 2.6) although it can be inserted without cement in narrow femoral canals. It has a narrower and shorter stem than the Austin Moore prosthesis and does not have the holes in the stem. There is no hole proximally for extraction.

Currently used cemented hemiarthroplasty implants allow better cementing with the use of appropriately sized broaches to prepare the femoral canal (Fig. 2.7).

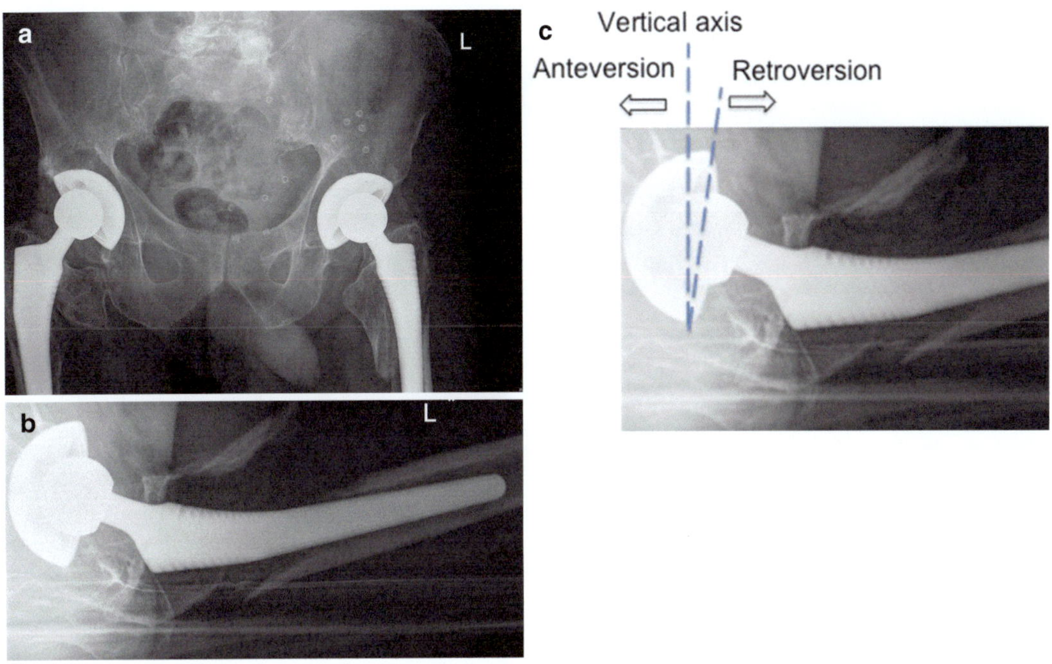

Fig. 2.3 (**a**) Bilateral cementless total hip replacement. On the right side, there was a previous periprosthetic fracture involving the lesser trochanter, which was managed nonoperatively. On the left side, there is a periprosthetic fracture involving the femoral shaft. The acetabular component on the left side appears to have an acceptable version. (**b**) A shoot-through lateral radiograph shows retroversion of the component. This illustrates the importance of shoot-through lateral radiograph in assessing anteversion. (**c**) Assessment of version on the shoot-through lateral radiograph of the hip. The image shows retroversion, while a tilt of the acetabular component on the other side of the vertical axis would denote anteversion

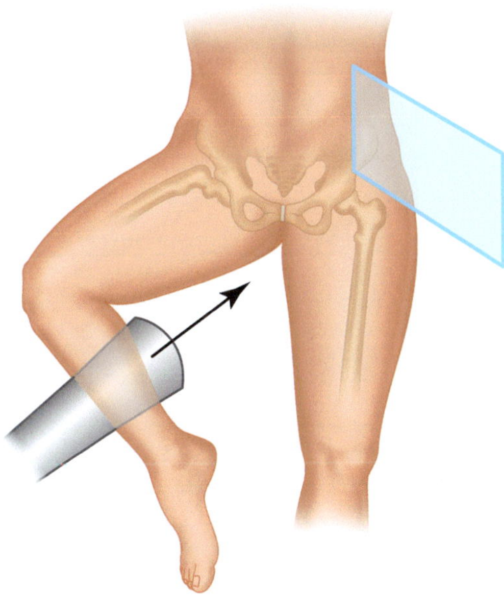

Fig. 2.4 The method for obtaining a shoot-through lateral radiograph

The bipolar prosthesis (Fig. 2.8) has an articulation within the head, which allows an additional interface for motion, hence reducing the motion at the metal articular cartilage interface. This may reduce erosion of the acetabular articular cartilage. The implant should match the natural anatomy of the patient as closely as possible.

Figure 2.9 shows a hemiarthroplasty placed in excessive anteversion. In the AP radiograph, the lesser trochanter is more prominent implying excess external rotation of the femoral shaft in the resting position. The offset appears reduced, and this is also due to the excess anteversion. This hemiarthroplasty implant has a bipolar design, which means there is an additional articulation with the femoral head. The excess anteversion led to anterior instability and required revision to a total hip replacement, whereby the version of the femoral stem was corrected.

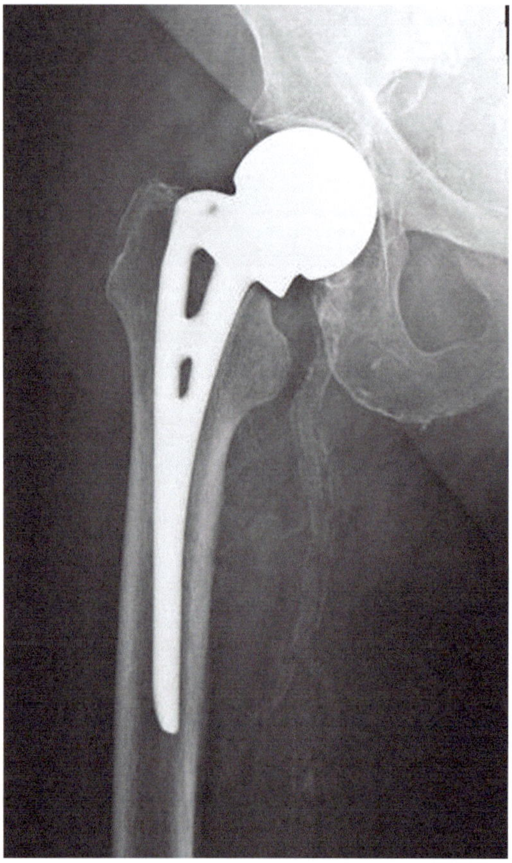

Fig. 2.5 The Austin Moore hemiarthroplasty prosthesis. The prosthesis is inserted without cement

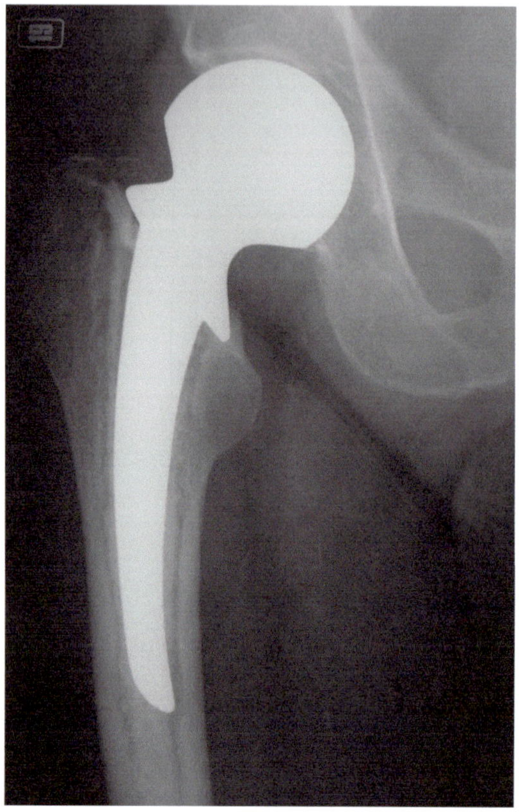

Fig. 2.6 The Thompson hip hemiarthroplasty prosthesis. This is a cemented prosthesis

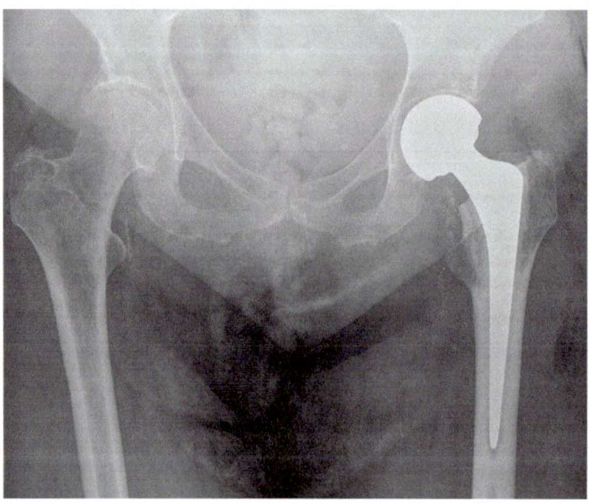

Fig. 2.7 A cemented monoblock (unipolar) hip hemiarthroplasty prosthesis. The prosthesis has a distal centraliser (lucency at the tip of the stem) and a cement plug (at the distal extent of the cement mantle) for obtaining a circumferential cement mantle

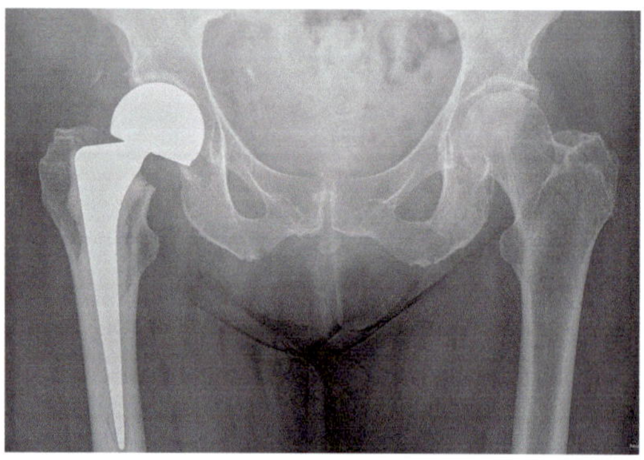

Fig. 2.8 A bipolar cemented hemiarthroplasty prosthesis. There is an additional articulation within the femoral head

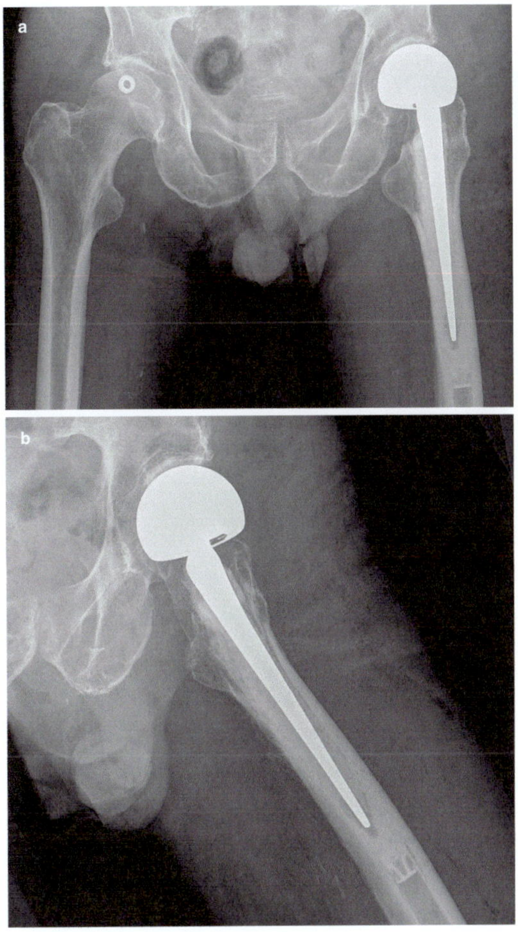

Fig. 2.9 AP (**a**) and attempted lateral (**b**) view of a left hip showing over anteversion of cemented bipolar hemiarthroplasty prosthesis. On both views, the lesser trochanter is more prominent

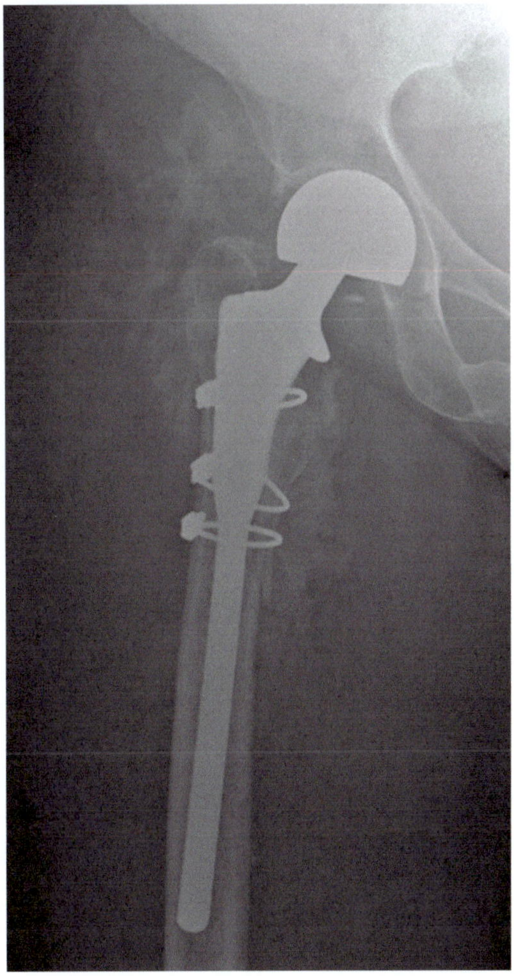

Fig. 2.10 A hydroxyapatite-coated long-stem bipolar hemiarthroplasty. This is the Furlong hemiarthroplasty (JRI, Sheffield, UK). The stem is longer than the standard stem, and this was used to manage the periprosthetic fracture at the proximal femur, which was around an uncemented Austin Moore prosthesis. This image was obtained 7 weeks following the revision operation and shows satisfactory alignment and callus formation. There is evidence of heterotopic ossification in the soft tissues

Modern cementless hemiarthroplasty components have a special coating on the surface which allows for bone integration—either through ingrowth or ongrowth of bone. An example is shown in Fig. 2.10 which shows a cementless hemiarthroplasty. The femoral stem has a hydroxyapatite coating on its entire surface below the collar of the stem, and this encourages bone ongrowth. Additionally, the proximal end of the stem has a taper on which a modular femoral head can be attached. The femoral head has a polyethylene articulation within it, and this allows movement at that interface. Femoral heads used in hemiarthroplasty with an additional articulation within them are referred to as bipolar heads.

Total Hip Replacement

Total hip replacement prostheses can have a cemented or cementless acetabular component and femoral component. Prostheses in which only one of the two components is cemented and the other is cementless are known as hybrid hip replacements.

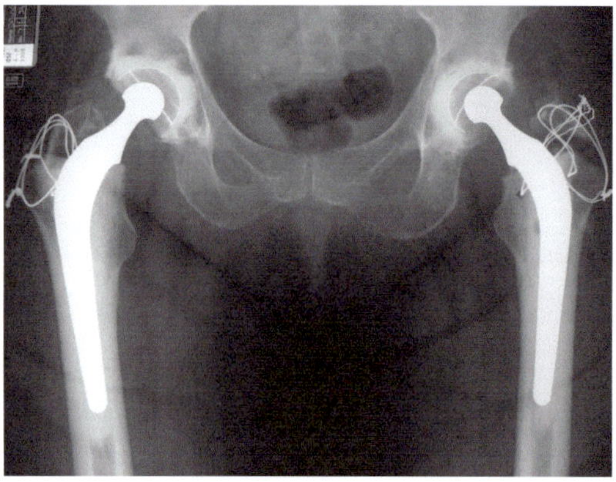

Fig. 2.11 Bilateral Charnley low-friction arthroplasty hip replacements. This implant has a cemented femoral component and a cemented acetabular component. Both operations were done through a trochanteric osteotomy, which has been fixed with wires. The wire markers in the acetabular component are helpful in assessing the alignment of the acetabular component. There is nonunion of the left trochanteric osteotomy fragment. The cement restrictor in this technique was a bone plug obtained from the cancellous bone of the proximal femur, and hence it is not clearly visible

The earlier designs of hip replacement were predominantly cemented—such as the Charnley low-friction arthroplasty (Fig. 2.11) and the Exeter hip replacement (Fig. 2.12). Charnley femoral stems are based on the principle of 'composite beam'' [1], which implies that subsidence of stem within the cement mantle is not intended, and represents loosening. On the contrary, the Exeter stems are based on 'sliding taper' principle, and the polished stems are expected to subside to a limited extent within the cement mantle (Fig. 2.13).

In earlier descriptions of the technique for hip replacement described by Charnley, the acetabular component was medialised to improve hip biomechanics and reduce the joint reaction force on the hip joint (Fig. 2.14). A hole was made in the medial wall where the reamers to prepare the acetabulum were seated. Prior to cementing, the hole was covered with a circular wire mesh. The approach for hip replacement was through a trochanteric osteotomy, which was fixed with wires at the end of the procedure. Current techniques no longer involve making the hole, and the acetabular component is placed at the level of the medial wall of the acetabulum or in a position to allow adequate superior coverage.

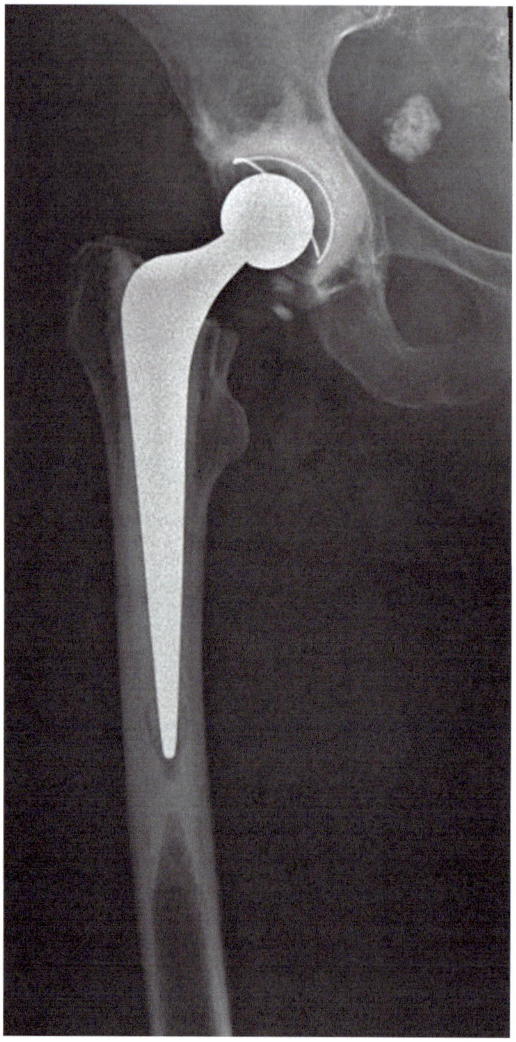

Fig. 2.12 A cemented total hip replacement. The femoral component in this hip has a polished surface, which allows subsidence within the cement mantle

The posterior lip augmentation device (PLAD) is a method to control recurrent dislocation of the hip in patients who are medically unwell to withstand revision surgery. It can only be used in all-polyethylene cemented cups which do not have a metal backing (Figs. 2.15 and 2.16). The device consists of a semicircular polyethylene component with a metal backing which is fixed to the acetabular component by five screws. The effect of the device is to increase the height of the posterior margin as well as a physical restraint, preventing posterior dislocation.

The zones of cementing around the femoral component were described by Gruen [2] and

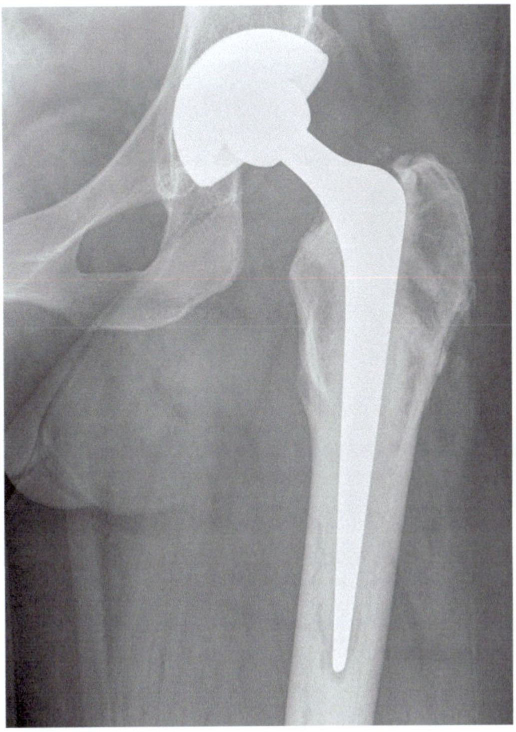

Fig. 2.13 Subsidence in a polished tapered stem. Radiolucency in zone 1 at the metal-cement interface represents subsidence of the stem. In a polished stem, this is expected and is not a cause for concern. This patient had fixation of the femoral neck fracture with cannulated screws prior to hip replacement. The screws were removed at the time of hip replacement, and there is ingress of cement in the screw holes

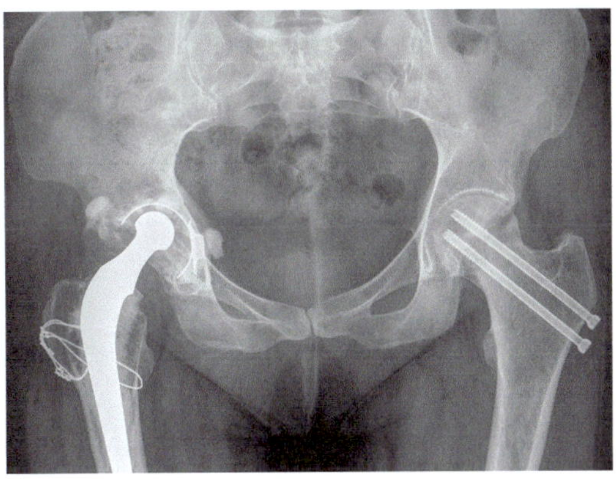

Fig. 2.14 A Charnley total hip replacement on the right side. There is evidence of cement in the pelvis, which has been pushed through the hole in the medial wall of the acetabulum at the time of pressurisation of acetabular cement. The wire mesh to cover the hole is visible against the medial wall. Note the superior migration of the femoral head within the acetabulum, which is due to eccentric wear of the polyethylene

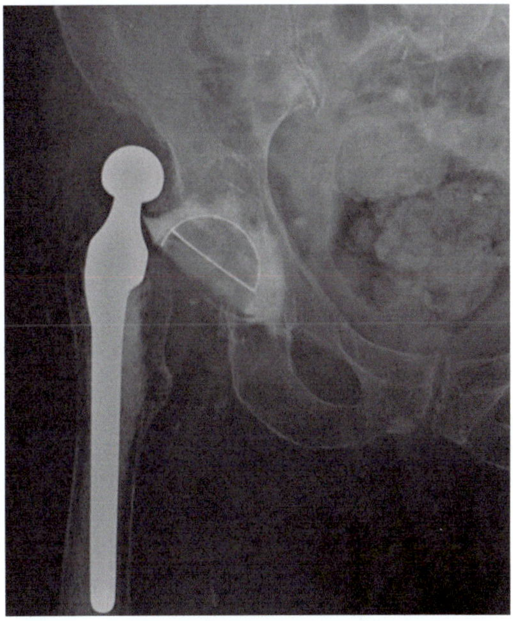

Fig. 2.15 A dislocated Charnley hip replacement with a cemented all-polyethylene acetabular component and a cemented femoral component

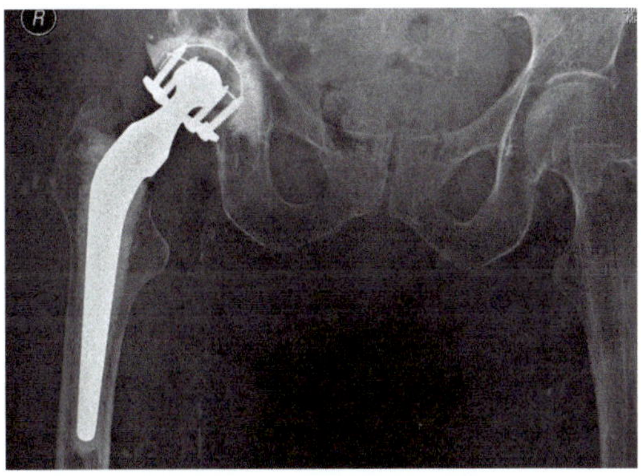

Fig. 2.16 The hip was reduced, and a PLAD was inserted to stabilise the hip. The polyethylene component is not visible radiographically, but the metal backing of the PLAD indicates its position on the acetabular component

those around the acetabulum by Charnley [3] (Figs. 2.17 and 2.18). Progressive radiolucency in these zones indicates loosening of the components. Absolute signs of loosening are progressive radiolucency at the cement bone interface seen on serial radiographs, migration of the component (Fig. 2.19a, b), fracture of the component or fracture of the cement mantle. Loosening of the femoral component appears as debonding

Fig. 2.17 Gruen zones to describe loosening around the acetabular component

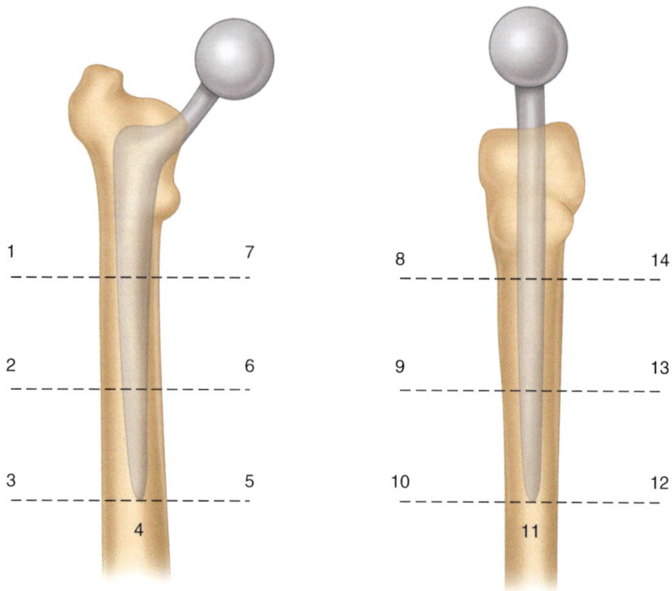

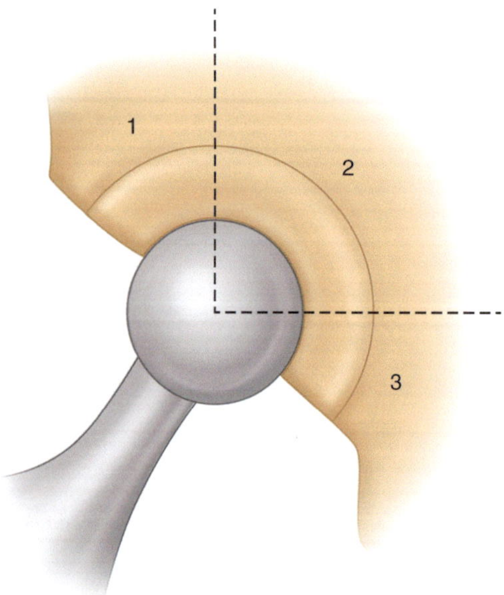

Fig. 2.18 DeLee Charnley zones to describe loosening around the femoral component

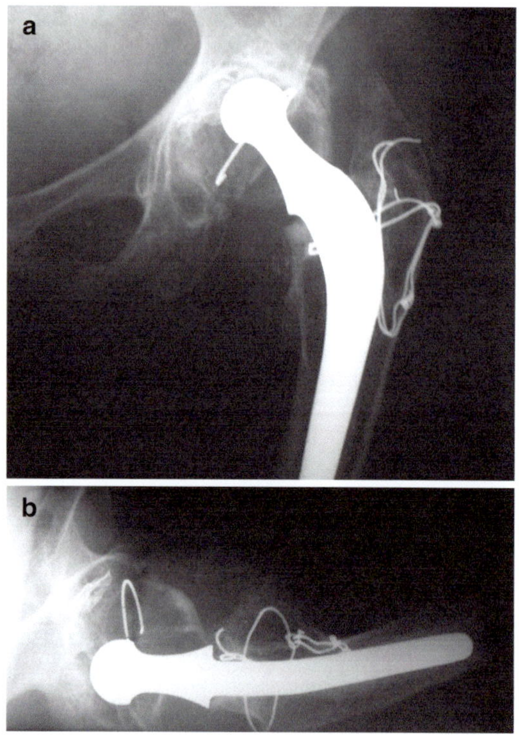

Fig. 2.19 AP radiograph (**a**) and lateral radiograph (**b**) of the pelvis showing displacement of the acetabular component outside the natural acetabulum. In the AP view, the round outline of the face of the acetabular component is visible. There is debonding of the femoral stem evidenced by the gap between the cement and the metal in zone 1—at the shoulder of the femoral stem. In the lateral view, the acetabular component can be seen anterior to the femoral head

(lucency at the cement metal interface at the shoulder of the femoral stem).

The all-poly cemented cups have a wire marker around the pole of the cup and often along

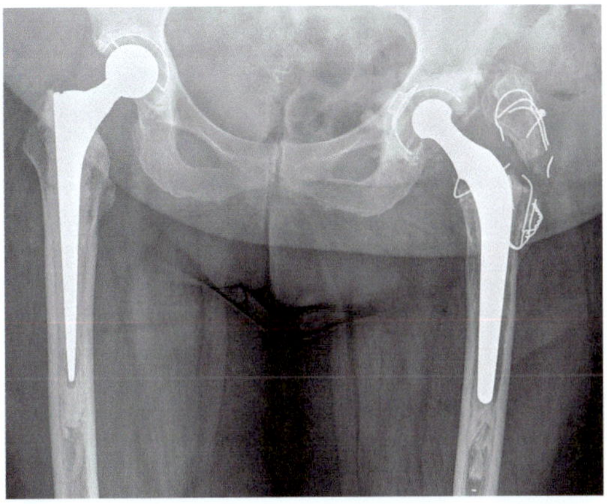

Fig. 2.20 Bilateral cemented total hip replacements. The surgical approach was through a trochanteric osteotomy for the left hip. The trochanter was wired back, but the fixation has failed. The trochanter has 'escaped'—proximal migration. There is wear in the superior part of the acetabulum, evidenced by reduced distance between the head and the wire marker superiorly, compared to the distance inferiorly. There is extensive osteolysis all along the stem of the femoral component. The acetabulum is not radiologically loose. On the right side, there is congruence of the femoral head and the acetabular wire marker

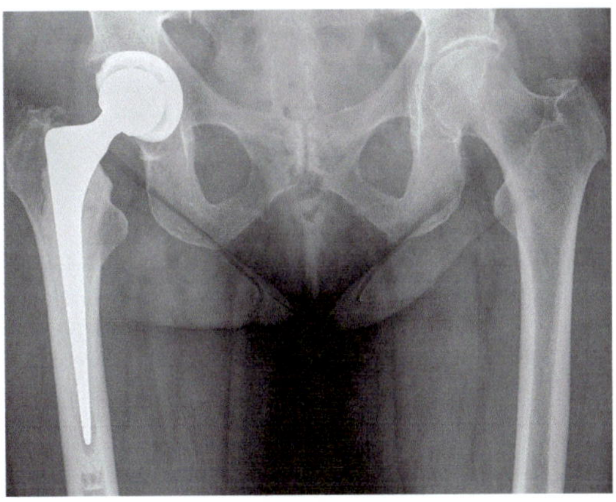

Fig. 2.21 A hybrid total hip replacement. The acetabulum is uncemented. On the femoral side, the stem is aligned with the femoral shaft, with good cementation. There are no voids in the cement mantle. This is grade A cementation

the face of the cup, which helps in assessing the alignment of the cup. Superior migration of the femoral head can also be assessed as a measure of wear of the polyethylene (Fig. 2.20).

Hybrid hip replacements have a cementless acetabular component and a cemented femoral component (Figs. 2.21 and 2.22). The grade of cementing around the femoral component was described by Barrack and Harris [4] (Table 2.1).

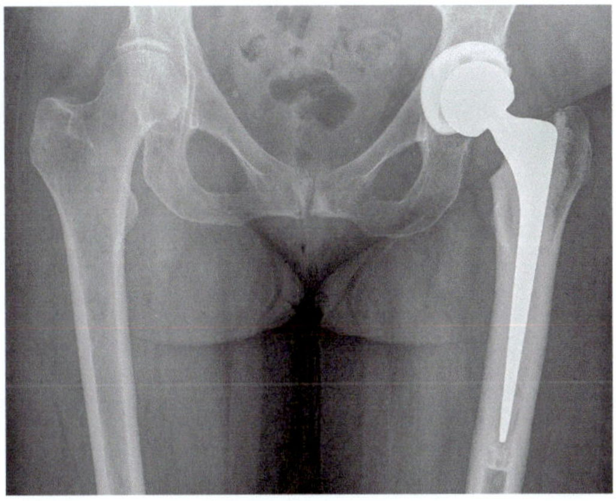

Fig. 2.22 A hybrid hip replacement similar to Fig. 2.21. Note the two small metal projections from the lateral margin of the acetabular component. These represent the locking mechanism, which holds the polyethylene within the metal acetabular shell. There are two small voids in the femoral cement mantle—one each in zones 2 and 3. These represent filling defects. Defects of this magnitude would not compromise the long-term survival of the femoral stem. This is grade B cementing

Table 2.1 Grades of femoral cementing

Grade A	Complete filling of the medullary cavity with cement. Also known as 'white out'
Grade B	Slight radiolucency of cement bone interface
Grade C	Radiolucency involving 50–99% of cement bone interface; or a defective or incomplete cement mantle
Grade D	100% radiolucency at cement bone interface in any projection; or failure to fill the canal with cement such that the tip of stem is not covered

Cementless hip replacements (Figs. 2.23 and 2.24) rely on primary stability, which is achieved by a press fit of the prosthesis and secondary stability, which is achieved by bone ingrowth or bone ongrowth. The prosthesis has a surface coating to encourage bone integration.

For stable fixation in cementless hips, firm primary stability and intimate host bone contact are desirable. Radiolucent lines along the metal-bone interface on the postoperative X-ray indicate inadequate contact (Fig. 2.25a). However, if the component is stable, the lucencies may resolve with progressive osseointegration (Fig. 2.25b).

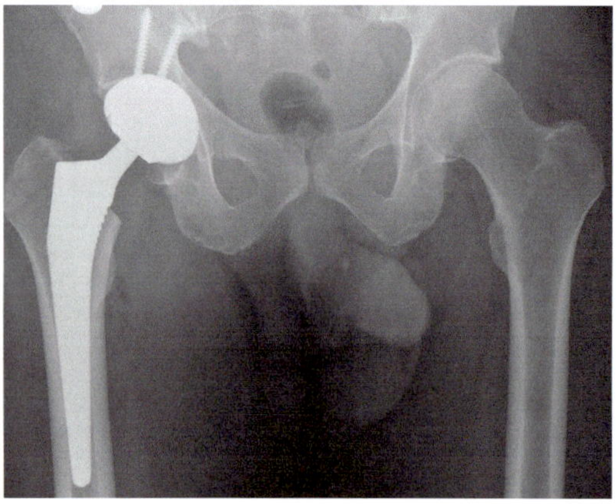

Fig. 2.23 Cementless total hip replacement. The acetabular component has two screws which help in primary stability of the acetabular shell, although screws are not always necessary. The femoral component fills the canal and has restored leg lengths and horizontal offset

Cementless augments can be used to fill defects in the acetabulum where there is extensive bone loss (Fig. 2.26). These are fixed into the pelvis with screws for primary stability, and bone integration leads to long-term stability.

Pedestals may form at the tip of cementless stems. These are bony trabeculae from the endosteum to the tip of the stem and may [5] or may not [6] be a sign of loosening of the stem (Fig. 2.27). Other signs of loosening of cementless femoral stems include radiolucent lines at the prosthesis bone interface (Fig. 2.28), calcar hypertrophy and poor implant-bone contact. Signs of well-fixed cementless stems (Figs. 2.29 and 2.30) are presence of spot welds, calcar atrophy and absence of radiolucency at the implant-bone interface. Spot welds are streaming trabeculae from the endosteum to the implant surface. The calcar participates in load bearing, but with a well-fixed stem, the load bearing bypasses the calcar, resulting in rounding or atrophy of the calcar.

Stress shielding in the proximal femur is seen where the load bypasses the proximal femur through an extensively coated stem. Cemented stems do not generally demonstrate clinically significant stress shielding. Bypassing the load can be minimised by using cementless stems which have a porous coating only in the proximal part (proximally coated stems). A thicker and consequently stiffer cementless stem is likely to cause more stress shielding. Variations in stem design have been tried to reduce stiffness and match the elasticity of the stem to that of the bone (Fig. 2.31). The elasticity of titanium is closer to that of cobalt-chrome, and hence titanium is the preferred material for cementless femoral stems.

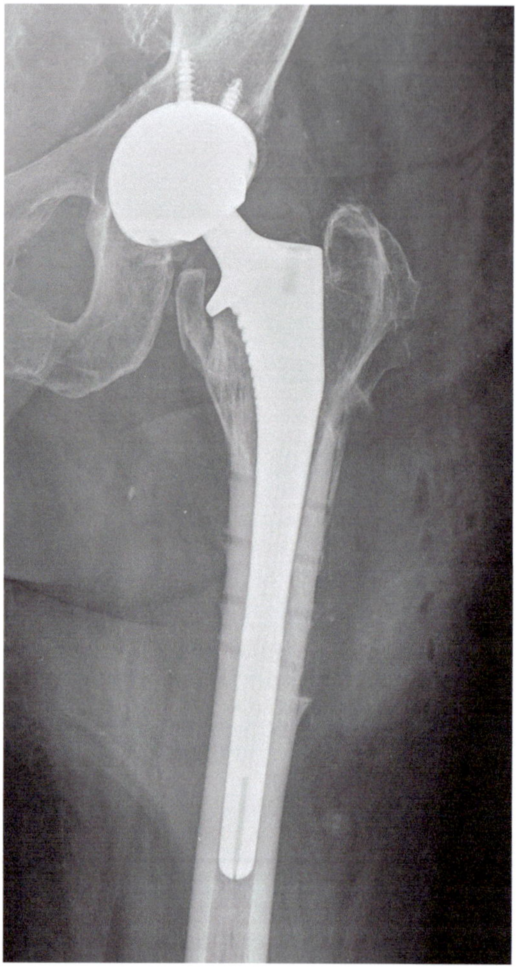

Fig. 2.24 Cementless total hip replacement after a failed dynamic hip screw. Evidence of previous metalwork is visible along the femoral shaft and proximal femur. The femoral stem bypasses the distal screw hole by two cortical diameters

The positioning of the acetabular component is important for stability, function and long-term survival of the prosthesis. The vertical (superior-inferior) positioning on the AP view is referenced from the teardrop. The medial margin of the acetabular component should be adjacent to the teardrop (Fig. 2.32).

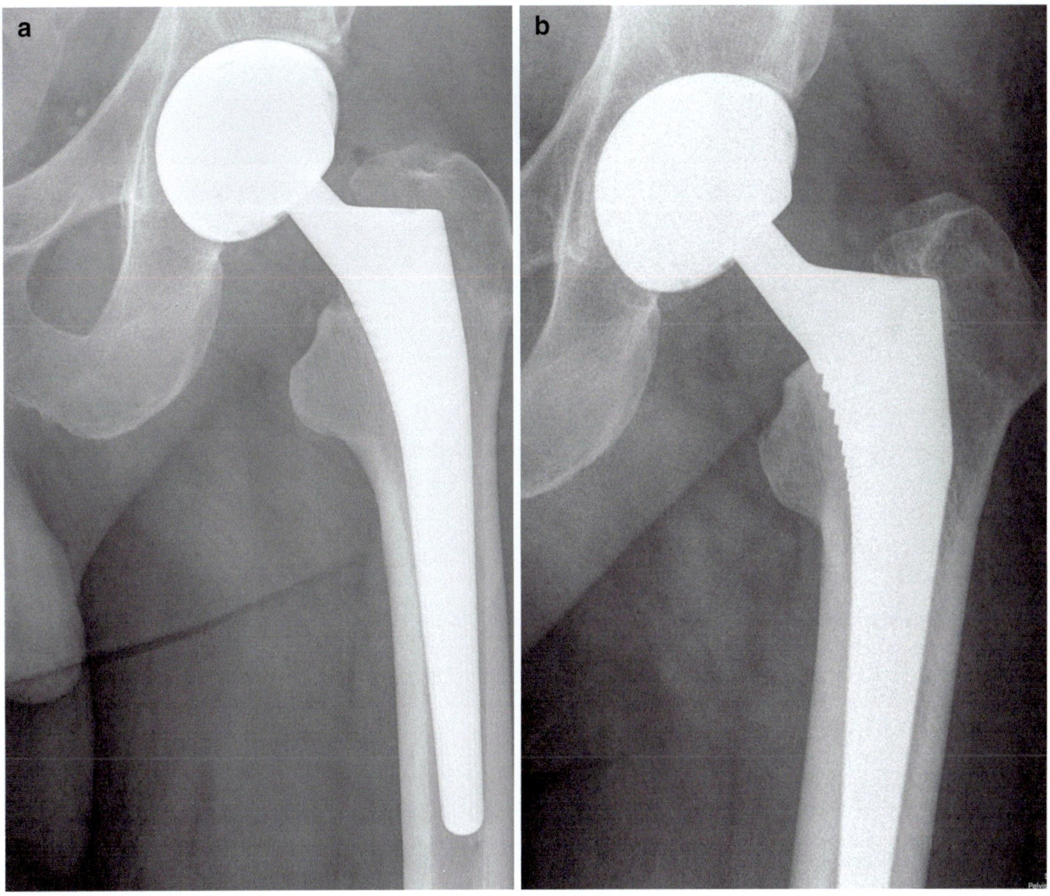

Fig. 2.25 Postoperative radiograph (**a**) of a cementless total hip replacement showing radiolucent line in zones 1 and 2 around the acetabular component. After 14 months (**b**), the lucency has disappeared with a well-fixed stable acetabular component. Osseointegration can lead to resolution of thin radiolucencies in stable cementless acetabular components

The version of the acetabulum can be described as radiologic, anatomic or operative version [7] (Fig. 2.33). Operative anteversion is the angle between the acetabular axis on the sagittal plane and the longitudinal axis of the patient. It is achieved by flexion of the acetabular component in relation to the transverse axis of the patient. Radiographic anteversion is the angle between the acetabular axis and the coronal plane. Anatomic anteversion is the angle between the acetabular axis and the transverse axis of the patient.

An estimate of anteversion (or retroversion) can be made on the AP radiograph. There are various methods (Fig. 2.34) described to measure anteversion on plain radiographs, and these are summarised in Table 2.2.

The shoot-through lateral view can be used to directly measure version [12]. A line is drawn along the face of the acetabular component in the lateral view and the angle which this makes with the vertical is the version of the cup (Figs. 2.35 and 2.36). This method will distinguish between anteversion and retroversion, which would not be possible with methods using only the AP view of the pelvis. However, any pelvic tilt will affect the measurement of version with this method.

Increased anteversion may predispose to anterior instability (Fig. 2.37).

The superior-inferior positioning of the acetabular component was described by Pagnano et al. [13]. The acetabular component is approximately 20% of the vertical height of the pelvis.

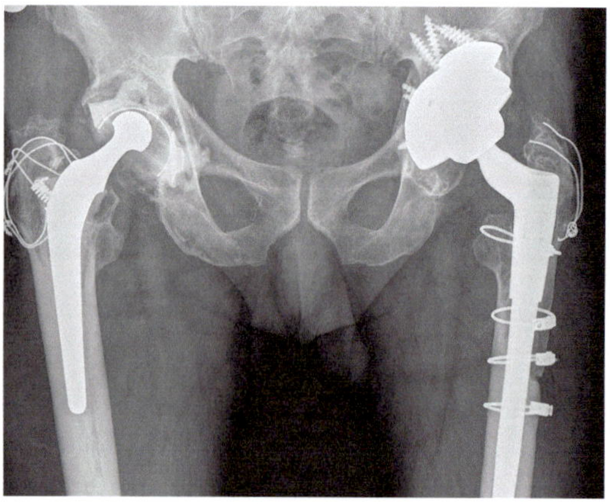

Fig. 2.26 Revision of the left hip using trabecular metal augments to fill defects in the acetabulum. The augment has been fixed to the pelvis using two screws. The cementless acetabular component is then placed and fixed with multiple screws. On the femoral side on the left side, a long modular cementless stem has been used. Evidence of extended trochanteric osteotomy (ETO) is visible, which was done for exposure and removing the previous femoral component. The ETO has been stabilised with three cables, and fourth cable is around the femoral shaft. The wires in the left greater trochanter are from the primary hip replacement which was done through a trochanteric osteotomy. There is good bone contact on both the acetabulum and femoral side on the left hip. The right hip is a Charnley hip with a grossly loose acetabular component and extensive periacetabular osteolysis. There is marked wear of the polyethylene superiorly. Note the wire mesh medial to the acetabulum and small amount of cement in the pelvis. The greater trochanter has been wired using a spring-loaded wire, as described by Wroblewski and Shelley [16]. There is a long cement plug distal to the femoral stem, and the cement restrictor is not visible. Despite extensive wear, there is no loosening of the femoral component.

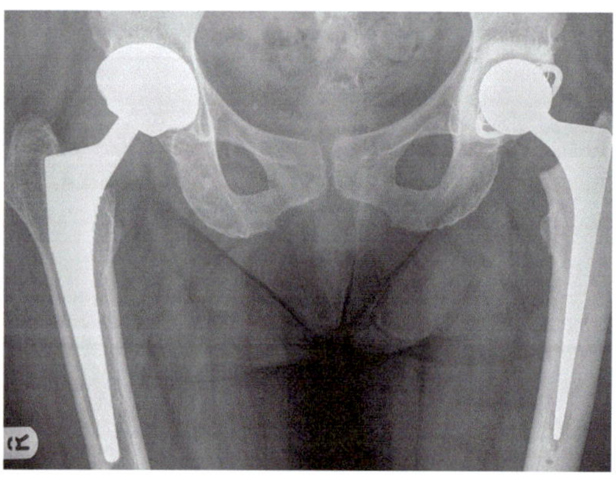

Fig. 2.27 Pedestal at the tip of a well-fixed femoral cementless stem right hip

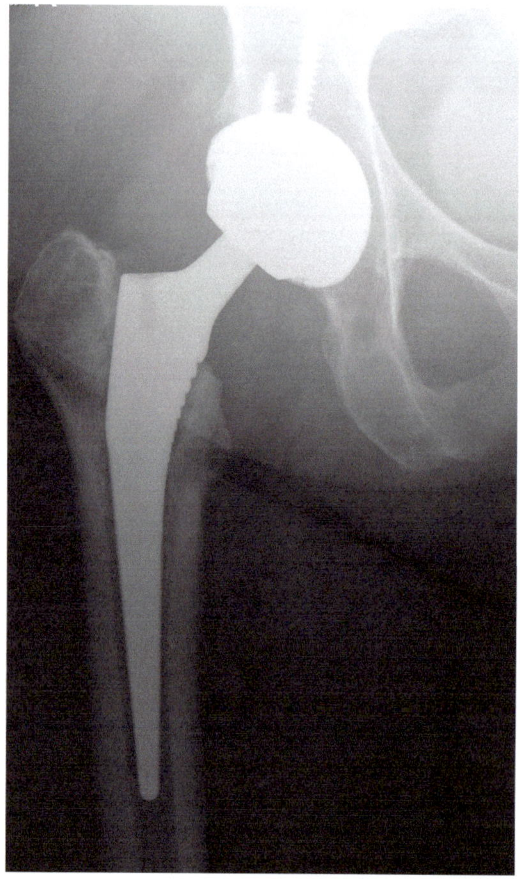

Fig. 2.28 An example of loosening of a cementless femoral component. This was secondary to infection. A continuous radiolucency is noticeable at the implant-bone interface of the femoral component

The inferior margin of the acetabular component is at the level of the teardrop. The approximate femoral head centre can be predicted by drawing an isosceles triangle which is 20% of the height of the pelvis as shown in Fig. 2.38a. The centre of the femoral head is at the centre of the hypotenuse. Proximal migration of the acetabulum (Fig. 2.38b) can be assessed by this method.

The angle of the acetabular component with the horizontal axis should be between 40 and 45°. Excess vertical placement (Fig. 2.39) or horizontal placement (Fig. 2.40) may adversely affect the survival of the hip prosthesis.

Another feature to note on postoperative radiographs is lengthening or shortening of the limb (Fig. 2.41).

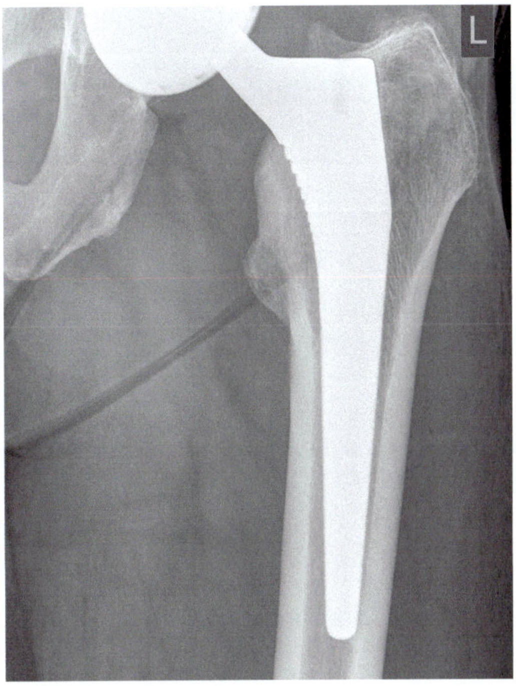

Fig. 2.29 A well-fixed cementless hip replacement with streaming trabeculae from the endosteum to the implant interface, seen best in zone 2

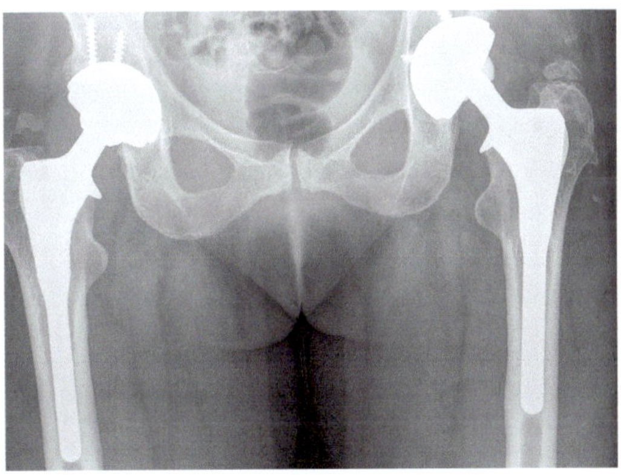

Fig. 2.30 Pedestal at the tip of a well-fixed cementless femoral stems on both sides. Note the spot weld on the lateral aspect of the femoral stem. There is cortical thickening at the tip of the femoral stems due to increased load transfer at this level. Note the calcar rounding (atrophy) on the right side, but not on the left. The acetabular component on the left hip is more vertical (open), and there is stress shielding superior to the acetabulum. The femoral head on the left side is made of Zirconia ceramic, which is less radio-opaque compared to the delta ceramic head (as on the right side) or metal femoral heads. There are islands of heterotopic ossification superior to the greater trochanter bilaterally, and these may represent trauma to the abductor muscles. Both of these hip replacements were done through a Hardinge approach

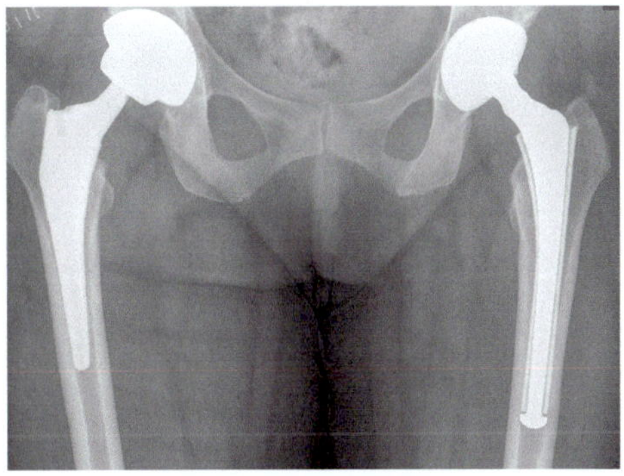

Fig. 2.31 An example of a stem developed to reduce stress shielding in the proximal femur (Epoch stem). The central core the femoral stem is made of cobalt-chromium-molybdenum for mechanical strength, and the outer covering is made of titanium fibre metal which provides cementless fixation and elasticity similar to the cortical bone. Note the endosteum along the lateral cortex where the reamer has made an indentation during preparation of the femoral canal

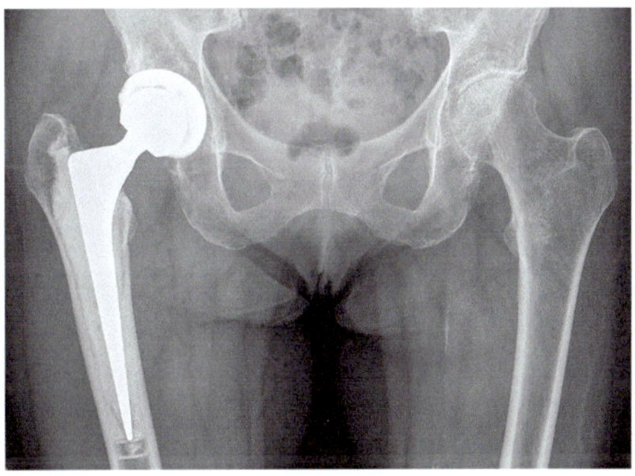

Fig. 2.32 A well-positioned acetabular component with the medial margin adjacent to the distal margin of the teardrop

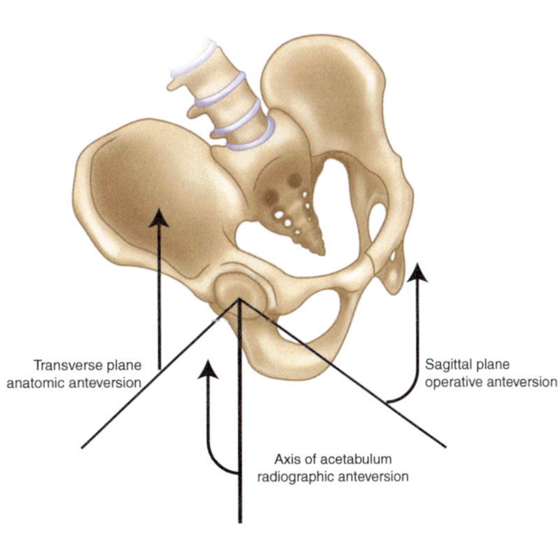

Fig. 2.33 Descriptive types of anteversion of the acetabular component

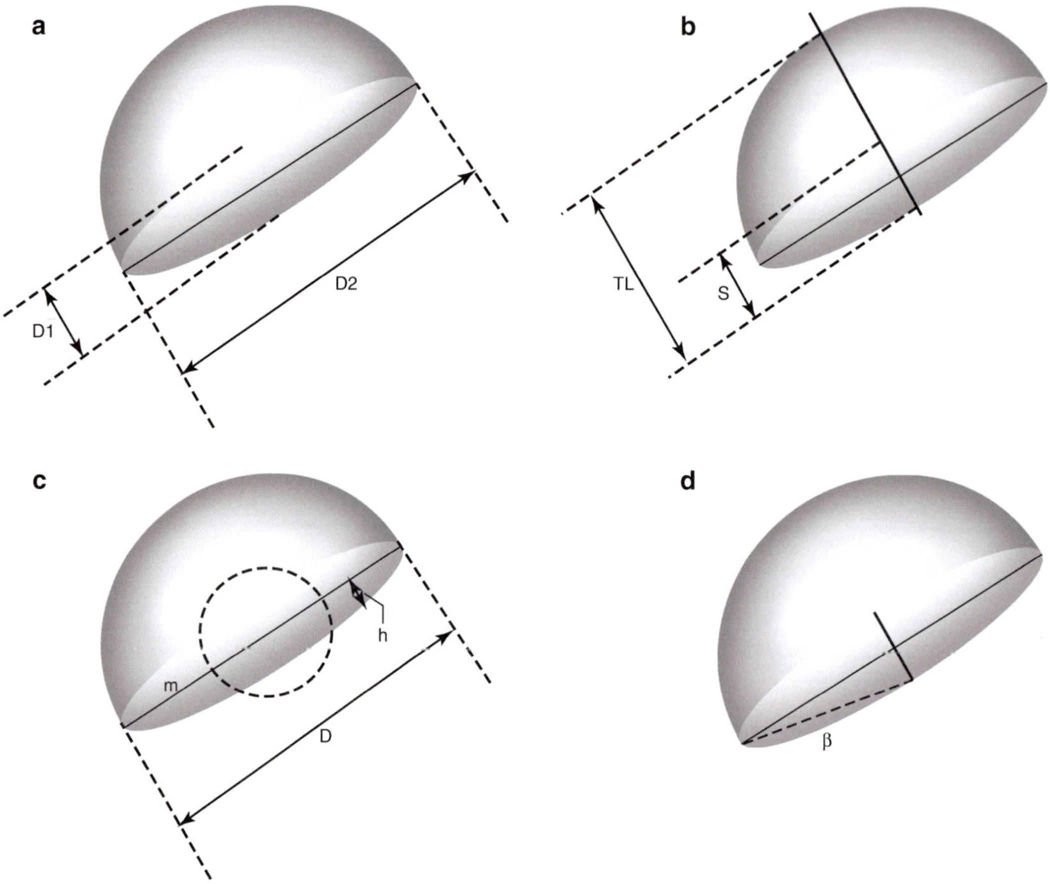

Fig. 2.34 (**a–d**) Various methods for measuring anteversion of the acetabular component in the AP radiograph. Lewinnek's method (**a**), Widmer's method (**b**), Hassan method (**c**) and Liaw's method (**d**)

Table 2.2 Methods of determining acetabular version

Lewinnek's method [8]	Version = arcsin $(D1/D2)$	$D1$—Length of short axis of ellipse $D2$—Distance of long axis
Widmer's method [9]	Version = Arcsin (Short axis S)/(Total length (TL)	S—Short axis length (same as $D1$) TL—entire length of the projected cross section of acetabular component
Hassan method [10]	Version = Arcsin $[(h/D)/\sqrt{[(m/D)-(m^2/D^2)]}$	D—maximum diameter of acetabular component m—distance along D which is not obscured by femoral head h—perpendicular from m to acetabular rim
Liaw's Method [11]	Version = $\sin^{-1} \tan\beta$	β is the line joining the long axis of the acetabular component to the end of the ellipse

A line can be drawn along identical fixed points on each side, and the level of the lesser trochanter is assessed in relation to this line. Murphy [14] described measurement of femoral lengths on the AP radiograph, which can serve as a surrogate marker for leg lengths. A line is drawn along the inferior aspects of the teardrop, and the vertical distance is measured on either side from this line to the superior aspect of the lesser trochanter.

A CT scanogram will provide a more accurate measurement and is useful in preoperative planning for revision surgery (Figs. 2.42 and 2.43).

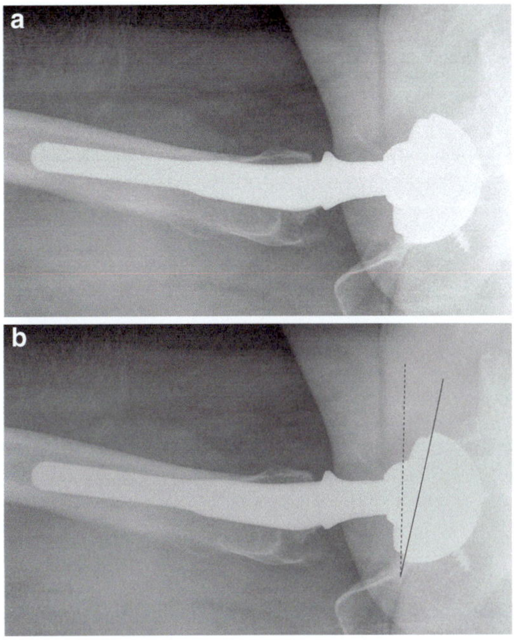

Fig. 2.35 Measurement of anteversion on the shoot-through lateral view. One line is drawn along the face of the acetabular component (solid line), and the other line is vertical (broken line). The version measures 15° in this patient and led to posterior instability

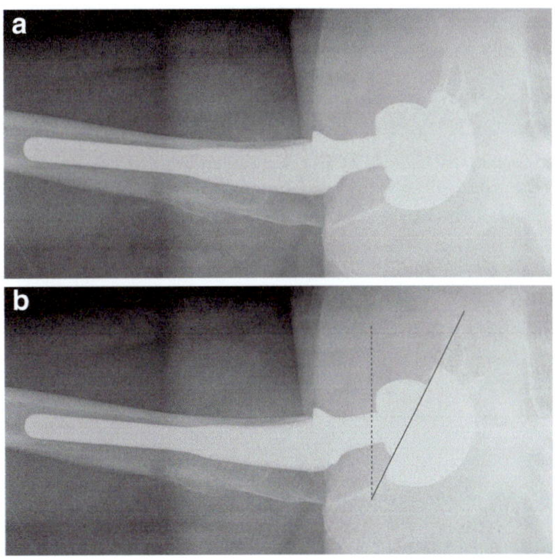

Fig. 2.36 Radiographs after revision of the same patient as shown in Fig. 2.35. The version of the acetabulum has been increased to achieve posterior stability. The head size has been increased as well

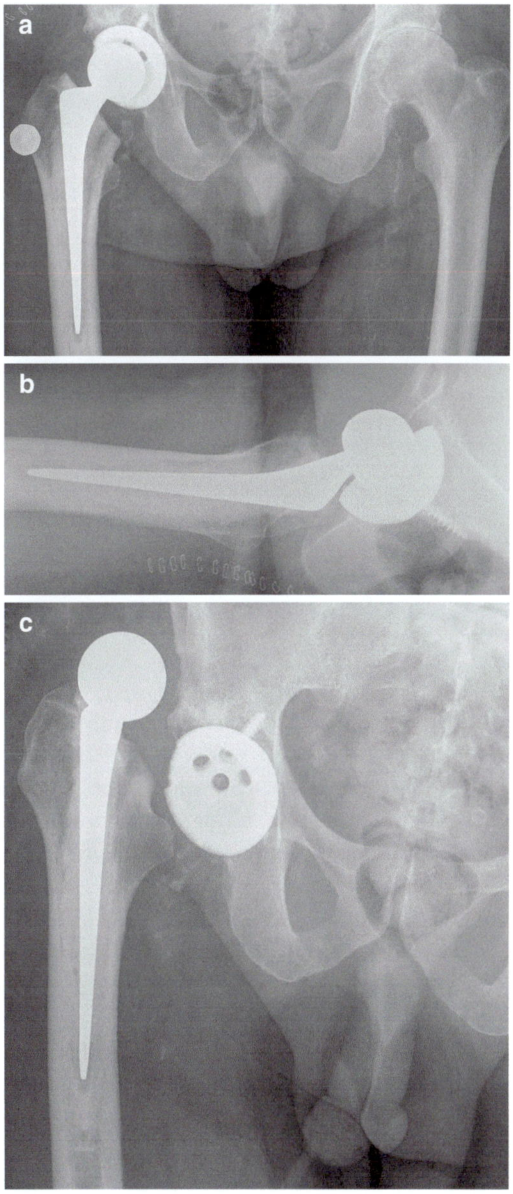

Fig. 2.37 Postoperative radiograph showing an excessively anteverted acetabular component (**a**, **b**) resulting in anterior dislocation (**c**). Revision to correct acetabular alignment reducing the excess anteversion (**d**, **e**)

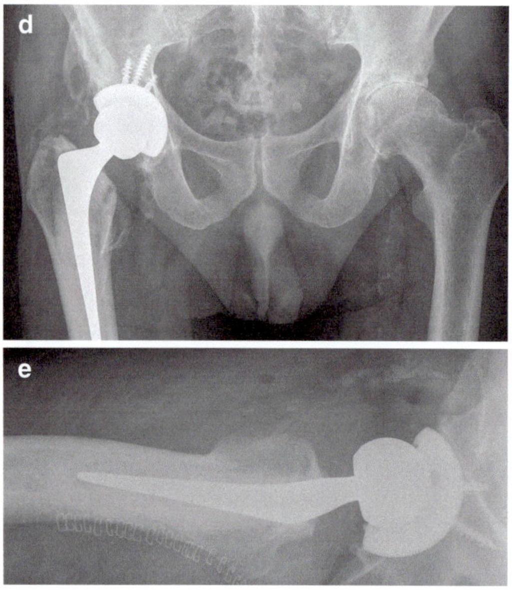

Fig. 2.37 (Continued)

Dislocations following total hip replacement (Fig. 2.44) can be early or late. Early dislocations are usually related to technical factors, which may require addressing through revision surgery. In patients with abductor deficiency, proximal or total femoral replacement or neurological conditions, constrained liners may be indicated (Figs. 2.45, 2.46 and 2.47). In these, the polyethylene arc is greater than a hemisphere and hence prevents the head from dislocating out of the liner. These have a metal reinforcement ring along the face of the liner, and various designs have been developed. Disadvantages of using constrained liners include increased stress at the fixation interface, accelerated wear, component failure and restriction of range of movement.

While the constrained liners reduce the risk of dislocation, it is still possible for the entire liner to be pulled out (Fig. 2.48) or indeed for the head to dislocate despite the ring (Fig. 2.49). Another type of constrained liner is designed such that the head has a flattened shape along the equator. This allows the head to be reduced within the liner but prevents dislocation in the physiological hip position (Figs. 2.50 and 2.51).

Infection in hip replacements is a rare but serious complication. In late stages, endosteal scal-

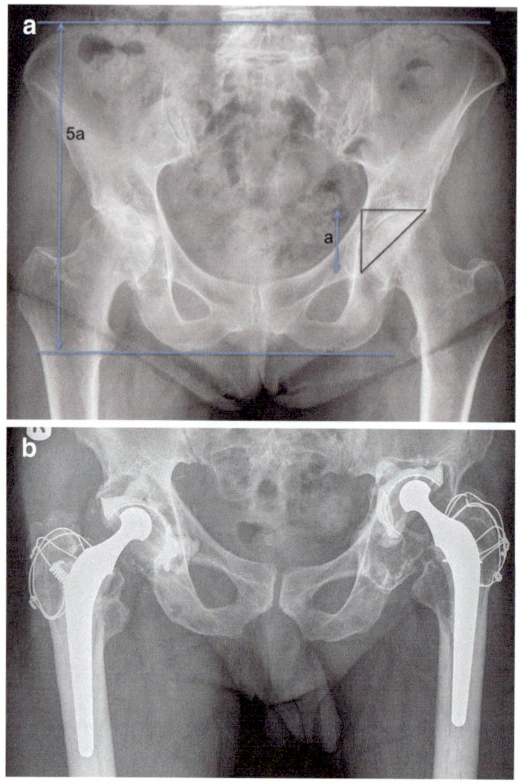

Fig. 2.38 (**a**) Positioning of the acetabular component as described by Pagnano et al. [13]. The vertical height of the acetabulum is one fifth of the vertical height of the pelvis. The femoral head corresponds to the centre of the hypotenuse. (**b**) Proximal migration of left acetabular component with bilateral extensive osteolysis. The spring-loaded wires for trochanteric reattachment on the right hip were described by Wroblewski and Shelley. There is eccentric wear of the acetabular polyethylene with superior migration of the femoral head. There is extensive bilateral pelvic osteolysis with loosening of acetabular components. The left acetabular component has migrated proximally. The femoral components are well fixed. Note the lack of cement restrictor in the femoral canal

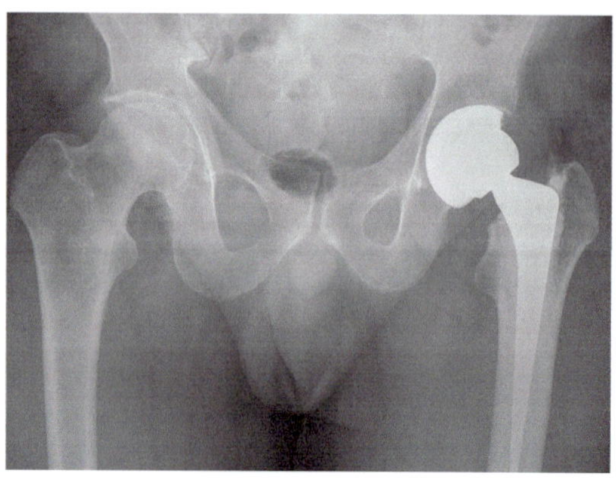

Fig. 2.39 Vertical placement of the acetabular component

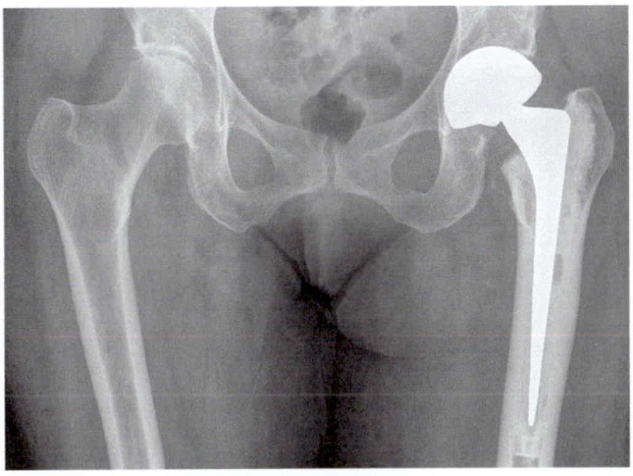

Fig. 2.40 Horizontal placement of the acetabular component

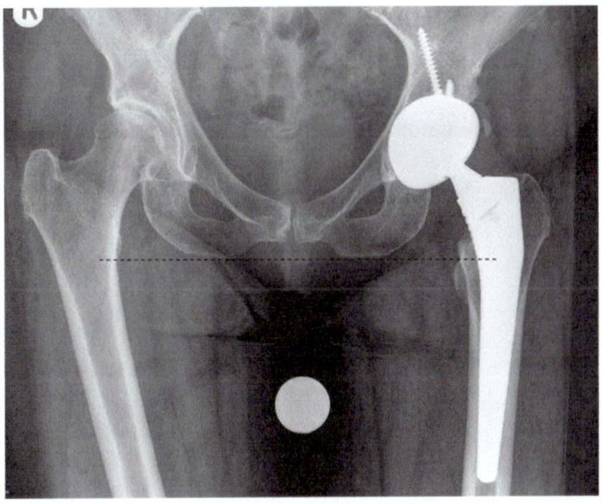

Fig. 2.41 Postoperative radiograph showing significant lengthening of the left side as evidenced by the difference in level of the lesser trochanter. The radiolucency in the proximal part of the femoral component is the junction of the modular neck segment with the femoral stem

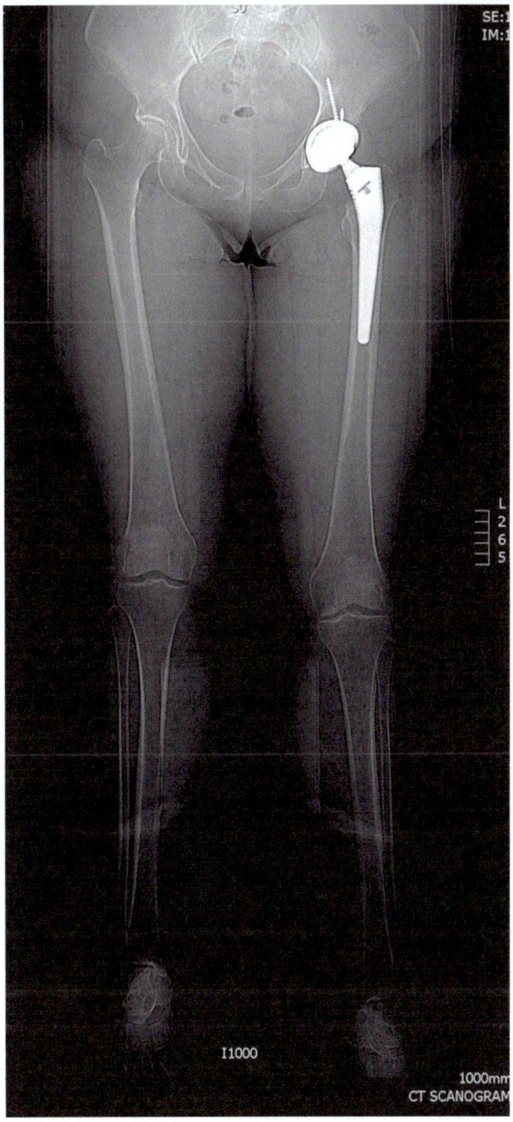

Fig. 2.42 A CT scanogram of the same patient as Fig. 2.41 showing the lengthening of the left side

loping may be observed, but is not diagnostic for sepsis. Periosteal new bone formation is highly specific but is observable in less than one in five patients (Fig. 2.52). Ultrasound scanning may reveal fluid in the hip and collection in the muscle and perimuscular fat, with a very high positive predictive value. Radioisotope scanning may provide further evidence of infection.

Heterotopic bone formation (Fig. 2.53) around hip replacements is commoner after muscle dividing approaches, hypertrophic arthritis and previous acetabular trauma. It is classified radiologically on the AP radiograph of the pelvis using the Brooker classification [15] (Table 2.3).

Failure of components is rare with modern implants. Cases of ceramic fracture involving the head or the acetabular liner have been reported (Fig. 2.54a, b). Failure of the femoral stem is even more rare (Fig. 2.55) with modern implants.

Resurfacing of the hip (Fig. 2.56) has been a popular procedure but has declined in use in recent years due to concerns about metal ion release in the local tissues and potential for adverse reaction to metal debris. Similar concerns have been associated with large diameter

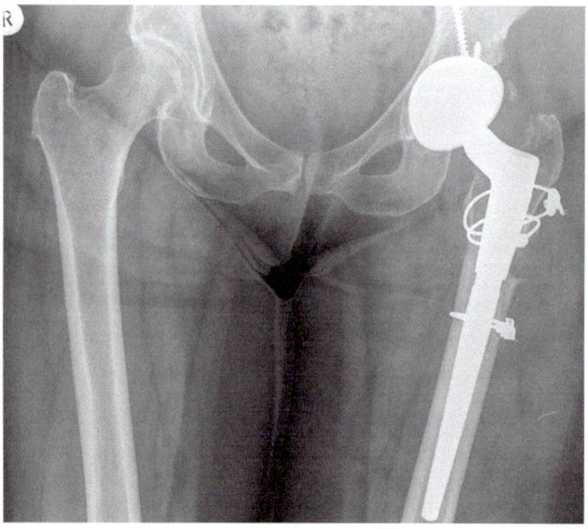

Fig. 2.43 Radiograph after revision of the left hip to restore difference in leg lengths

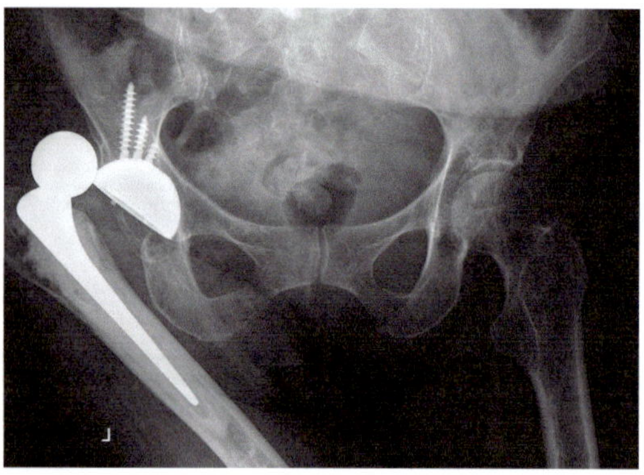

Fig. 2.44 Posterior dislocation following hybrid total hip replacement

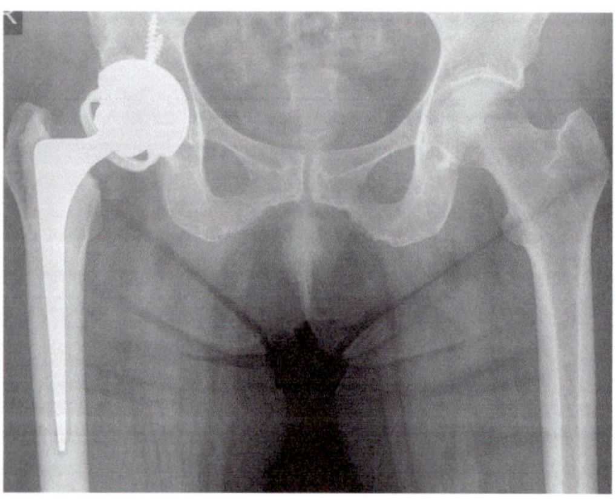

Fig. 2.45 Revision of the patient in Fig. 2.44 using a constrained ring acetabular component. The ring reinforces the polyethylene, and the head is captured by the extended polyethylene liner preventing dislocation

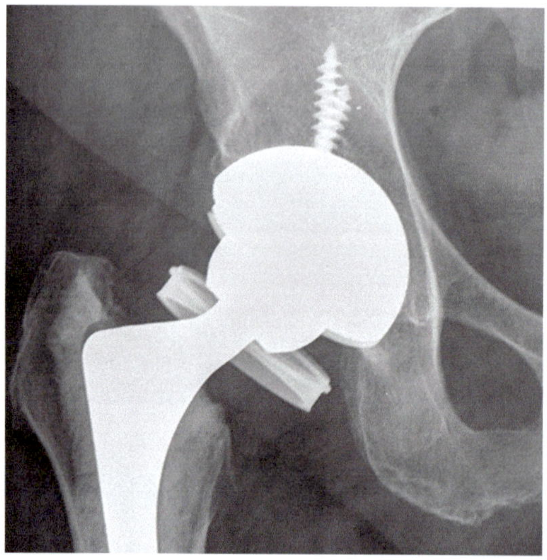

Fig. 2.46 Follow-up on the same patient as Figs. 2.44 and 2.45. The polyethylene liner has fractured along the ring after 14 months, and the ring has displaced distally. Note the increased separation between the ring and the acetabular shell

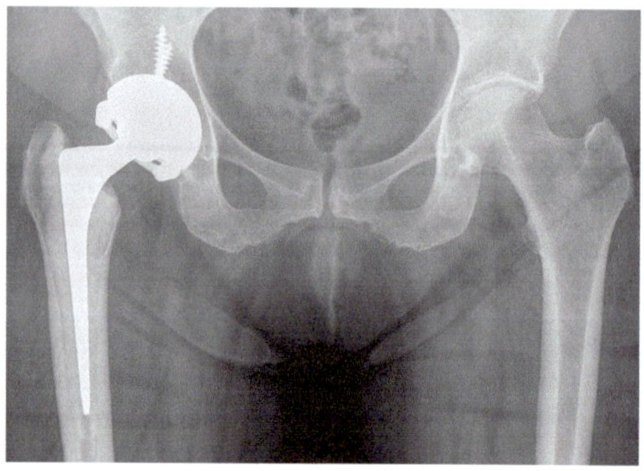

Fig. 2.47 Revision of the hip for the same patient (Figs. 2.44–2.46). A new type of constrained liner has been cemented in the original acetabular shell. This type has two extended polyethylene lips reinforced by a metal ring. Note the femoral stem has been revised as well but the cement mantle is largely preserved—a 'cement-in-cement' revision for the femur

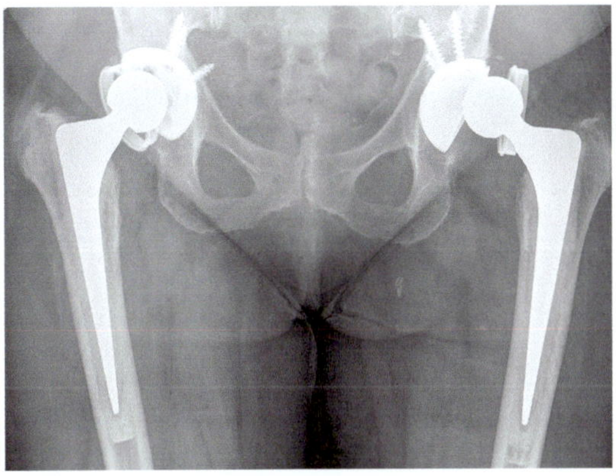

Fig. 2.48 Pulling out of the polyethylene constraining liner from the acetabular shell on the left hip

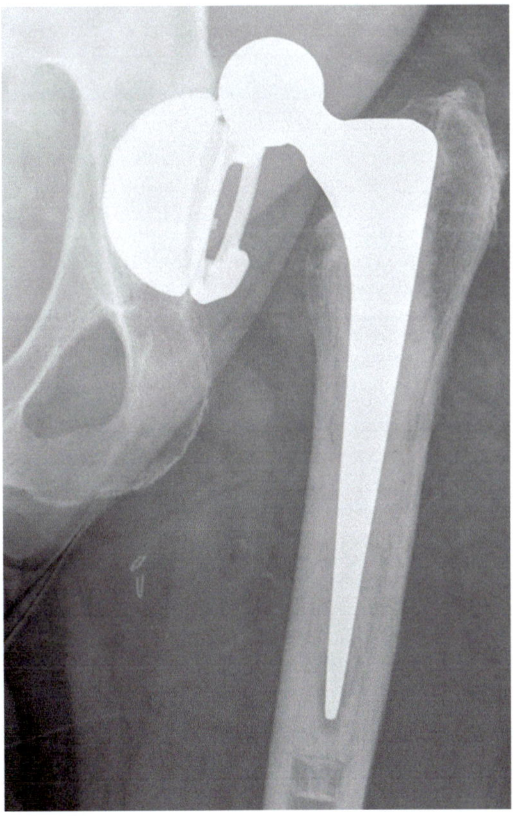

Fig. 2.49 Dislocation of the femoral head on the left side in the same patient as Fig. 2.48. The constraining mechanism has been changed, but the vertical position of the acetabulum predisposes to dislocation

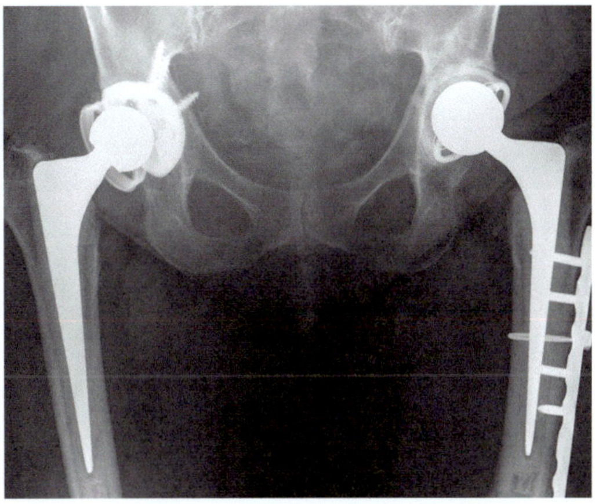

Fig. 2.50 Same patient as Figs. 2.48 and 2.49. The new constrained component has been placed, correcting the excess vertical placement of the previous acetabular component

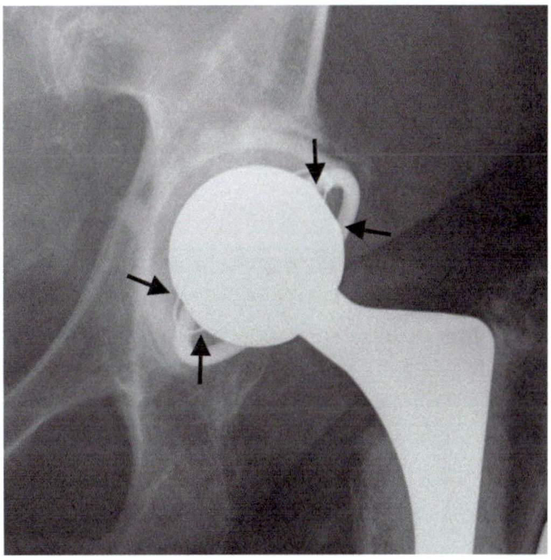

Fig. 2.51 Same patient as Figs. 2.48–2.50. The femoral head in this system is flattened at the equator, between the two sets of arrows. This allows reduction of the femoral head through the constraining ring intraoperatively but prevents dislocation in the physiological hip position

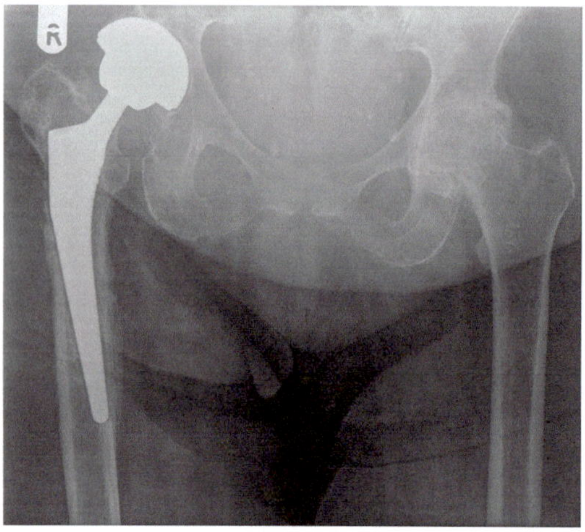

Fig. 2.52 Chronic infection around a cementless total hip replacement. There is a continuous radiolucency around the femoral stem with cortical erosion in zones 5 and 6. Extensive periosteal reaction is seen in this area. There is thinning of the femoral cortex in zones 1 and 2. The acetabulum has a near-complete radiolucency at the metal-bone interface and is proximally placed

metal on metal articulation hip replacements (Figs. 2.57 and 2.58).

Resurfacing hip replacements are considered to be more stable on account of larger head size, although dislocations are still reported (Fig. 2.59). Fractures of the intertrochanteric area are possible following resurfacing hip replacements (Fig. 2.60).

Various techniques have been evolved to reconstruct bone loss in revision hip replacement. For the acetabulum, impaction grafting and trabecular metal augments are the mainstay of reconstruction. In impaction grafting, the defect is converted to a contained defect, and bone graft is impacted before cementing (Figs. 2.61 and 2.62). Metal augments, which integrate with the cancellous bone, can be used to reconstruct uncontained defects or to fill contained defect (Figs. 2.63 and 2.64).

On the femoral side, long cementless stems can be used to gain fixation in the femoral diaphysis where proximal migration is compromised. These stems can gain fixation through a tight fit in the femoral shaft where the canal has good bone quality (Figs. 2.65 and 2.66). Alternatively, distal locking stems (Fig. 2.67) provide fixation in the distal third of femur where the canal is too wide.

For fractures in between two well-fixed implants, fixation is an option instead of revision of prosthesis (Fig. 2.68).

Replacement of the proximal femur (Fig. 2.69) or entire femur (Fig. 2.70), along with the hip and knee joint, is needed where there is extensive bone loss, or the femur is removed in tumour surgery. Extensive reconstruction of the acetabulum is needed for defects following tumour excision (Fig. 2.71).

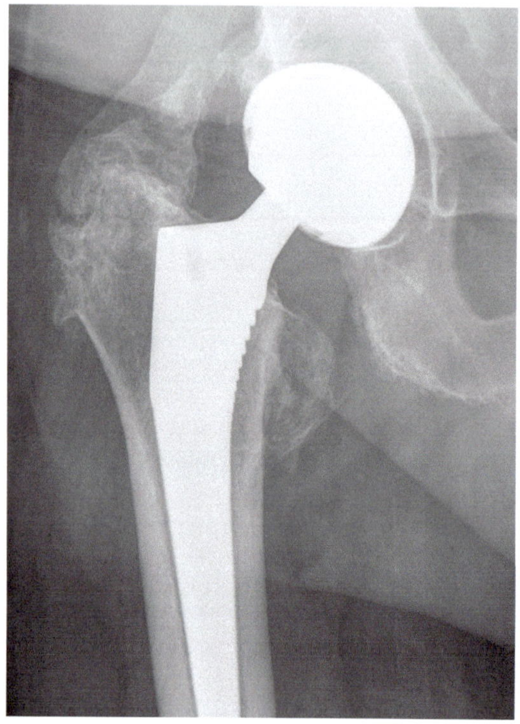

Fig. 2.53 Heterotopic ossification following total hip replacement. This procedure was done through a lateral approach (Hardinge approach)

Table 2.3 Brooker classification

Grade 1	Isolated islands of bone
Grade 2	Bone spurs with a gap of at least 1 cm between the opposing surfaces
Grade 3	Near complete bone bridging (gap less than 1 cm)
Grade 4	Apparent ankylosis

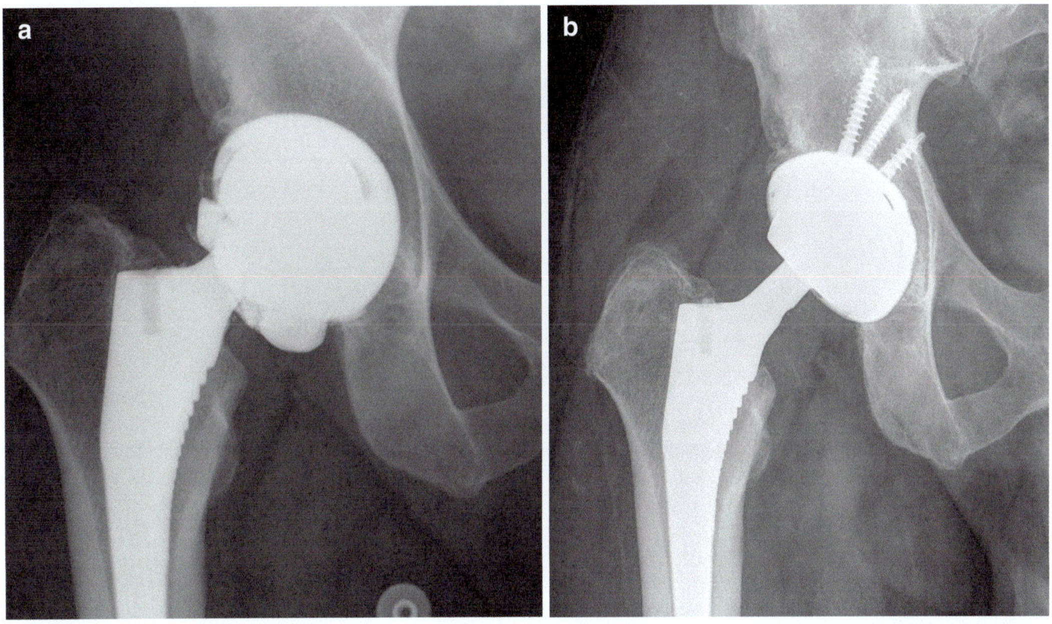

Fig. 2.54 (**a**) Fracture of the ceramic head 16 months after primary total hip replacement. (**b**) Revision of the hip shown in (**a**) using a ceramic on ceramic articulation

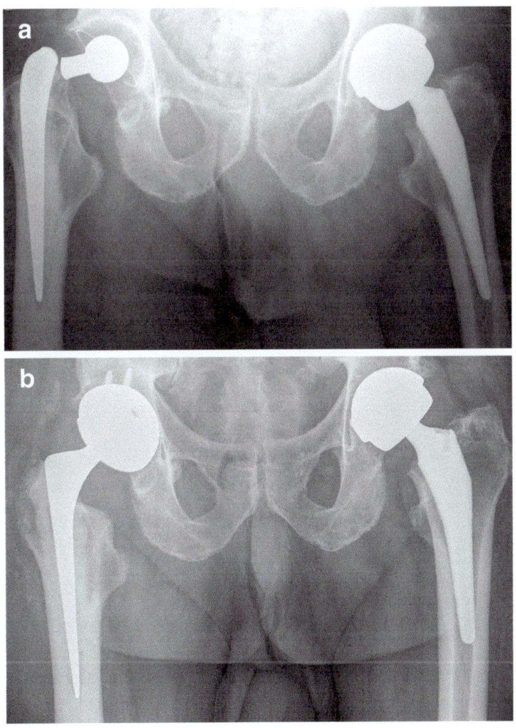

Fig. 2.55 (**a**) Fracture of the femoral stem 15 years after primary total hip replacement. (**b**) The stem has been revised using a 'cement-in-cement' technique. Most of the existing cement in the femoral canal was not removed as it was well fixed. The acetabulum has been revised to achieve adequate stability

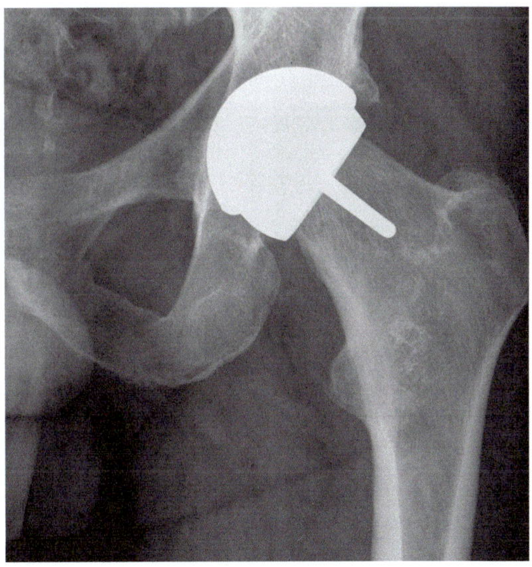

Fig. 2.56 Left hip resurfacing

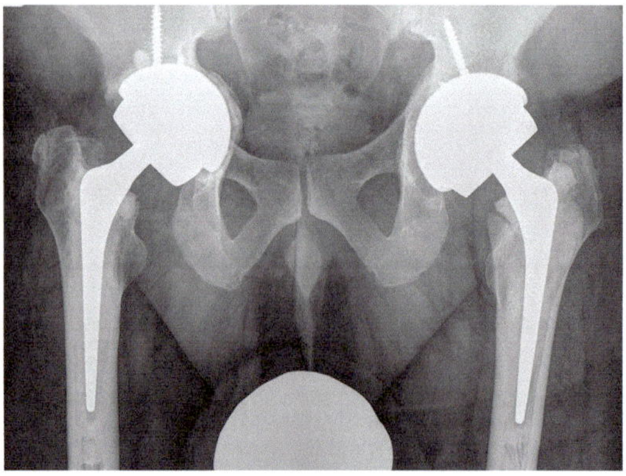

Fig. 2.57 Bilateral large diameter metal on metal hip replacement. The acetabular component is cementless and has additional screw for stability. It has a metal liner. Femoral components have large diameter metal heads and cemented stems

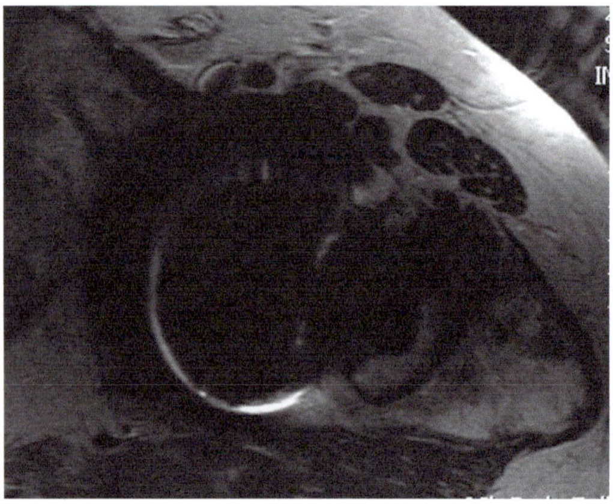

Fig. 2.58 MR scan of the patient in Fig. 2.57. There is a fluid collection in the region of the greater trochanter from the adverse reaction to metal debris (ARMD)

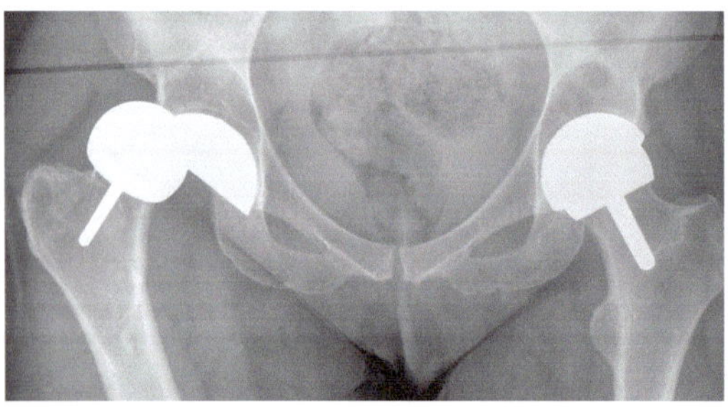

Fig. 2.59 Bilateral hip resurfacing with posterior dislocation on the right side

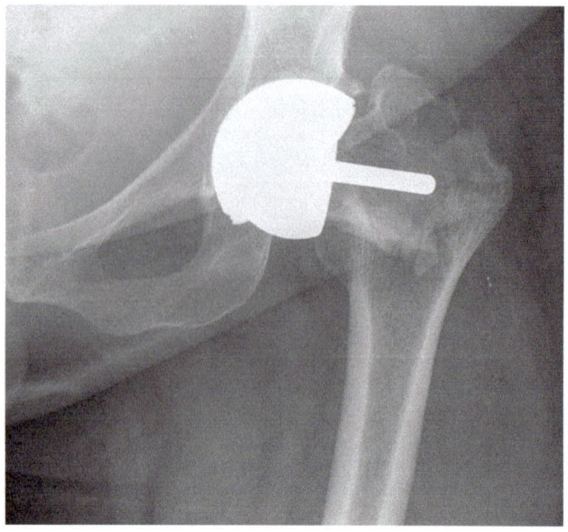

Fig. 2.60 Left hip resurfacing with intertrochanteric fracture of the proximal femur. The fracture was the result of trauma 4 years after the index operation

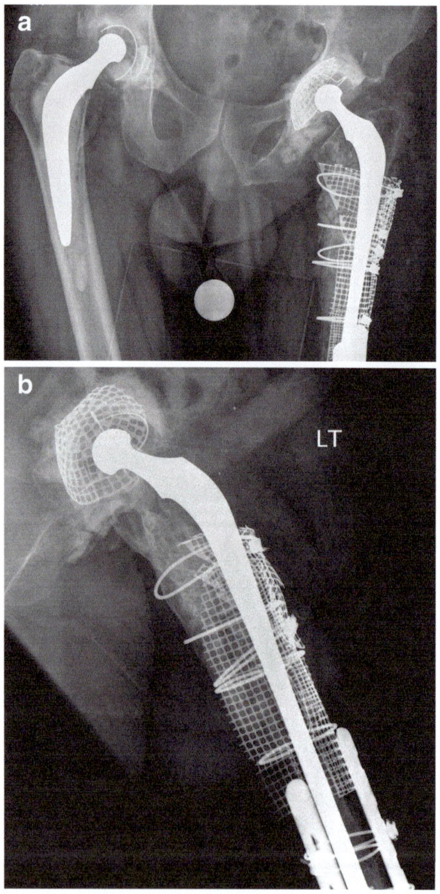

Fig. 2.61 Extensive impaction grafting of the acetabulum and femur. The wire mesh has been used to convert an uncontained defect to a contained defect. An all-polyethylene acetabular component is cemented into the bone graft. The femoral component is long stem and is cemented

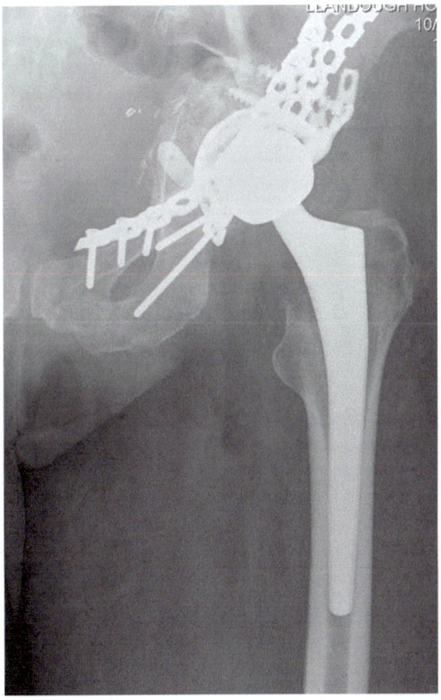

Fig. 2.62 Impaction grafting of the acetabulum to reconstruct a post-traumatic defect. Some of the metalwork used to reconstruct the anterior and the posterior column is in situ. The bone graft is visible medial to the original medial wall of the acetabulum. An acetabular cage has been used to reinforce the impaction grafting, and an all-polyethylene liner has been cemented into the cage. The technique helps restore bone stock

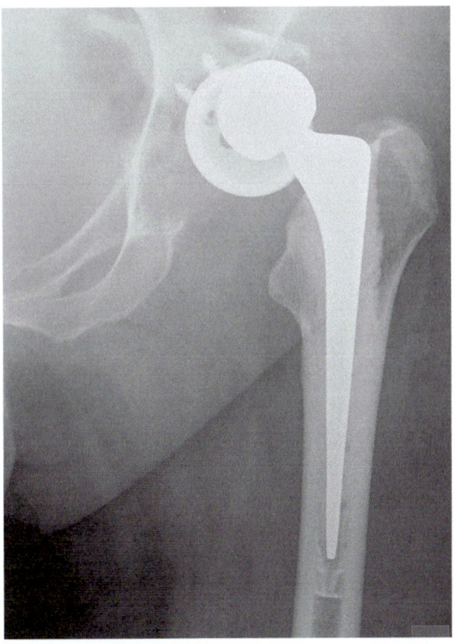

Fig. 2.63 Periprosthetic fracture of the acetabulum with displacement of the component

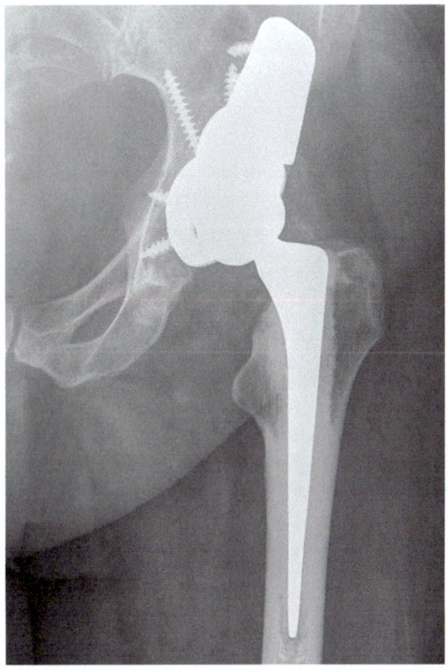

Fig. 2.64 Reconstruction of the uncontained defect of the posterior buttress using a trabecular metal augment. The augment is fixed to ilium with screws and provides primary stability. The cementless acetabular component is then fixed in place. Secondary stability is achieved through bone integration

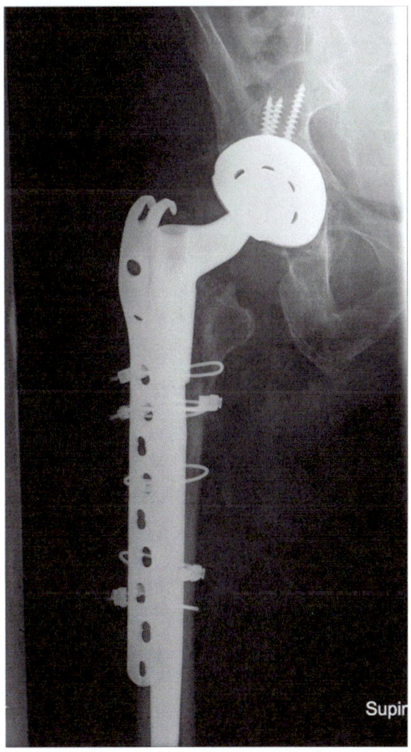

Fig. 2.65 Cementless modular stem used to stabilise a periprosthetic femoral fracture. The plate provides fixation to the greater trochanter fragment

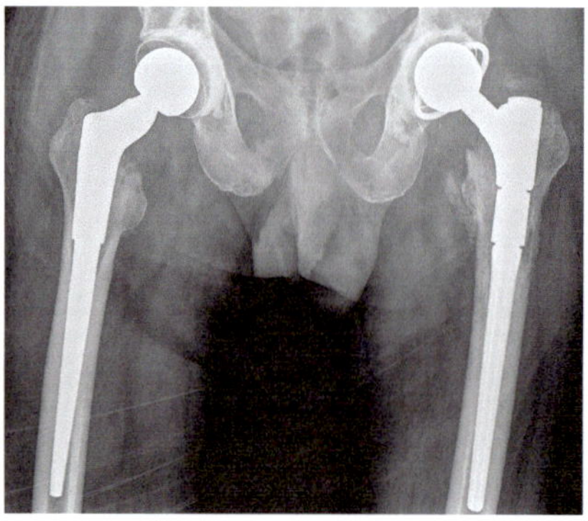

Fig. 2.66 Bilateral long-stem cementless femoral components for pathologic fracture of the neck of femur with proximal femoral involvement. A constrained acetabular component has been used on the left side. The femoral components are modular, which allows matching different proximal bodies and distal stems so as to achieve maximum contact with host bone without removing excess bone

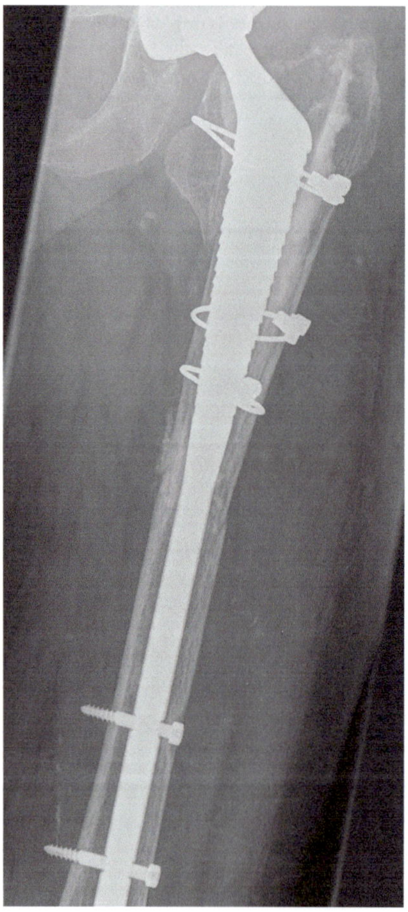

Fig. 2.67 Cementless femoral prosthesis with distal locking screws. These are suitable where inadequate bone stock precludes fixation in the proximal part of femur

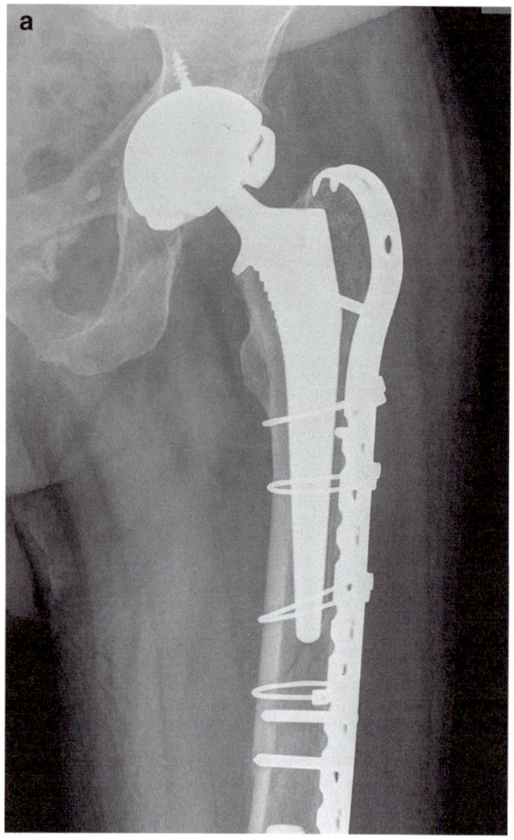

Fig. 2.68 Fixation of a femoral fracture between a revision hip replacement and a revision knee replacement. Presence of stemmed implants on either side produces a risk of fracture of the bone in the middle unsupported segment

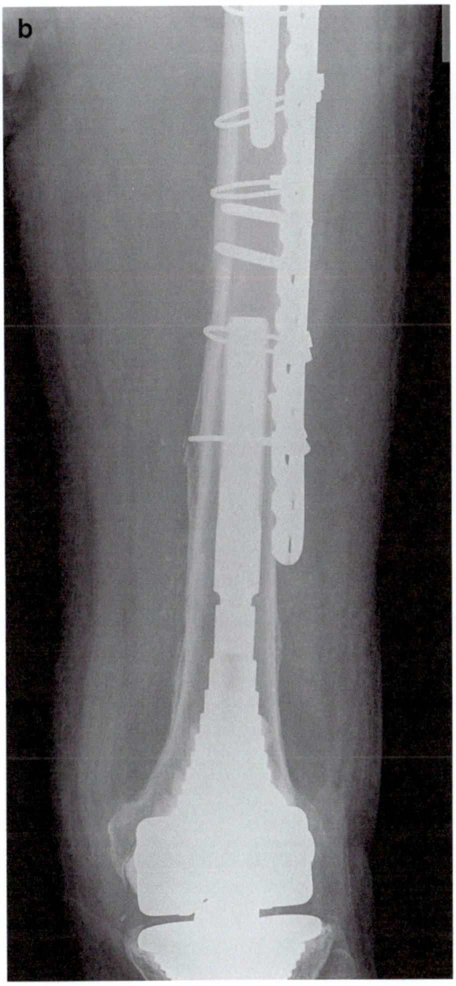

Fig. 2.68 (Continued)

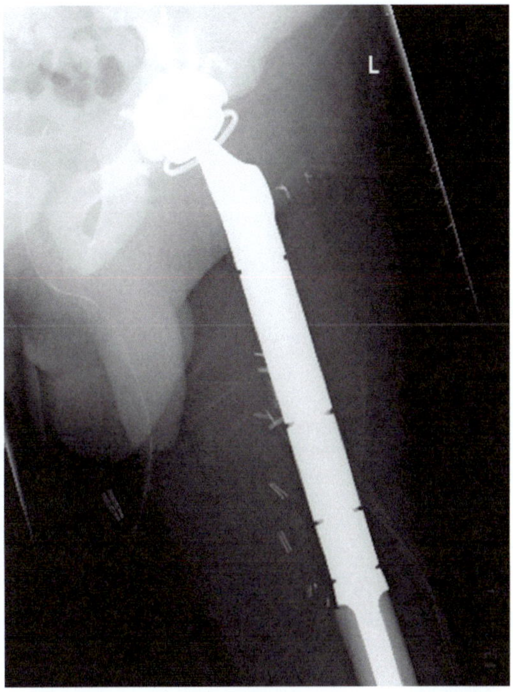

Fig. 2.69 Proximal femoral replacement. The acetabular component has a constrained liner to reduce the risk of dislocation. With the loss of trochanters, soft tissue tension in the hip is often inadequate for stability of the joint, and hence constrained liners are usually needed in these situations

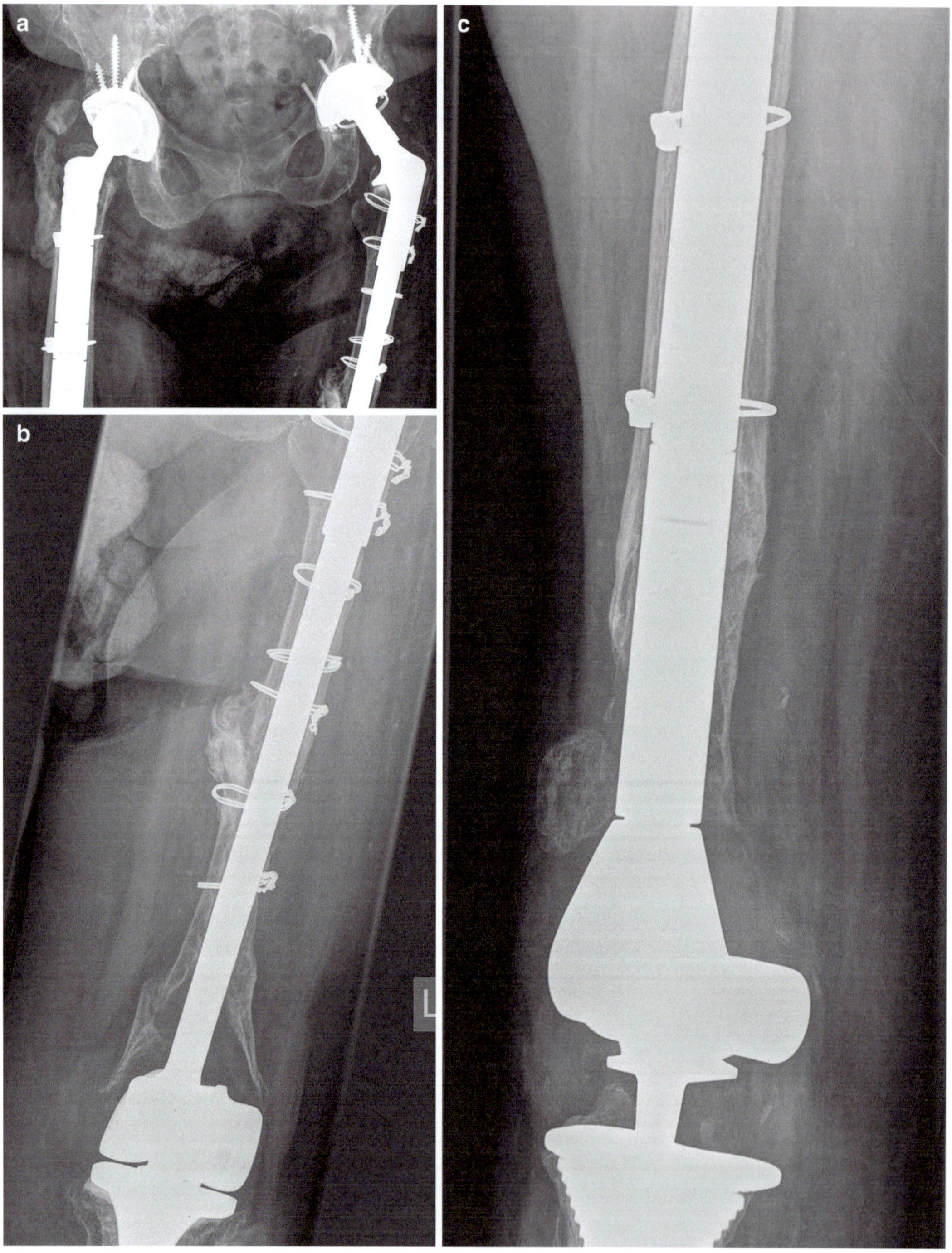

Fig. 2.70 Bilateral total femur replacement. Radiograph of the pelvis (**a**) and femoral shafts (**b**, **c**) are shown. The remaining part of femoral shaft allows some degree of soft tissue attachment

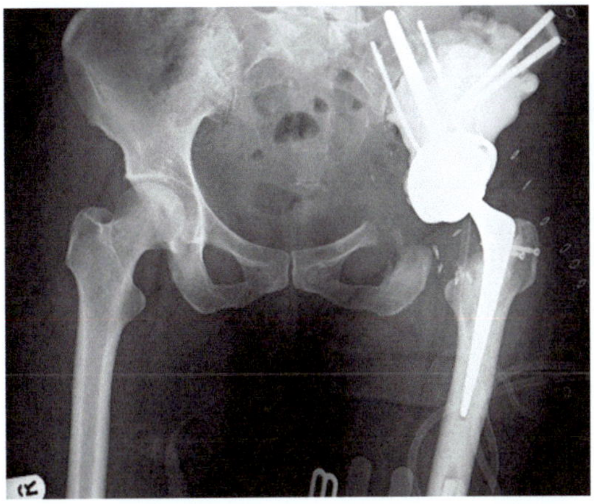

Fig. 2.71 Reconstruction of the acetabulum using cement reinforced with metal pins and a cemented acetabular component following tumour excision. Fixation has been achieved in the remaining part of the ilium and ala of the sacrum. There is no distal fixation or support for the acetabulum. The screws adjacent to the femoral component were used to fix the trochanteric osteotomy

References

1. Shen G. Femoral stem fixation: an engineering interpretation of the long term outcome of Charnley and Exeter stems. J Bone Joint Surg Br. 1998;80:754–6.
2. Gruen TA, McNeice GM, Amstutz HC. Modes of failure of cemented stem type femoral components. A radiographic analysis of loosening. Clin Orthop. 1979;141:17–27.
3. DeLee JG, Charnley J. Radiological demarcation of cemented sockets in total hip replacement. Clin Orthop. 1976;121:20–32.
4. Barrack RL, Mulroy RD Jr, Harris WH. Improved cementing techniques and femoral component loosening in young patients with hip arthroplasty. A 12 year radiographic review. J Bone Joint Surg Br. 1992;74:385–9.
5. Vresilovic EJ, Hozack WJ, Rothman RH. Radiographic assessment of cementless femoral components. Correlation with intraoperative mechanical stability. J Arthroplasty. 1994;9(2):137–41.
6. Takatori Y, Nagai I, Moro T, Kuruta Y, Karita T, Mabuchi A, Ninomiya S. Ten year follow up of a proximal circumferential porous coated femoral prosthesis: radiographic evaluation and stability. J Orthop Sci. 2002;7(1):68–73.
7. Murray DW. The definition and measurement of acetabular orientation. J Bone Joint Surg Br. 1993;75:228–32.
8. Lewinnek GE, Lewis JL, Tarr R, Compere CL, Zimmerman JR. Dislocations after total hip replacement arthroplasties. J Bone Joint Surg Am. 1978;60:217–20.
9. Widmer KH. A simplified method to determine acetabular cup anteversion form plain radiographs. J Arthroplasty. 2004;19:387–90.
10. Hassan DM, Johnston GH, Dust WN, Watson LG, Cassidy D. Radiographic calculation of anteversion in acetabular prosthesis. J Arthroplasty. 1995;10: 369–72.
11. Liaw CK, Hou SM, Yang RS, Wu TY, Fuh CS. A new tool for measuring cup orientation in total hip arthroplasties from plain radiographs. Clin Orthop. 2006;451:134–9.
12. Woo RY, Morrey BF. Dislocations after total hip arthroplasty. J Bone Joint Surg Am. 1982;64:1295–306.
13. Pagnano MW, Hanssen AD, Lewallen DG, Shaughnessy WJ. Superior placement of the acetabular component on the rate of loosening after total hip arthroplasty. J Bone Joint Surg Am. 1996;78(7):1004–14.
14. Murphy SB, Ecker TM. Evaluation of a new leg length measurement algorithm in hip arthroplasty. Clin Orthop Relat Res. 2007;463:85.
15. Brooker AF, Bowerman JF, Robinson RA, Riley LH. Ectopic ossification following total hip replacement. Incidence and method of classification. J Bone Joint Surg Am. 1973;55(8):1629–32.
16. Wroblewski BM, Shelley P. Reattachment of the greater trochanter after total hip replacement. J Bone Joint Surg Br. 1985;67(5):736–40.

3 Knee Implants

Sanjeev Agarwal, Mark Forster,
and Gaurav Jyoti Bansal

Knee replacement is an increasingly common operation with over 80,000 performed in the UK annually (UK National Joint Registry 12th Annual Report, 2015). The vast majority are cemented implants. Unicompartmental knee replacements account for about 8% of all knee replacements, and patellofemoral replacements are 1% of the total.

A large variety of implants are currently in use. In most primary knee replacements, the femoral component and polyethylene insert articulate without any mechanism to provide stability for collateral ligaments.

Knee replacement implants used in primary knee surgery may be cruciate retaining or posterior stabilised. In the cruciate-retaining implants, the posterior cruciate ligament is preserved during surgery (Fig. 3.1). On the other hand, in posterior-stabilised implants (Fig. 3.2), the posterior cruciate ligament is removed and substituted by a cam and post mechanism within the implant. The articulation between the post and the cam provides posterior femoral rollback. In patients with lateral ligamentous insufficiency, semi-constrained implants which provide some degree of varus and valgus support are used. If the medial collateral ligament is lax/non-functional, a hinged implant is generally needed to achieve a stable knee.

The assessment of knee replacement radiographs is based on the anteroposterior (AP), lateral and the skyline views.

On the AP view, the features to note are:

1. Femoral component varus/valgus alignment (alpha angle)
2. Femoral component overhang medially/laterally
3. Gap between femoral component and tibial tray on medial and lateral side
4. Tibial component varus/valgus alignment (beta angle)

S. Agarwal (✉) · M. Forster
University Hospital of Wales, Cardiff, UK
e-mail: mcforster@doctors.org.uk

G. J. Bansal
Cardiff and Vale University Health Board,
Cardiff, UK

S. Agarwal, G. J. Bansal (eds.), *Radiology of Orthopedic Implants*,
https://doi.org/10.1007/978-3-319-76009-4_3

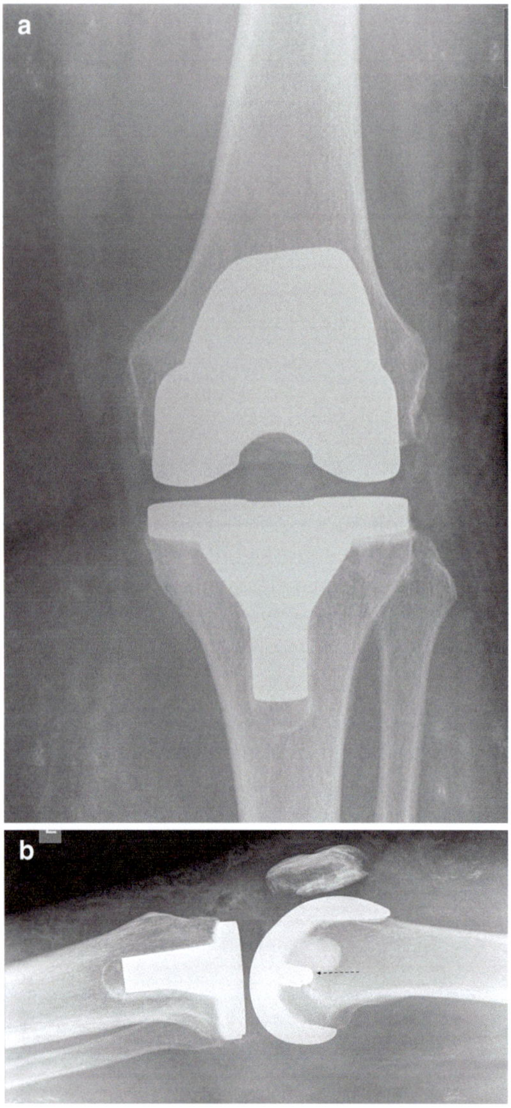

Fig. 3.1 Cruciate-retaining cemented total knee replacement. AP (**a**) and lateral (**b**) views. On the lateral view, there is no box for cam and post mechanism. There are two pegs (arrow) on the femoral component which appear superimposed on the lateral projection

5. Tibial component overhang medially/laterally
6. Relative angle between anatomical axis of the femur and anatomical axis of tibia
7. Any periprosthetic fracture
8. The level of joint line—compared to preoperative radiograph
9. Quality of cementation of the tibial component
10. Any retained cement

On the lateral view, the features to note are:

1. Femoral component positioning—flexion/extension compared to femoral anatomical axis.
2. Anterior flange of femoral component collinear with anterior cortex of the femur—evidence of notching of the femur or overstuffing of the patellofemoral joint.
3. Posterior condyle of the femur should blend with the outline of the femoral condyle.
4. Posterior condylar offset and posterior condylar offset ratio.
5. Patellar height.
6. Tibial slope—anteriorly sloping, posteriorly sloping or perpendicular to the anatomical axis of the tibia.
7. Tibial component anterior/posterior positioning.
8. Cementation of femoral and tibial component in cemented knee replacements.
9. Osseointegration/bone apposition in cementless knee replacements.
10. Any periprosthetic fracture.
11. Any retained cement.

In medium- to long-term follow-up, further features are:

1. Evidence of osteolysis
2. Loosening of components
3. Migration of components
4. Fracture of cement mantle
5. Thinning of the polyethylene
6. Metallosis in the soft tissues
7. Periosteal reaction

A major impediment to successful comparison of knee replacement radiographs is lack of reproducibility. Radiolucent lines under the tibial component would be best demonstrated if the beam is parallel to the under surface of the component.

One method to improve comparability is through fluoroscopy-guided radiographs. However, this method is labour intensive and is not practical for routine use.

The alpha angle is the angle between the longitudinal axis of the femur and a line tangential to

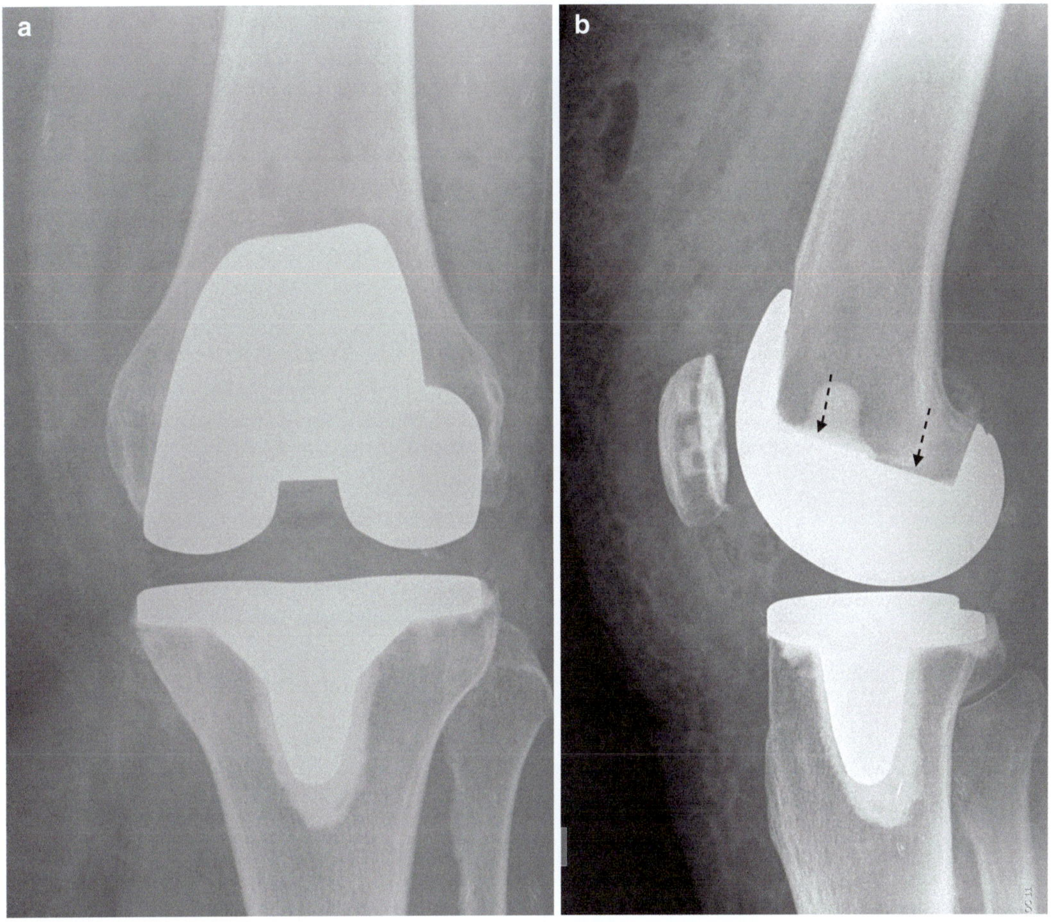

Fig. 3.2 Cruciate substituting (posterior stabilised) cemented total knee replacement. AP (**a**) and lateral (**b**) views. On the lateral view, there is a box (arrows) on the femoral component, which accommodates the cam and post mechanism

the distal aspect of femoral condyles (Fig. 3.3) in the AP view. Ideally this should correspond to the angle between the mechanical axis and anatomical axis of the femur. For most patients, it is between 3 and 7 degrees of valgus.

The beta angle is the angle between the longitudinal axis of tibia and a line tangential to the flat surface of tibial component (Fig. 3.3). The tibial component should be perpendicular to the mechanical axis of the tibia to avoid shear force at the tibial metal—bone interface.

Standard postoperative radiographs include only the knee joint, and hence measurement of axis of the femur and tibia is not accurate. Internal or external rotation of the limb may also affect accurate determination of longitudinal axis.

To determine the longitudinal axis of the femur, the midpoint of the femoral shaft is marked furthest from the knee joint, and another mark is made 10 cm proximal to the joint line. The axis is assumed to pass midway between two corresponding points on the cortex. Similarly, on the tibia, the point chosen is 10 cm distal to joint line and another point as far distal on the tibia as the radiograph allows.

On the lateral view, the longitudinal axis of the femur is marked out and compared to the axis of the femoral component. The axis of femoral component on the lateral view is determined by the longitudinal axis of the pegs or perpendicular to the box (in posterior-stabilised knees) or parallel to anterior/posterior flange of the femur. In implants with diverging flanges, the line bisecting the angle between the flanges is the femoral axis. The angle between the femoral axis and the axis of the implant is the gamma angle (Fig. 3.4).

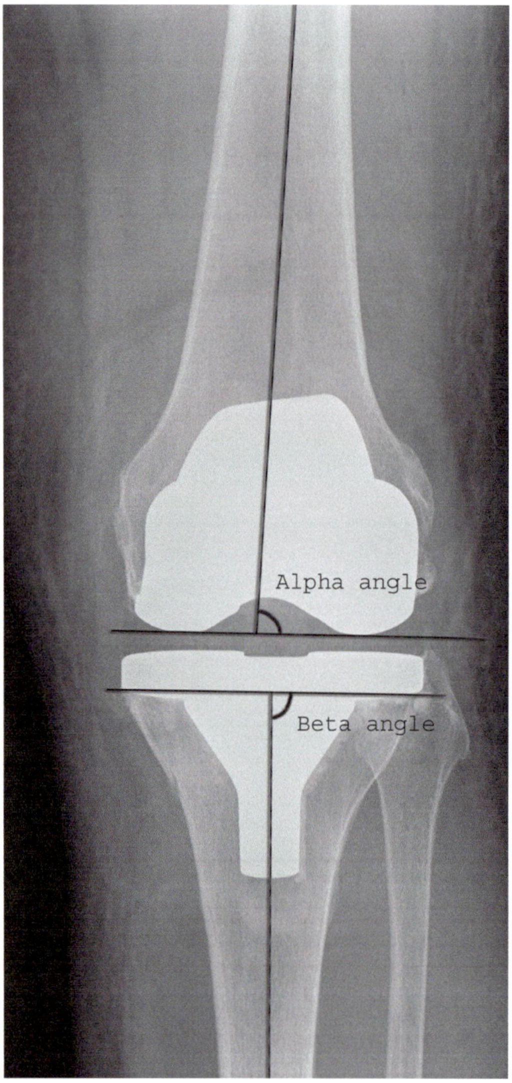

Fig. 3.3 Determination of the alpha angle and beta angle on the AP radiograph of the knee

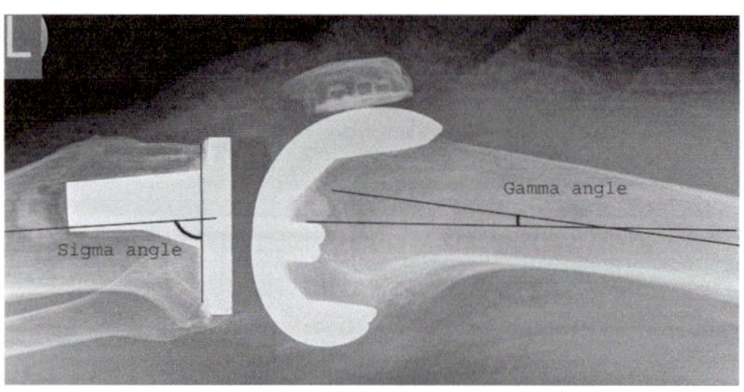

Fig. 3.4 Determination of the gamma angle and sigma angle on the lateral radiograph

The axis of femoral component should be collinear with the femoral axis.

On the lateral view of the tibia, the tibial axis is along the keel of tibial component. The angle between the tibial component and the tibial axis is sigma angle. Posterior slope on the tibia is desirable in most implants. Anterior slope on the tibia should be avoided as it impedes posterior femoral rollback and leads to restricted knee flexion.

The Knee Society has developed a scoring system [1] for knee replacement radiographs (Fig. 3.5). The presence of radiolucency at cement-bone or implant-bone interface can be described based on the radiologic zones.

In the AP view (Fig. 3.5a), seven zones have been defined for the cement interface of the tibial component. Zones 1, 2, 3 and 4 are along the tibial base plate, and 5, 6 and 7 represent the keel of the tibial component. For the femoral component fixation, seven zones are defined in the lateral view (Fig. 3.5b), with the peg represented by zones 5, 6 and 7. The patellar fixation is determined on the skyline view, with the pegs on the patellar component designated as zones 3, 4 and 5. Further derivations of numeric system to define loosening of the component have been reported, which is based on zones with radiolucency and the width of the radiolucent line in millimetres.

The main advantage of this system lies in its definition of zones of fixation.

While this is an elaborate attempt to introduce comparability in knee radiographs, the overwhelming limitations of this system are lack of reproducibility of knee radiographs and lack of clinical correlation of the numeric system.

A nonprogressive radiolucent line, less than 2 mm wide at the cement-bone interface, is fairly common, and does not signify loosening of the implant [2].

Asymmetry of the extension gap has been associated with increased postoperative pain following total knee replacement. This assessment is based on the routine postoperative radiograph (Fig. 3.6). The distance between the femoral condyle and tibial component is compared between the medial side and the lateral side. Presence of a medial opening extension

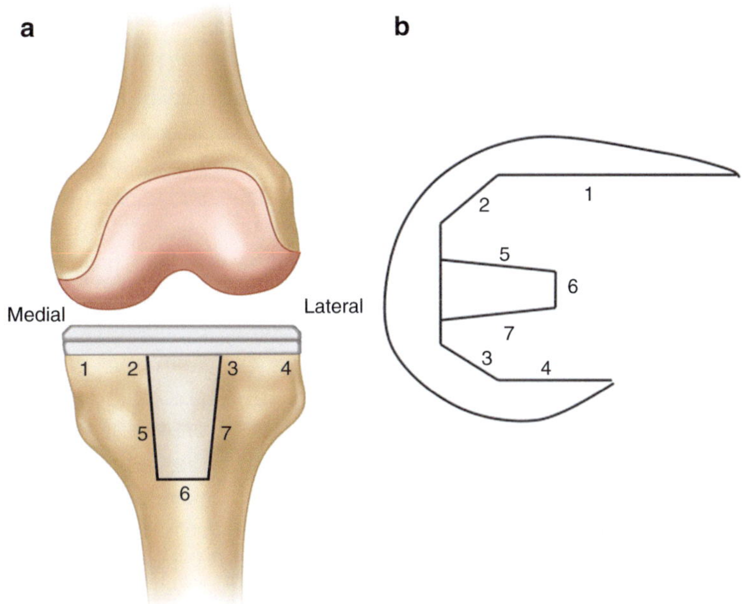

Fig. 3.5 Knee society scoring system for knee radiographs. The numeric system describes zones on the femoral and tibial interface. The zones on the tibia are demonstrated on the AP view (**a**), and the femoral zones are shown in the lateral view (**b**)

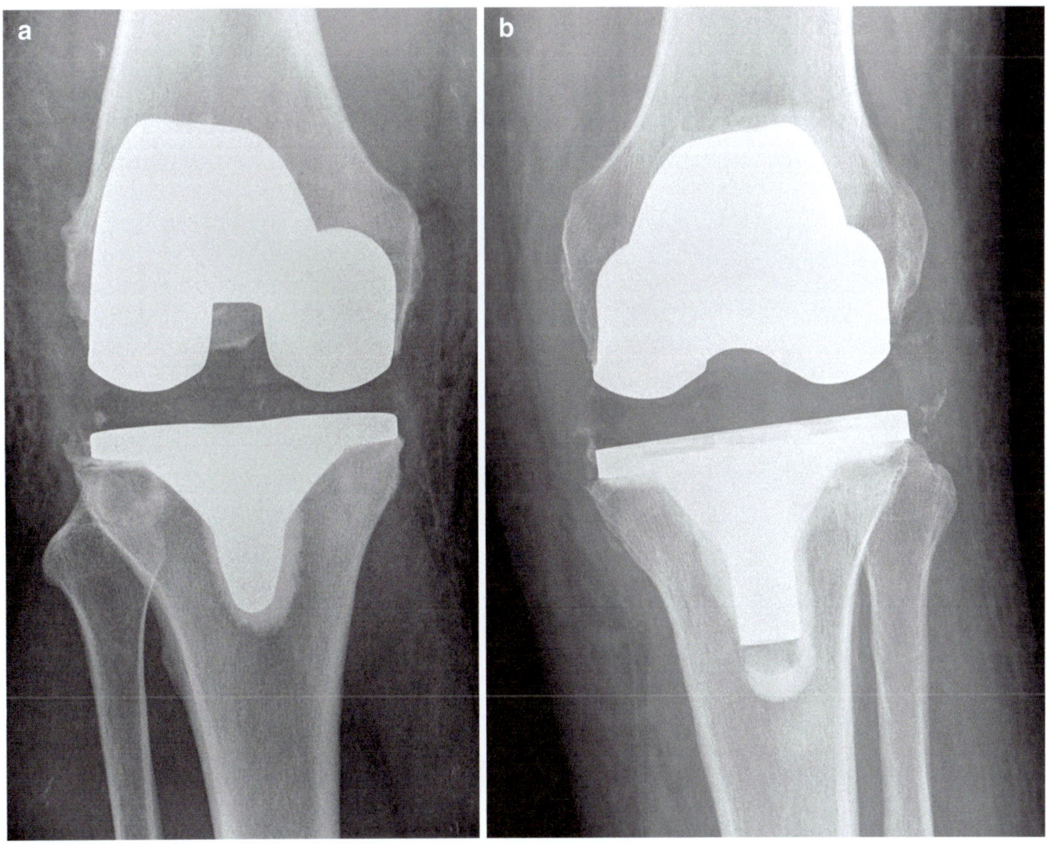

Fig. 3.6 (**a**) Asymmetric gap on postoperative radiograph. Lateral widening indicates lateral ligamentous laxity. (**b**) An example of medial gap widening

gap (wider space on the medial side compared to lateral side of the joint) may be associated with increased incidence of pain postoperatively [3]. Patients with lateral opening of the joint had better improvement in pain compared to those with medial opening.

In effect, asymmetry of the joint on non-weight-bearing postoperative radiographs indicates ligamentous imbalance. This may not be evident on the weight-bearing AP radiograph as the femur and tibial components are compressed together. Weight-bearing radiographs are helpful to detect gross ligamentous insufficiency in malaligned knees, but minor degrees of imbalance may be masked on weight bearing.

Varus or valgus malalignment of the femoral component will affect the axis of the limb. A tilted joint line may lead to postoperative pain (Figs. 3.7, 3.8, and 3.9).

Overhang of the tibial or femoral component may be a cause of pain postoperatively due to soft tissue irritation (Fig. 3.10). Medial tibial overhang impinges on the medial collateral ligament, and lateral overhang can impinge on the iliotibial band.

The posterior condylar offset is measured (Fig. 3.11) from the posterior aspect of the femoral condyle to a line extended along the posterior cortex of the femur on the lateral view. The posterior condylar offset ratio can be measured on the lateral radiograph. A straight line is drawn on the lateral view as an extension to the posterior cortex of the femur. The posterior offset ratio is the maximum projection of the posterior condyle posterior to the line compared to

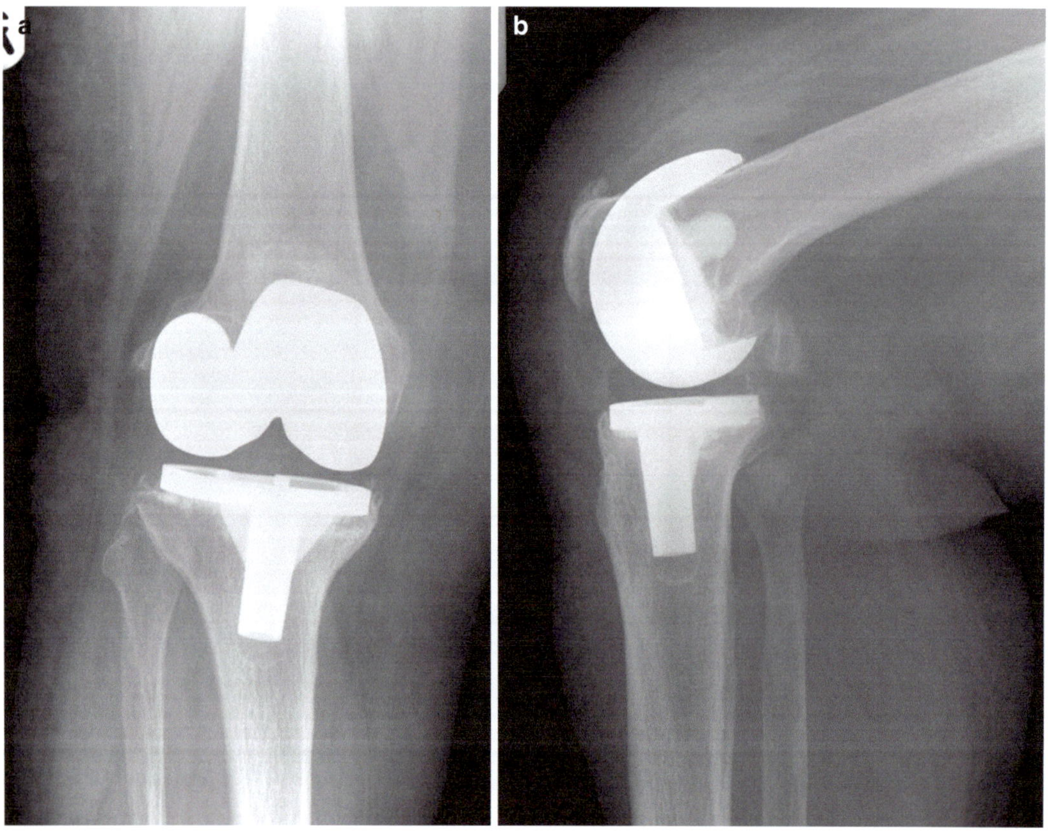

Fig. 3.7 Excess valgus positioning of the femoral component along with varus malalignment of the tibial component leading to a tilted joint line evident on the AP view (**a**). Note the anterior slope on the tibia on the lateral view (**b**), which may lead to restricted flexion range post operatively

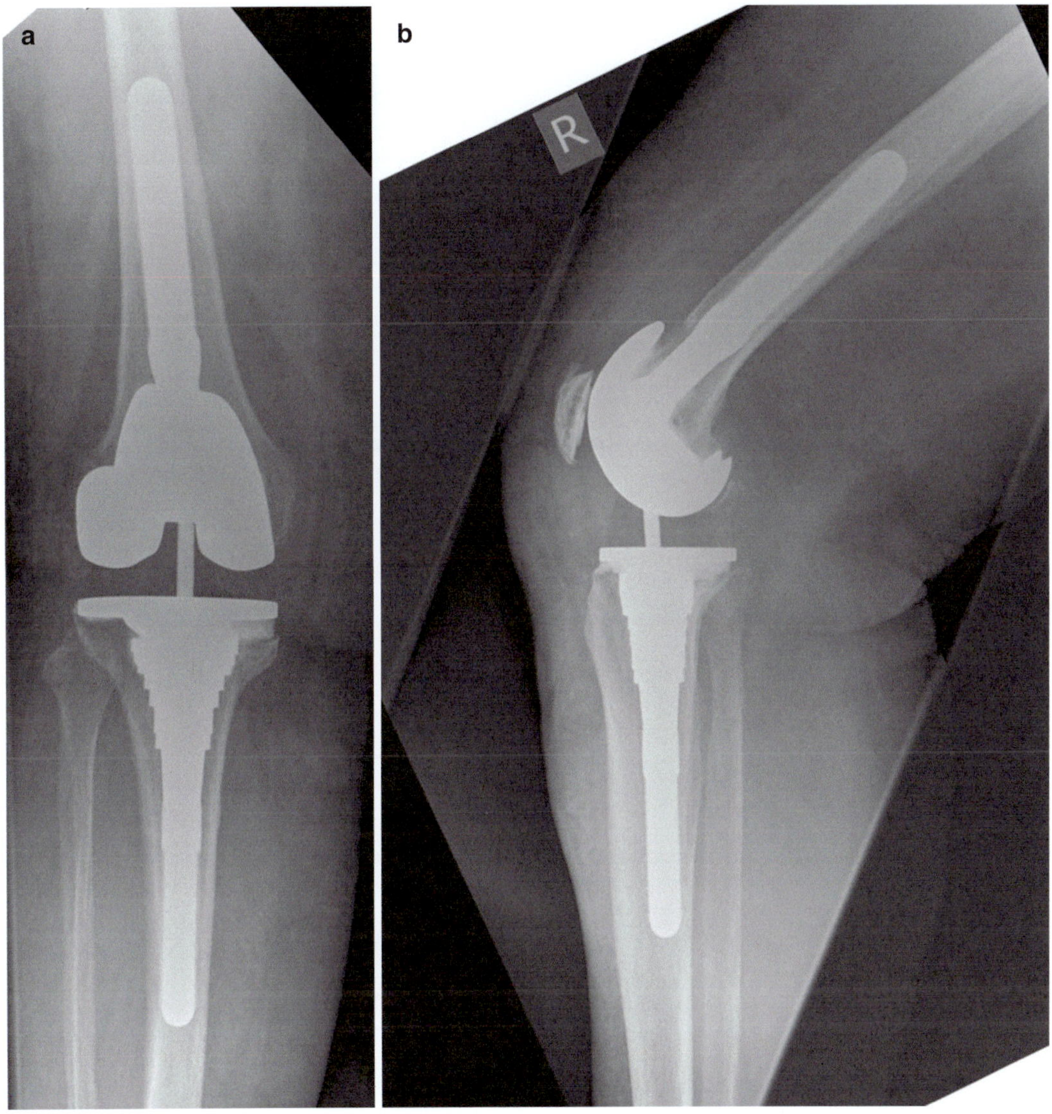

Fig. 3.8 Radiographs after revision showing restoration of normal femoral valgus angle. The tibial varus has been corrected on the AP view (**a**). Stem and sleeve have been used to augment fixation on the tibia. There is bone loss on the medial margin of tibia which has been filled with cement. Tibial fixation has been achieved predominantly through the use of metaphyseal sleeve with good contact in the AP and lateral view (**b**). The femoral component has a stem. An augment (not visible on radiographs) was used to fill the defect in distal part of lateral femoral condyle

the distance from the anterior femoral cortex to the tip of posterior condyle at that level [4]. Inadequate restoration of posterior condylar offset can lead to flexion instability (Fig. 3.12), while increasing the posterior offset can lead to a tight flexion gap and restriction of flexion postoperatively.

Postoperative radiographs should be carefully scrutinised for iatrogenic fractures, especially in the osteopenic bone (Fig. 3.13).

Cementless total knee replacements were 4% of all knee replacements done in the UK in 2011. The metal implants have a porous coating to allow bone ingrowth. Some implants have a tra-

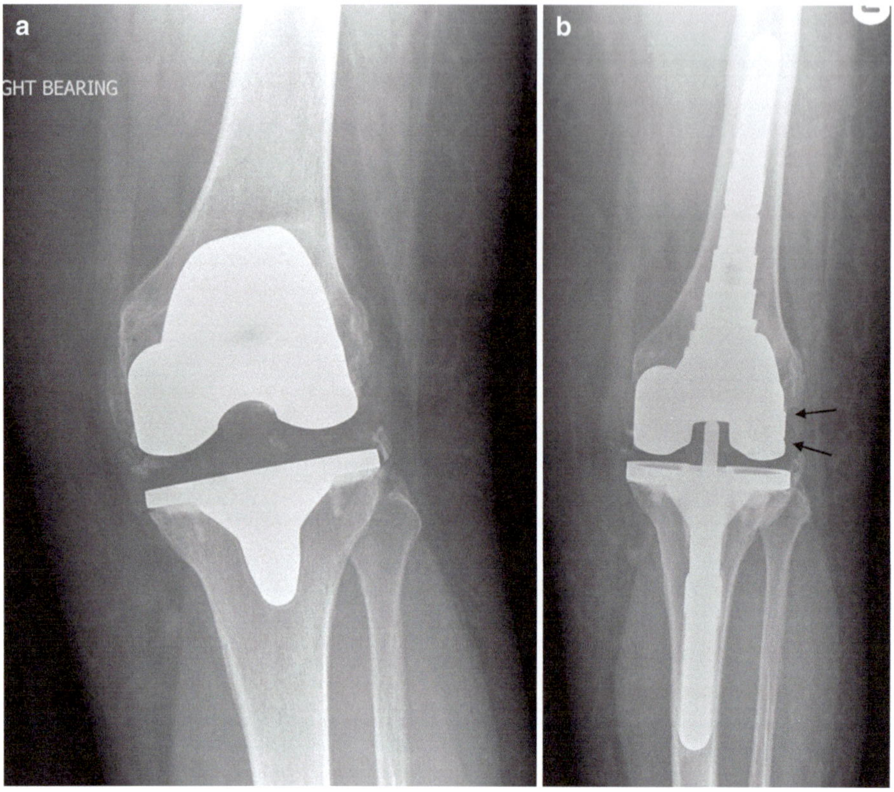

Fig. 3.9 Excess valgus of the femoral component evident in the AP view (**a**) corrected through revision surgery (**b**). The augment on the lateral side of femoral component is visible on post-revision radiograph (**b**). The augment, shown by the arrows, fills the gap between the femoral component and the distal lateral femoral condyle

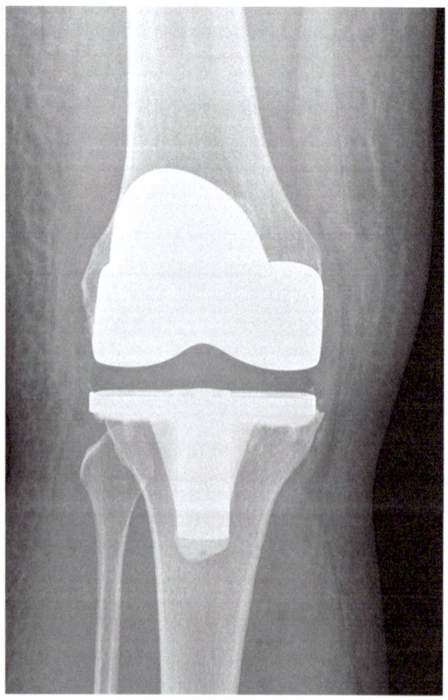

Fig. 3.10 Overhang of the tibial component on the lateral side. Medial overhang should be avoided as it impinges on the medial collateral ligament and may lead to attrition rupture of the tendon

becular metal interface on the tibial side (Fig. 3.14).

All-poly tibial components are made entirely of polyethylene and are in the same shape as the combination of metal and polyethylene insert (Fig. 3.15). They lack the modularity, which is present in metal-backed tibial components, but survival of all-polyethylene tibial components is similar to metal-backed tibial components.

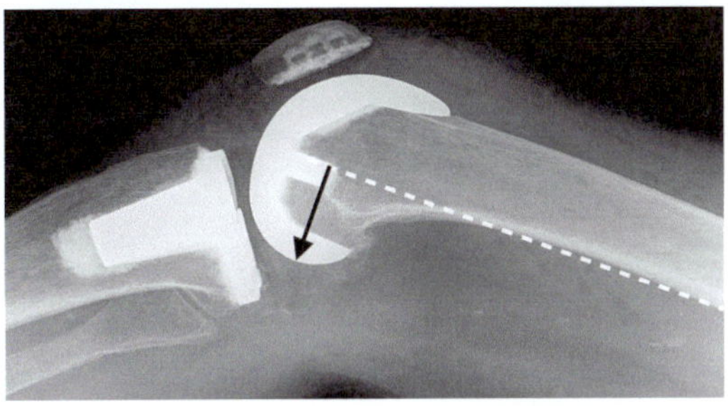

Fig. 3.11 Measurement of posterior condylar offset. The white dotted line is the projection along the posterior cortex of the femur, and the black arrow denotes the posterior condylar offset

Mobile-bearing knee replacements have been developed in an effort to reduce the wear of the polyethylene insert. These allow flexion-extension and some gliding on the superior surface of the insert, and rotation occurs on the under surface of the insert. As the insert is free to rotate on the tibial component, accurate balancing of the gaps is essential to minimise risk of bearing spinout (Figs. 3.16 and 3.17).

Unicompartmental knee replacements comprised 8% of all knee replacements in the UK in 2015 (12th Annual report, National Joint Registry, UK). The medial, the lateral or the patellofemoral compartments can be replaced individually, thereby preserving the other two compartments.

Medial replacements comprise the vast majority of unicompartmental replacements. The Oxford design (Fig. 3.18) is the commonest mobile bearing in use in the UK. In the mobile-bearing version, the superior surface of tibial component is smooth and highly polished, allow-

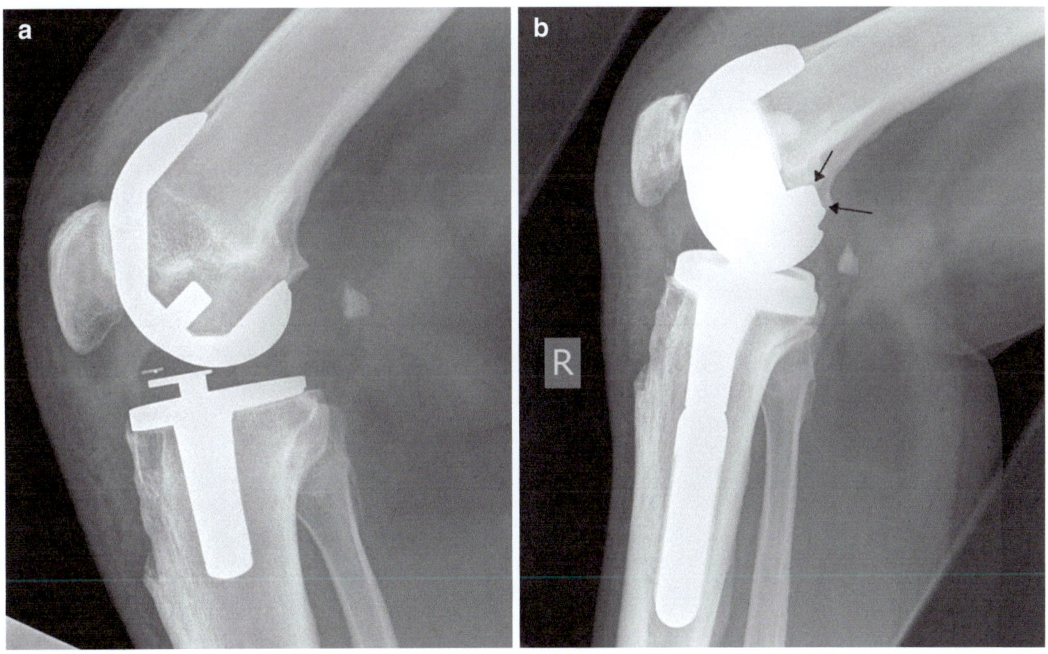

Fig. 3.12 (**a**) Lateral view of the knee showing excess posterior resection on the femoral condyle, which led to a loose flexion gap and flexion instability. (**b**) At revision the posterior femoral condyle was built up using 8 mm augments on both medial and lateral femoral condyles. Note the augment just below the tip of the flange of the femoral component posteriorly between the two arrows

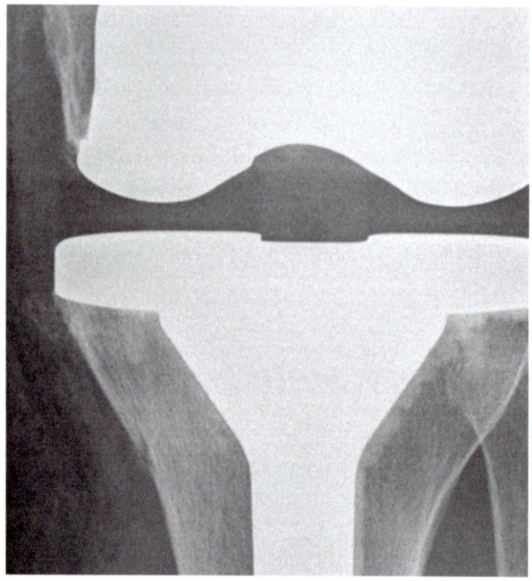

Fig. 3.13 Discontinuity along the proximal medial tibial cortex noted on postoperative images. This could be due to iatrogenic fracture sustained during tibial preparation or impaction. Alternatively, this could be from the tip of a pin used to fix the tibial preparation tray. The pins are inserted vertically, and due to the conical shape of the proximal tibia, they may sometimes penetrate the medial tibial cortex. Further imaging (CT scan) may be helpful to determine the cause and extent of this discontinuity

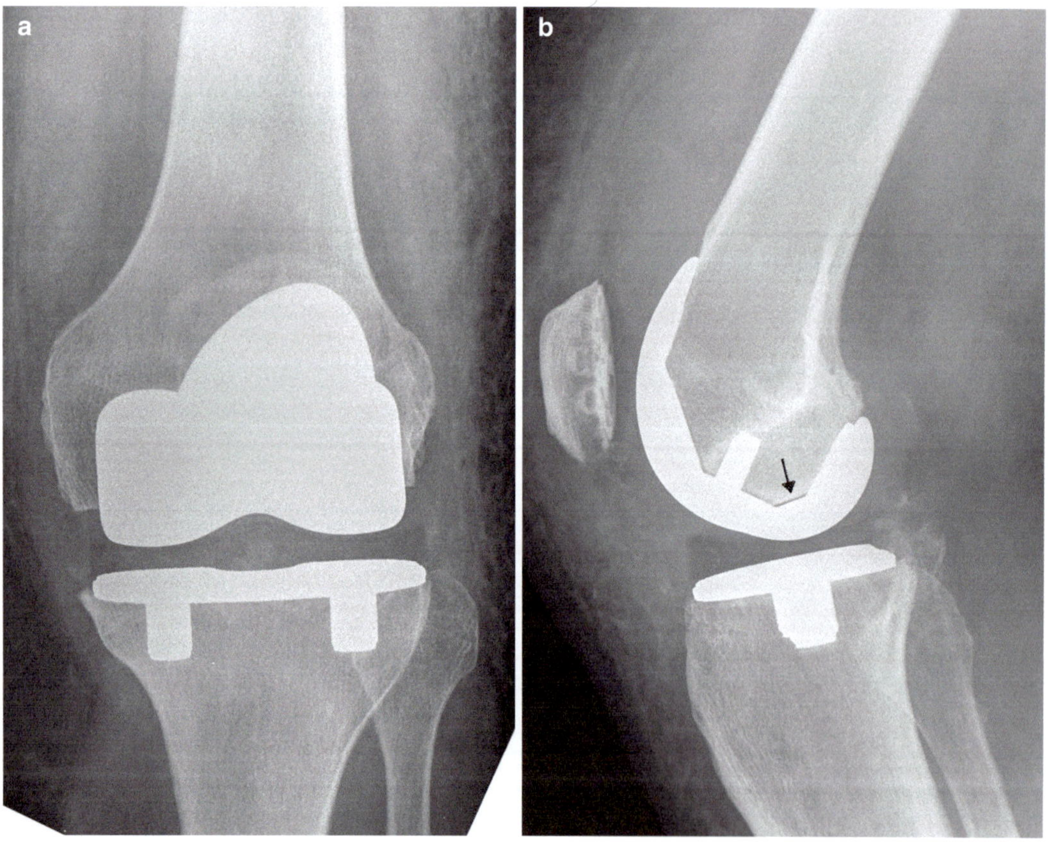

Fig. 3.14 AP (**a**) and lateral (**b**) view of cementless total knee replacement. In this implant, the tibial interface is trabecular metal. On the femoral side in lateral view, there is radiolucency along the posterior chamfer (arrow). This was present on the first postoperative radiograph and was nonprogressive on serial radiographs. It implies lack of contact between the metal and bone, while seating the implant, but does not indicate loosening

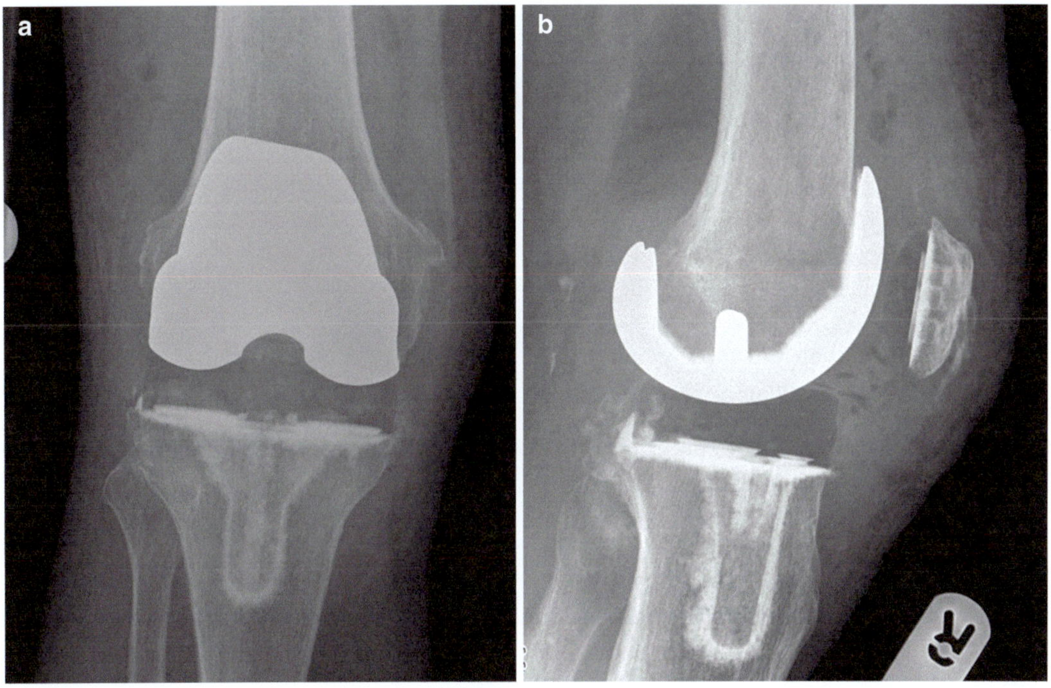

Fig. 3.15 All-polyethylene tibial component with a cemented cruciate-retaining femoral component in the AP (**a**) and lateral (**b**) view. Only the cementation is visible on the tibial side

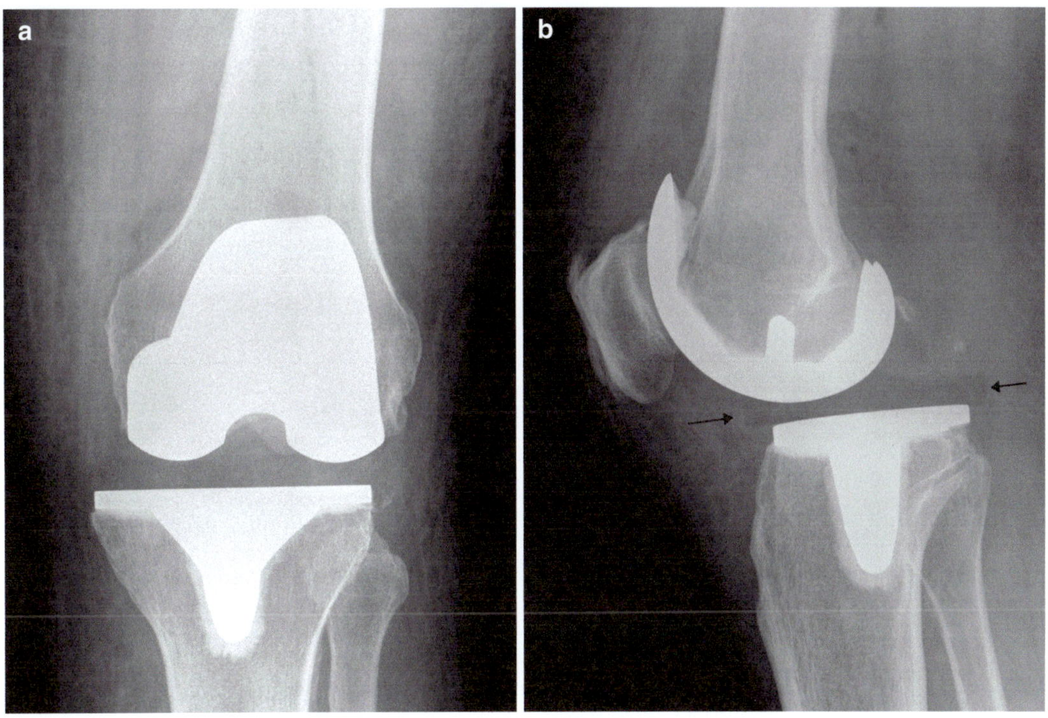

Fig. 3.16 A cruciate-retaining mobile-bearing insert which has 'spun out'. On the AP view (**a**), there is malalignment between the femoral and tibial component. On the lateral view (**b**) of the knee, the insert is visible as if it is in an anteroposterior projection (between the black arrows)

ing the highly conforming polyethylene insert to move freely over the tibial component. The superior surface of the insert is concave and matches the shape of the spherical femoral component. Accurate sizing and positioning of the component (Fig. 3.19) and optimum tension in the soft tissues are essential for good outcome. Excess valgus alignment of the knee will lead to over load of the lateral compartment and pain, requiring revision surgery.

In the fixed-bearing version (Fig. 3.20), the superior surface of the tibial component has a locking mechanism to engage the polyethylene insert. The insert remains fixed to the tibia.

As opposed to total knee replacements, the coronal plane restoration of alignment depends on the balancing of the soft tissues rather than the angle of bone resection. Increasing the tightness by using thicker insert will shift the mechanical axis of the limb to the contralateral side of the knee, resulting in increased loading of the unreplaced compartment. This can lead to accelerated wear of the unreplaced compartment, with subsequent need for total knee replacement.

Lateral unicompartmental replacements are less than 1% of all knee replacements. Most of the lateral replacement implants employ fixed-bearing design. The limb alignment should be few degrees of valgus to prevent overload on the medial side (Fig. 3.21).

Patellofemoral replacements are less than 1% of all knee replacements. The patellar components are all polyethylene and cemented. The femoral component resurfaces the trochlea and can be an onlay design (Fig. 3.22) or an inlay design (Fig. 3.23).

Bicompartmental knee replacements (Fig. 3.24) are intended to deal with two arthritic compartments while preserving the cruciate ligaments. Long-term survival of these is unproven at present.

The polyethylene insert may dislocate in mobile-bearing unicompartmental replacements. This is generally due to improper balancing (ten-

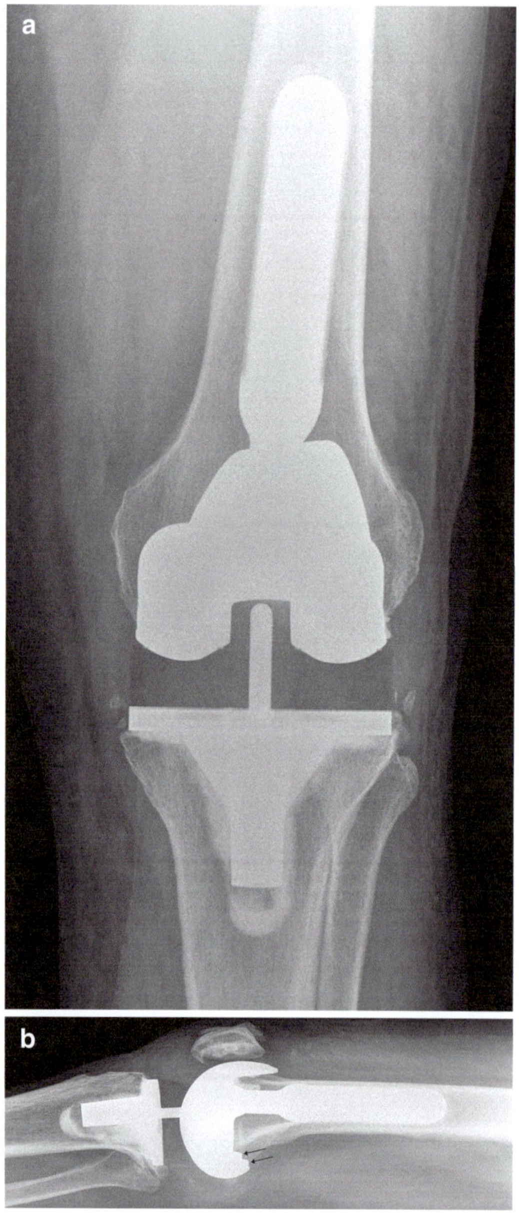

Fig. 3.17 Radiographs following revision surgery for spinout. The tibial component has been switched to a fixed-bearing tray (**a**), in which the insert is fixed to the tibial component. The gaps were accurately balanced, and posterior augments (arrows) are visible on the lateral view (**b**). A semi-constrained implant has been used to provide some degree of varus and valgus stability. The metal bar within the polyethylene insert is the reinforcement bar for the relatively longer polyethylene peg of the insert. A stem has been used on the femoral side for additional fixation

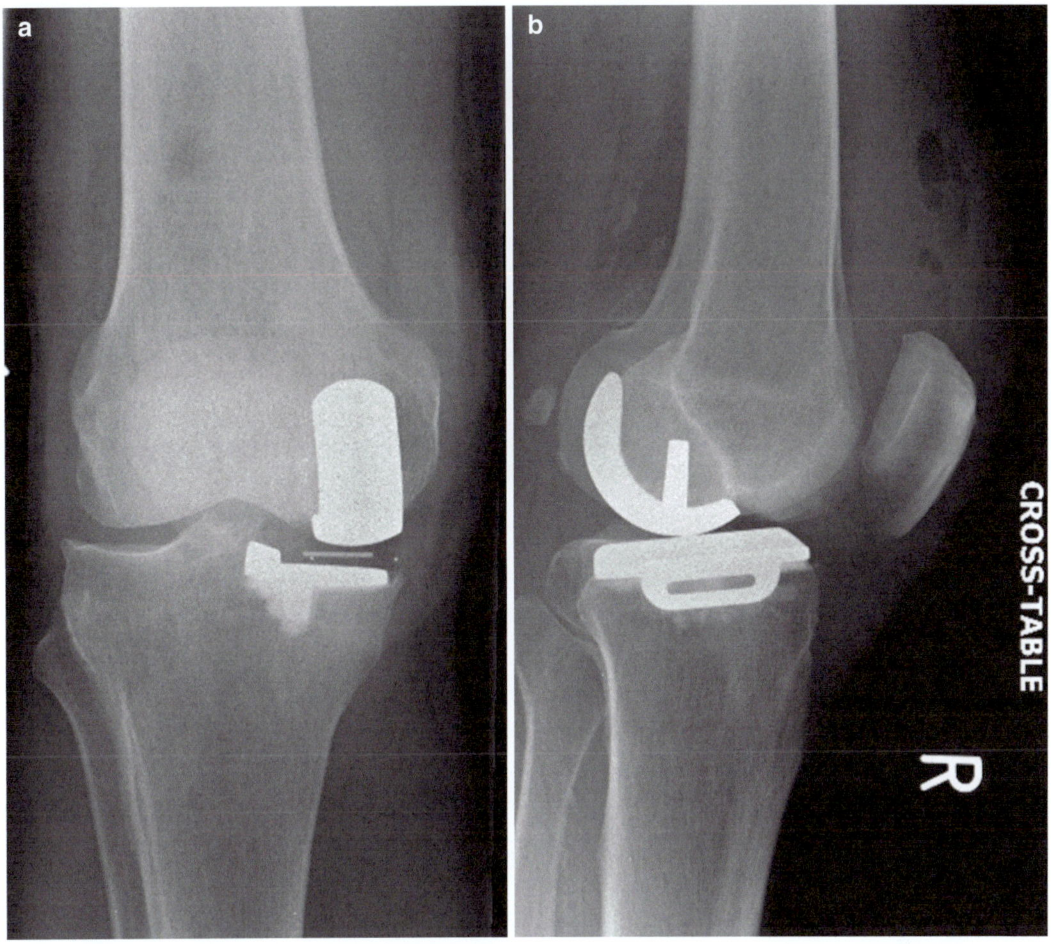

Fig. 3.18 Oxford medial unicompartmental replacement in the AP (**a**) and lateral view (**b**). The polyethylene insert is mobile (not fixed to the tibial component). The shape of the polyethylene matches the shape of the femoral component superiorly and is flat on the inferior surface to match the tibial component

sioning) of the knee with an excessive lax medial side (Fig. 3.25).

Notching of the anterior femoral cortex (Fig. 3.26) can predispose to supracondylar fracture of the femur. Ideally, the anterior flange of the femoral component should be along the anterior cortex of femur. Posterior translation of the femoral component will lead to notching. Excess anterior translation, conversely, will 'overstuff' the patellofemoral joint and may cause anterior knee pain (Fig. 3.27).

Bone loss in the proximal tibia may require the use of metal augments. These are fixed to the undersurface of the tibial component and can be either on one half (Fig. 3.28) or on the entire undersurface of the tibial component (Fig. 3.29). Overhang of the augments should be avoided, as medial overhang can lead to attrition rupture of the medial collateral ligament.

An alternative method to gain fixation in the compromised bone is through the use of metal metaphyseal sleeves (Fig. 3.30) [5]. These allow

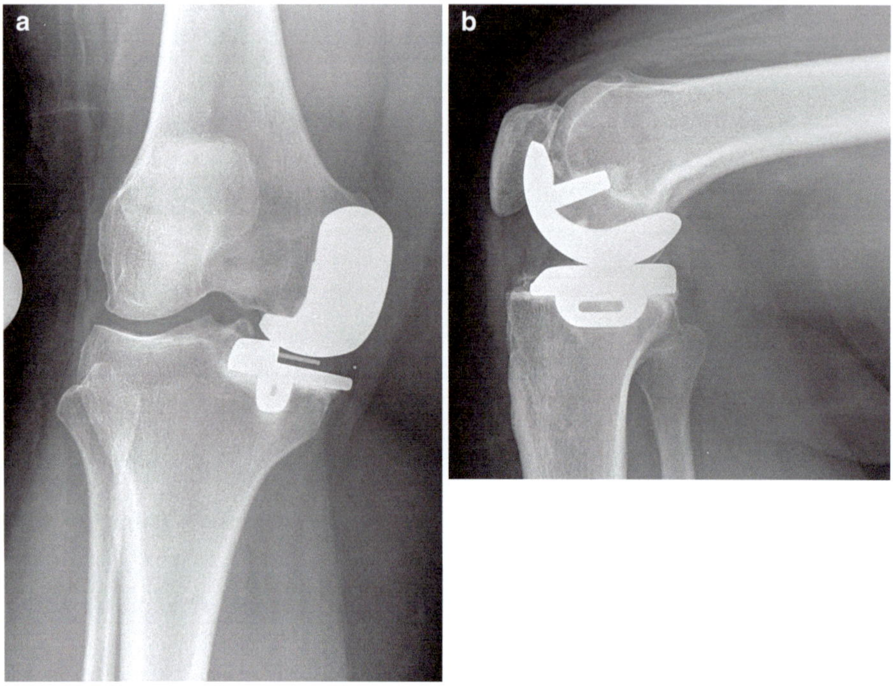

Fig. 3.19 An Oxford medial unicompartmental replacement with overhang of the tibial component on the medial side seen in the AP view (**a**). There is minimal posterior slope on the tibial component, and the tibial component is translated posteriorly in the lateral view (**b**). The femoral component appears oversized evident by the overhang posteriorly and prominence beyond the femoral condyle anteriorly. The alignment of the knee is excess valgus in the AP view, which would shift the weight-bearing axis laterally and overload the lateral compartment

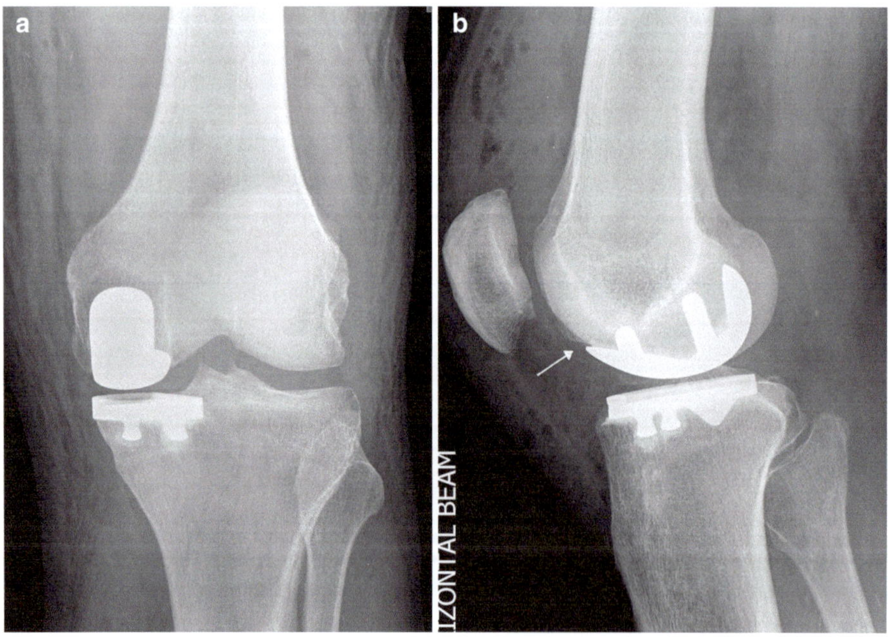

Fig. 3.20 A fixed-bearing medial unicompartmental knee replacement. There should not be any medial overhang of the tibial component on the AP view (**a**), as this can lead to pain and damage the medial collateral ligament. The tibial component should be perpendicular to the tibial mechanical axis. It is important to note the relative angle of the axis of femur and tibia. In this knee, the femur and tibia axis are collinear, implying a varus alignment of the knee. This prevents overloading of the lateral compartment. In the lateral view (**b**), the femoral component should not extend beyond the resected femoral surface (arrow), or this can impinge on the patella and lead to pain on patellar gliding

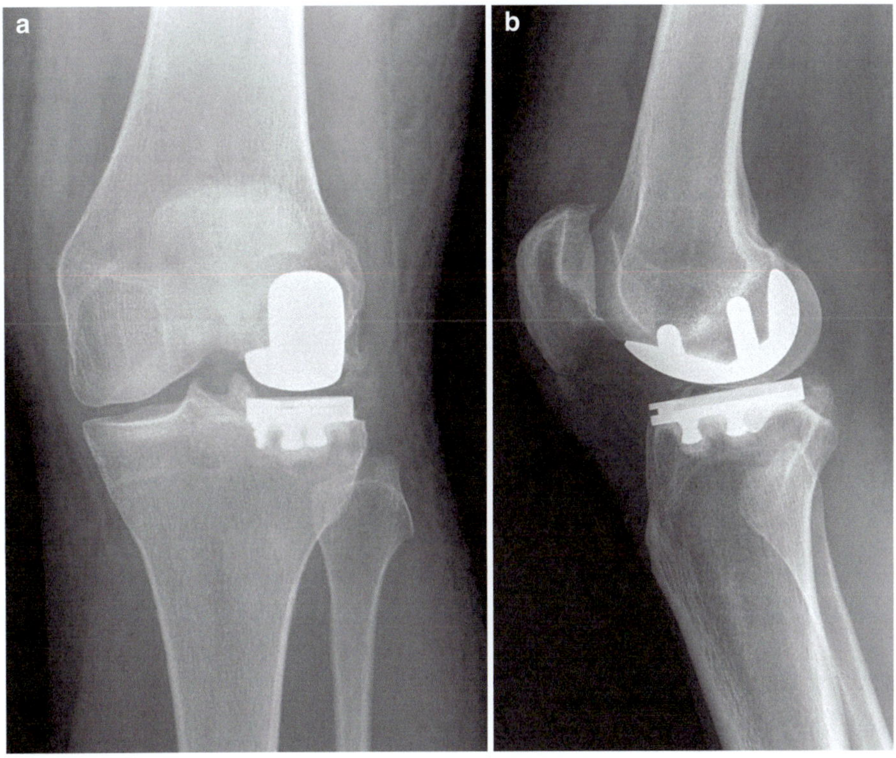

Fig. 3.21 Lateral unicompartmental replacement AP (**a**) and lateral (**b**) view using a fixed-bearing implant done for arthritis secondary to lateral meniscectomy. The limb alignment is valgus, which helps load the implant

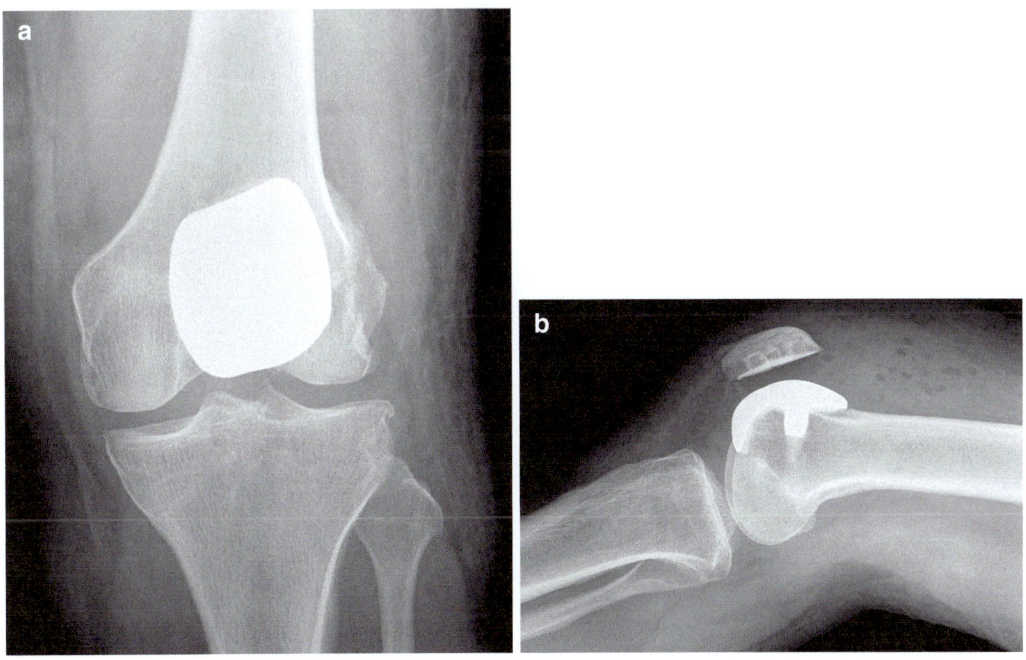

Fig. 3.22 AP (**a**) and lateral (**b**) radiographs following patellofemoral replacement. The joint space in the medial and lateral tibiofemoral joints is well preserved. The trochlear component is an 'onlay' design

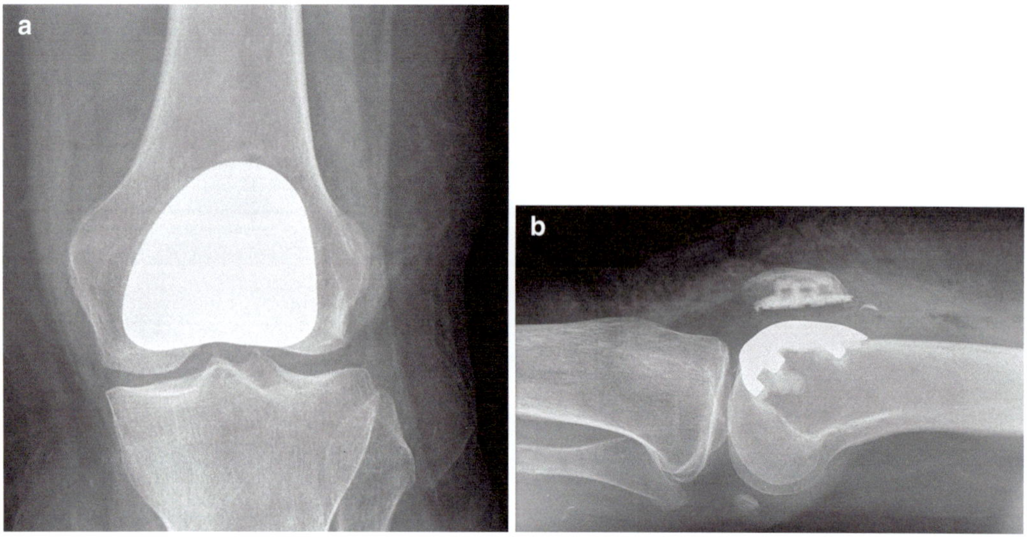

Fig. 3.23 A different patellofemoral replacement design. The AP view (**a**) is similar to the implant in Fig. 3.22; the femoral component has a lower profile on the lateral view (**b**). The femoral component is 'inlay' type and is placed into a milled area. Compare this to Fig. 3.22b where the femoral component in 'onlay' and the posterior aspect of the femoral flange are collinear with the anterior femoral cortex. The inlay implants cause less 'overstuffing' of the patellofemoral joint

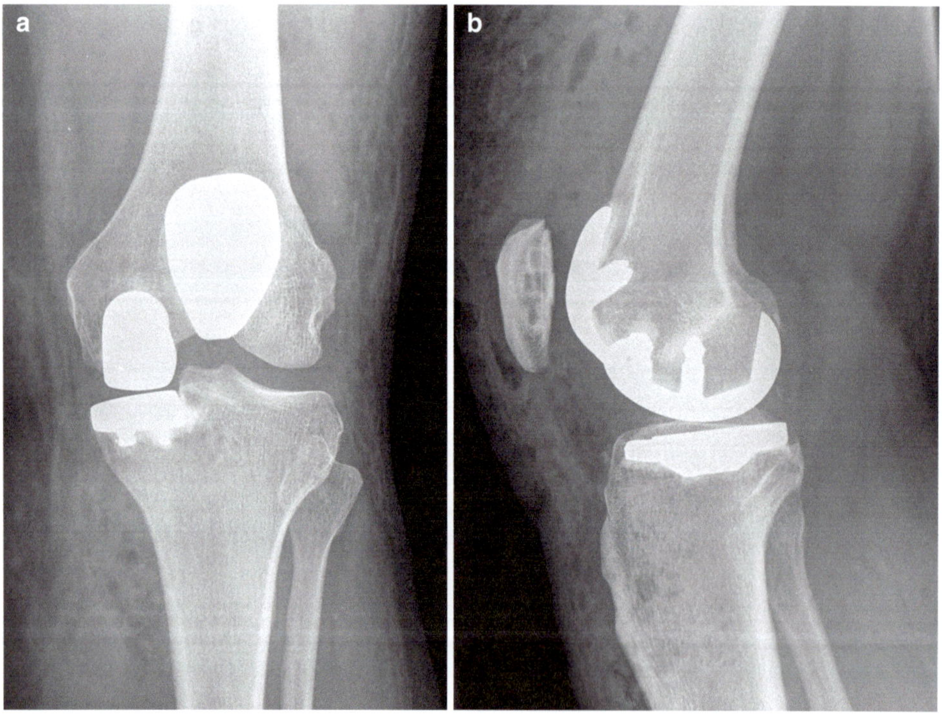

Fig. 3.24 Medial and patellofemoral compartment replacement. AP view (**a**) and lateral view (**b**) show replacement of the medial and patellofemoral compartment. The lateral compartment is preserved, and the cruciate and collateral ligaments are left intact

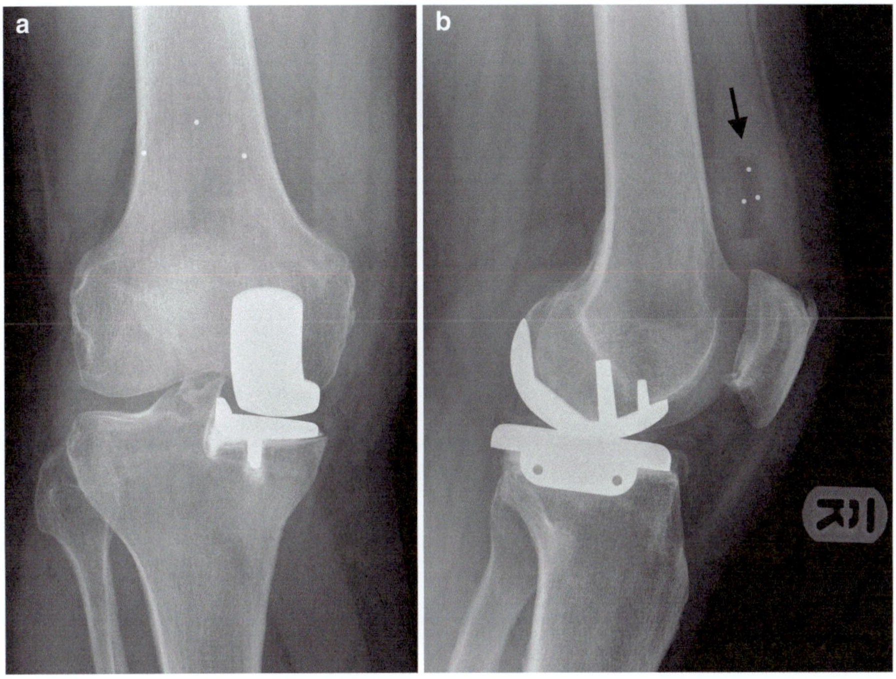

Fig. 3.25 Dislocated polyethylene from a medial unicompartmental replacement. The gap between the femoral and tibial component is reduced on the AP view (**a**). The polyethylene insert in this particular implant has three radio-opaque markers seen in both views. These are visible in the suprapatellar pouch within the radiolucency of the insert seen in the lateral view (**b**). This patient had revision of the mobile bearing to a fixed-bearing medial unicompartmental replacement

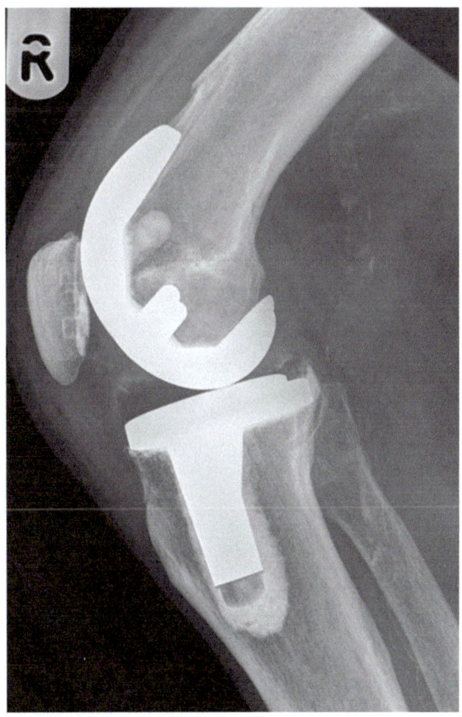

Fig. 3.26 Lateral radiograph after total knee replacement using a cruciate-retaining, fixed-bearing cemented implant. There is gross notching of the anterior femoral cortex. The tibial component has been placed in excess posterior slope, which can cause flexion instability

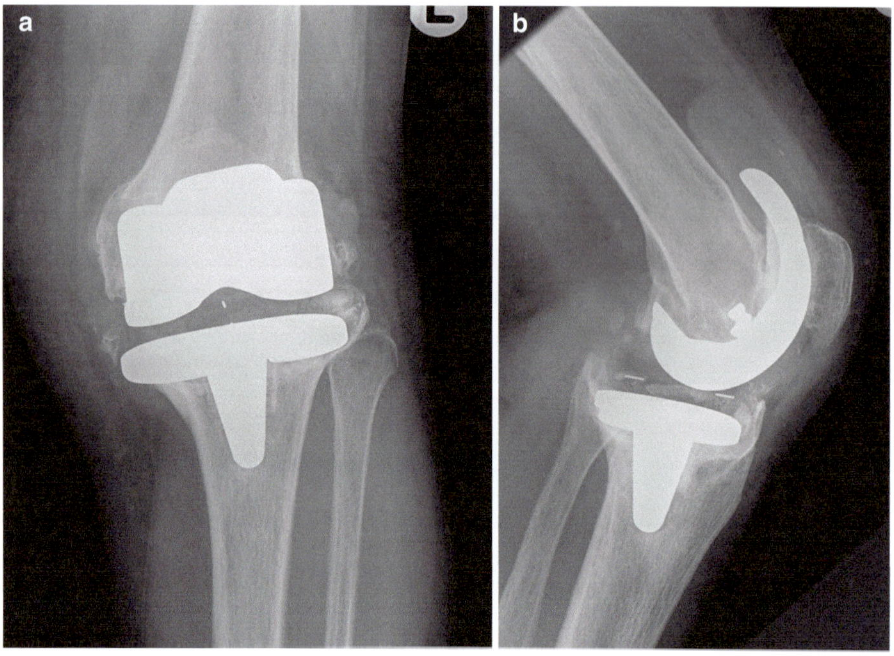

Fig. 3.27 Gross loosening and subsidence of the tibial component. There is proximal medial tibial bone loss, resulting in an uncontained defect seen in the AP view (**a**). The femoral component is oversized, with an anteriorly translated anterior flange, overstuffing the patellofemoral joint in the lateral view (**b**). Femoral component valgus measures 14°, as opposed to the usual 4–7° valgus. This would imply lateral femoral condyle bone loss. The polyethylene has a metal marker which identifies the position of the polyethylene insert

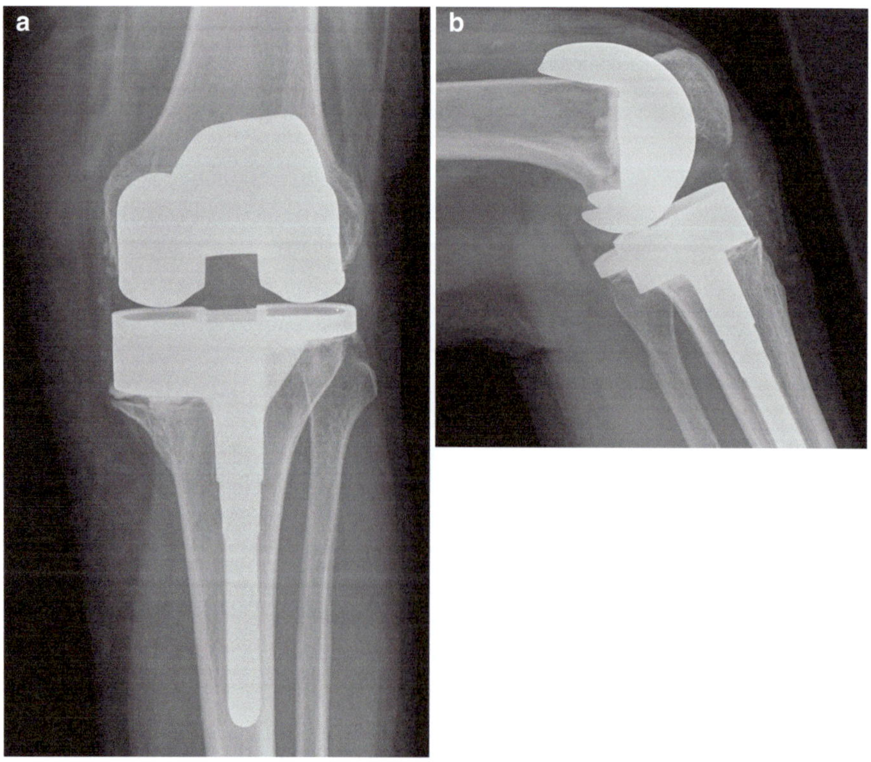

Fig. 3.28 AP (**a**) and lateral (**b**) view of knee prosthesis showing an augment on the under surface of the tibial component to manage medial tibial bone loss

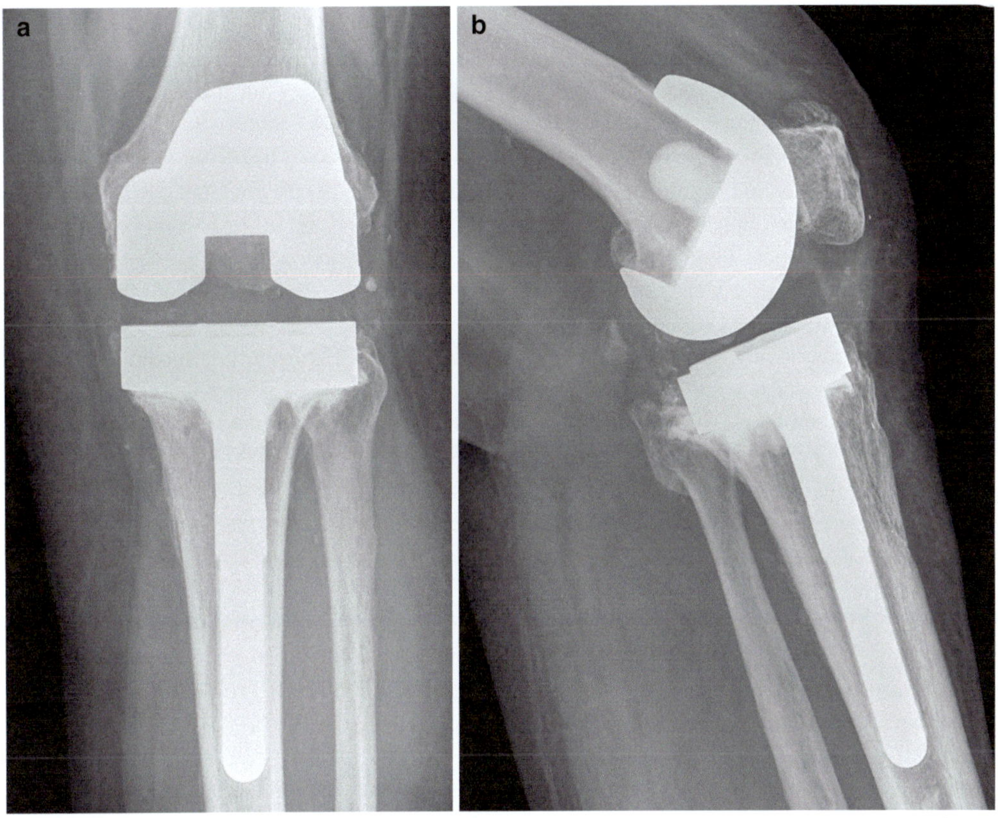

Fig. 3.29 A block augment on the under surface of the tibial component to manage proximal tibial bone loss. There is overhang of the augment on both medial and lateral cortices

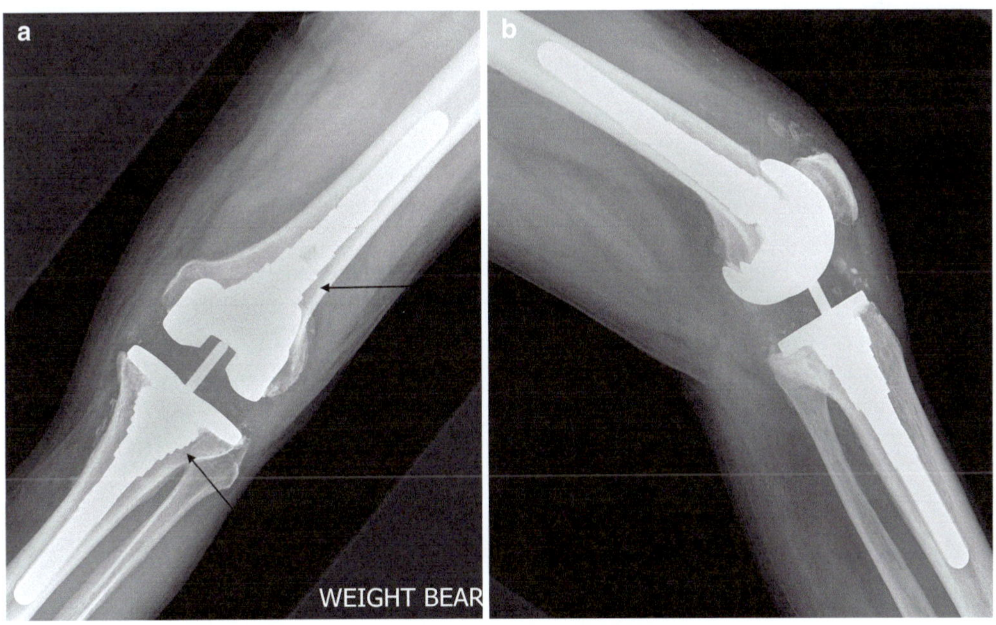

Fig. 3.30 Metal metaphyseal sleeves used to achieve cementless fixation in the proximal tibia and the distal femur. The metal sleeve (arrows) has stepped margins seen on the AP (**a**) and lateral (**b**) view and can be attached to the tibial and/or femoral component. Stems have been used on the femur and tibia. The metal in the polyethylene is for reinforcement of the peg, as this implant provides some degree of varus and valgus stability

cementless fixation in the metaphyseal bone of the proximal tibia and distal femur.

The degree of constraint used in the knee implant depends on the integrity of the knee ligaments. In unicompartmental knee replacements, the cruciate and collateral ligaments are preserved. In cruciate-retaining total knee replacement, the anterior cruciate ligament is removed, but posterior cruciate and both collaterals are preserved. Posterior-stabilised implants substitute for the posterior cruciate ligament but provide no stability against varus or valgus stress. Semiconstrained implants (Fig. 3.30) have greater conformity between the polyethylene peg and the box of the femoral component. These provide some degree of varus and valgus stability but are often inadequate for medial collateral ligament laxity. Deficiency of the medial collateral ligament is managed with the use of a hinged knee prosthesis (Fig. 3.31). Different designs are used in different situations (Fig. 3.32).

Osteolysis around knee replacements appears a number of years after initial surgery. The extent of osteolysis is often underestimated on plain radiographs, and CT scanning is more accurate in determining the degree of bone loss (Fig. 3.33).

An alternative method to reconstruct bone loss is through the use of trabecular metal shapes (Fig. 3.34). These are fixed to the host bone and achieve osseointegration. The knee prosthesis is cemented into the shapes. This differs from sleeves, as the sleeves are fixed to the prosthesis itself.

Failure of the components (Fig. 3.35) is rare with modern implants. The polyethylene insert wear may eventually lead to failure of the polyethylene (Fig. 3.36). In posterior-stabilised knee replacements, peg dislocation is a possible complication where the cam is dislocated anterior to the peg of the polyethylene (Fig. 3.37).

Extensive bone loss associated with periprosthetic fracture (Fig. 3.38) is a complex problem, and if the implants are loose, revision to a constrained implant may be the best option (Fig. 3.39). Loss of the distal femur through non-union (Fig. 3.40) or bone loss can be managed by replacement of the distal femur (Fig. 3.41).

Various options exist for the treatment of medial compartment arthritis of the knee. A common procedure is the high tibial osteotomy, which can be through a medial open wedge (Figs. 3.42 and 3.43) or a lateral closing wedge osteotomy. Another device aims to reduce the load on the medial compartment through distraction using a spring loaded system fixed to the medial side of the knee (Fig. 3.44). Currently, these have very limited utility.

Anterior cruciate ligament placement in the knee is described in relation to the femoral and tibial tunnels. The femoral reference is based on a grid described by [6] and known as the 'Bernard and Hertel grid' (Figs. 3.45 and 3.46). The grid 5 × 10 is based on tangent drawn along Blumensaat's line in the lateral view of the knee. Two perpendiculars are drawn at the intersection of this tangent with the shallow and the deep border of the lateral femoral condyle. The fourth line is parallel to Blumensaat's line and is tangent to the inferior border of the condyles. The centre of the femoral attachment of the ACL should be 27% in the deep-shallow direction and 34% in the high-low direction (Fig. 3.47).

In the AP view, the angle between the femoral tunnel and the femoral anatomical axis should be, on average, 39°. Angle below 17° may be associated with rotational instability.

For the tibial tunnel, the centre of the tibial tunnel should be 43% from the anterior cortex of the tibia, using the entire AP dimension of the tibia as a reference. The tibial tunnel should be

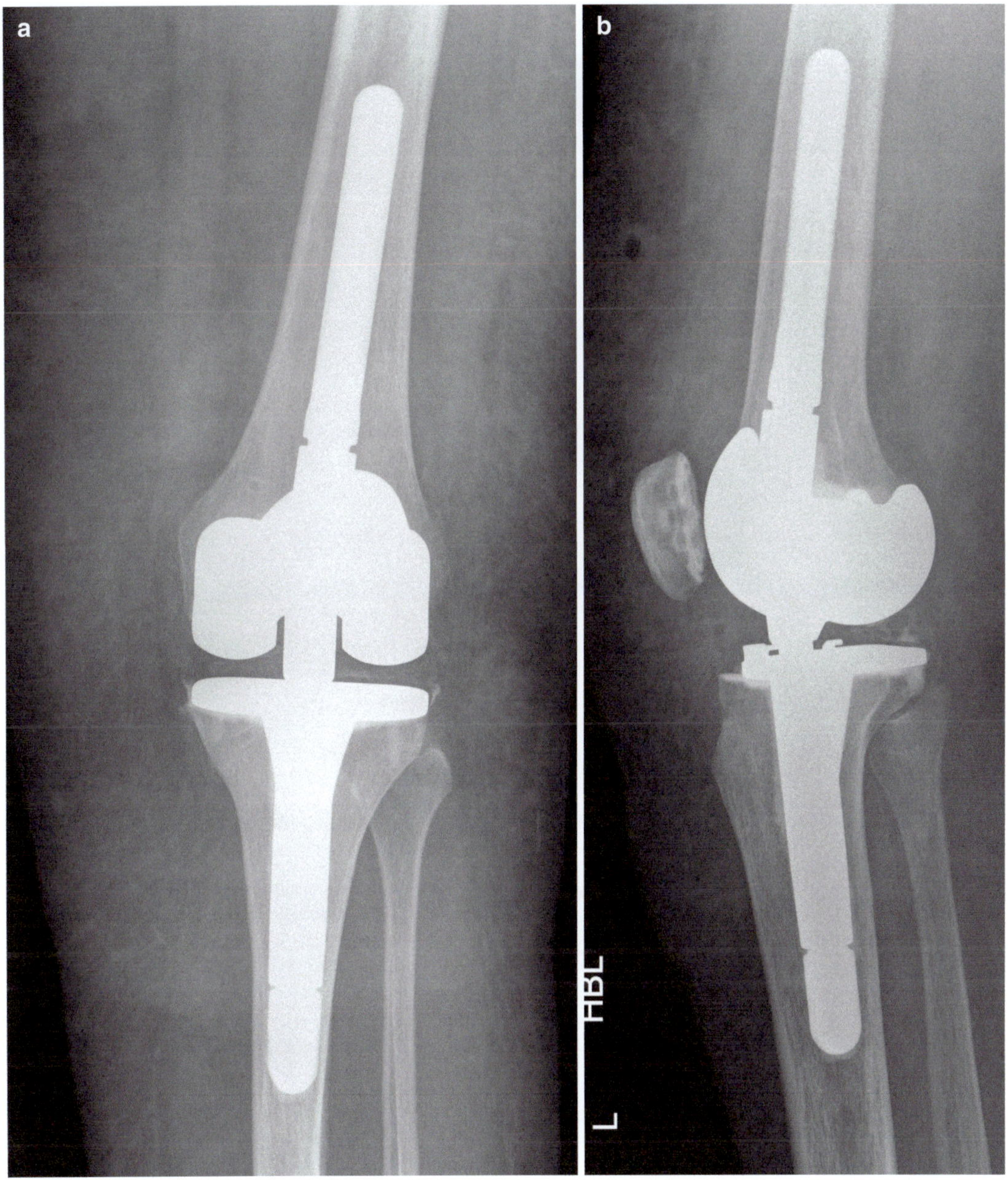

Fig. 3.31 A hinged knee replacement. The femoral and the tibial components are linked through a hinge, which prevents any varus/valgus movement. On the AP view (**a**), the link between the femoral component and tibial component is evident. On the lateral view (**b**), the hinge in this particular implant is central. This hinge allows rotation between the polyethylene insert and the tibial component, which reduces the stress at the fixation interface

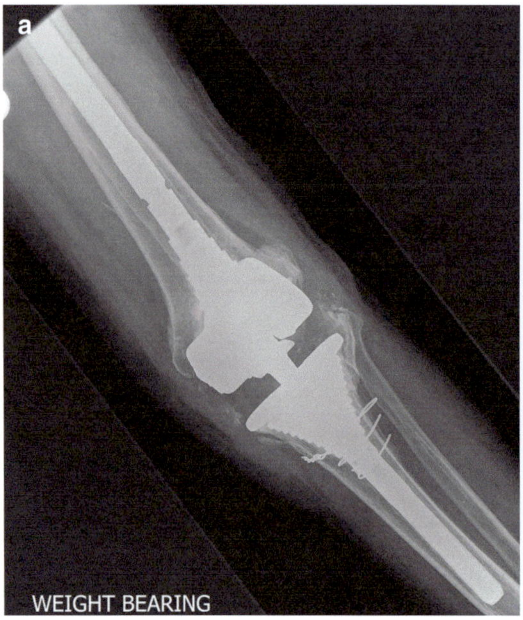

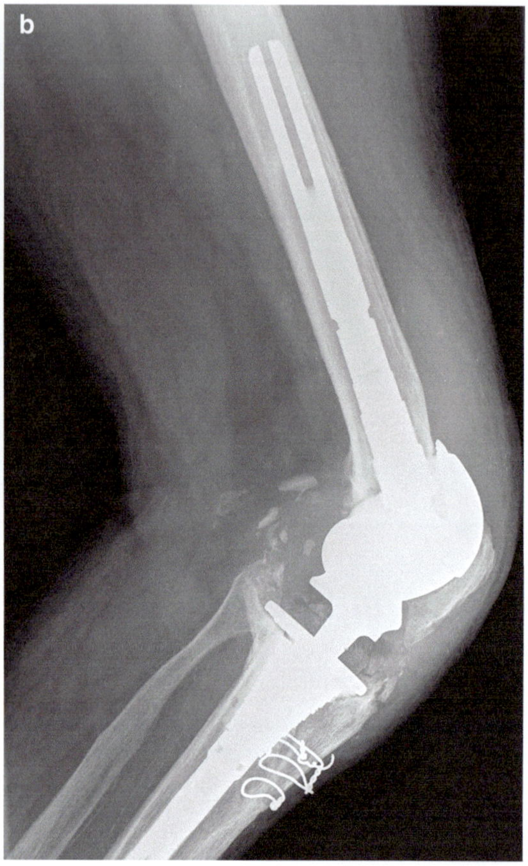

Fig. 3.32 Another example of a hinged knee replacement. There are stems in the femur and tibia along with metaphyseal sleeves (**a**). This design has a posterior location of the hinge (**b**), as opposed to the implant in Fig. 3.31, which has a central hinge. The wires in the anterior part of tibia are used to fix the tibial tubercle osteotomy, which was done for exposure of the knee joint for revision surgery

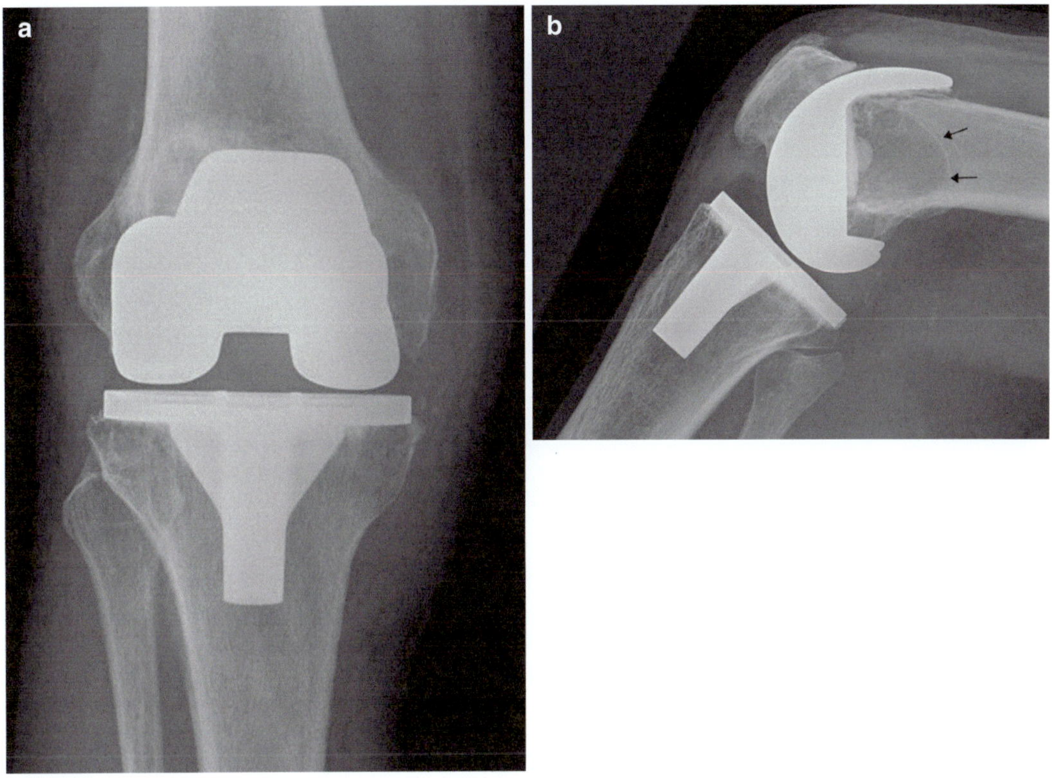

Fig. 3.33 Osteolysis in the distal femur which is largely obscured in the AP view (**a**) but visible in the lateral view (**b**) outlined by the arrows. (**c**) CT scan showing the extent of osteolysis in the distal femur. Metal metaphyseal sleeves have been used in revision surgery to gain fixation in the intact metaphysis in the distal femur. AP (**d**) and lateral (**e**) view shows the large sleeve required to achieve host bone contact. The tibial component has a stem but sleeves were not required

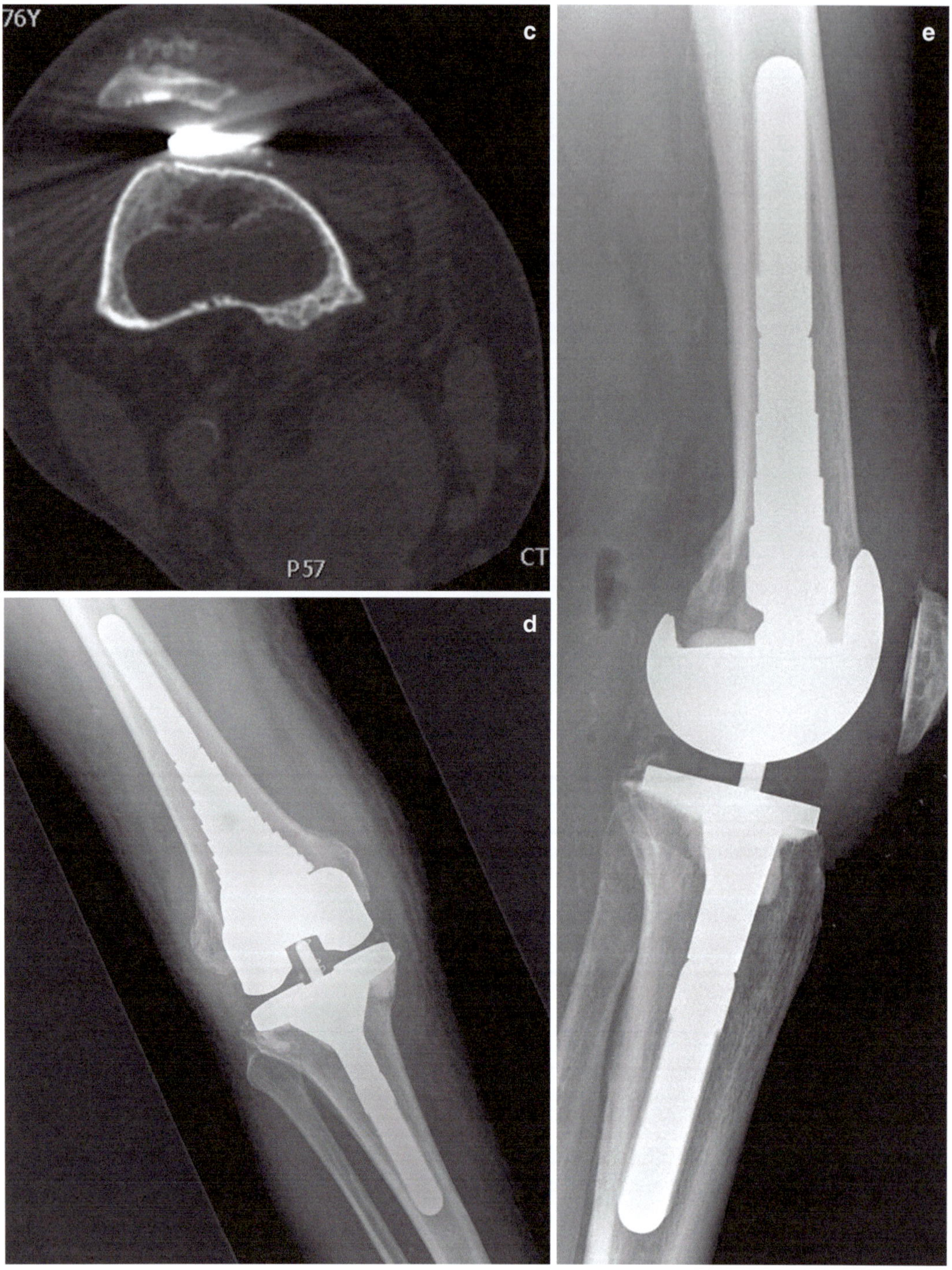

Fig. 3.33 (continued)

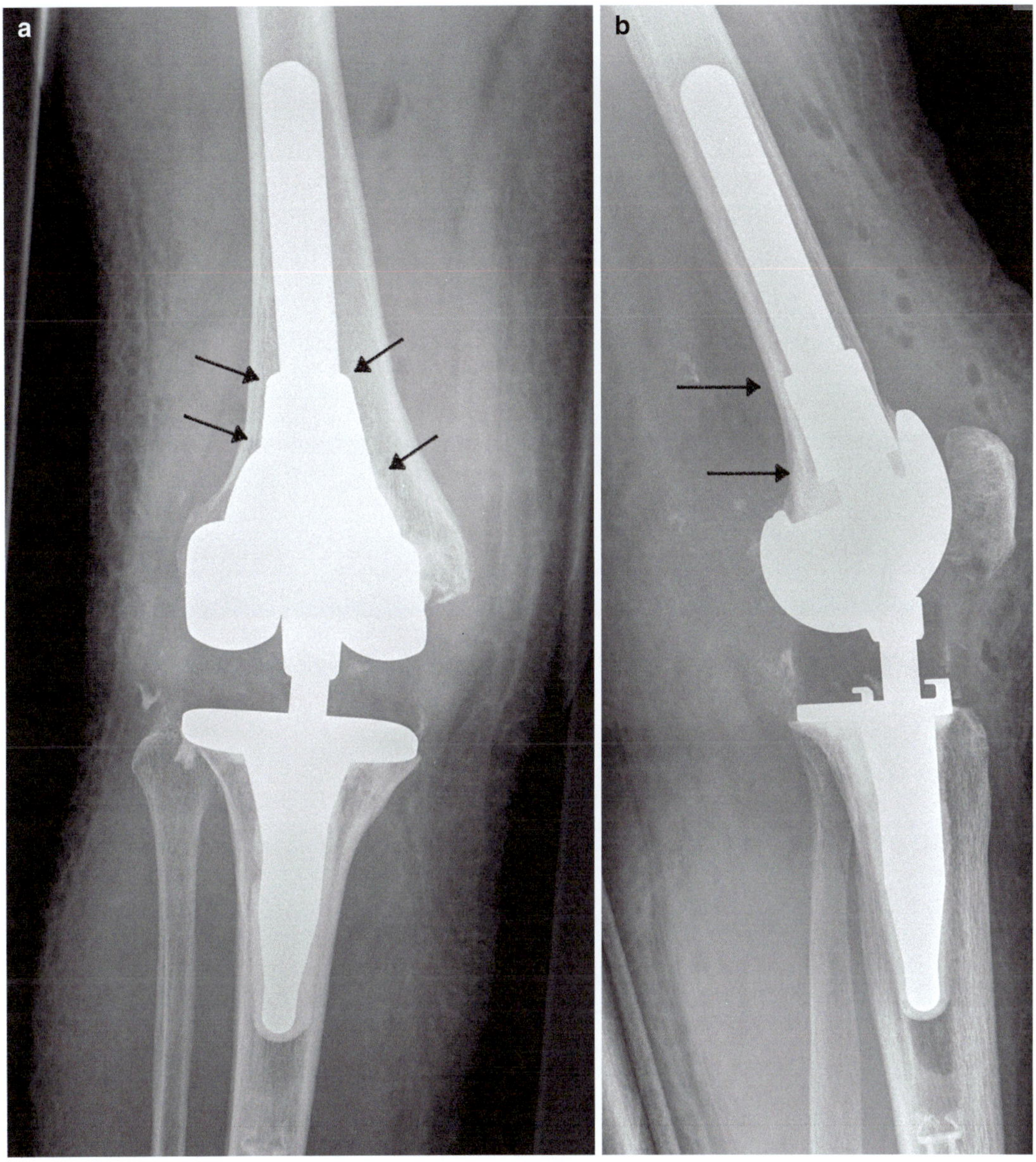

Fig. 3.34 Trabecular metal shape denoted by arrows in the AP (**a**) view and the lateral (**b**) view used to reconstruct bone loss on the femoral side

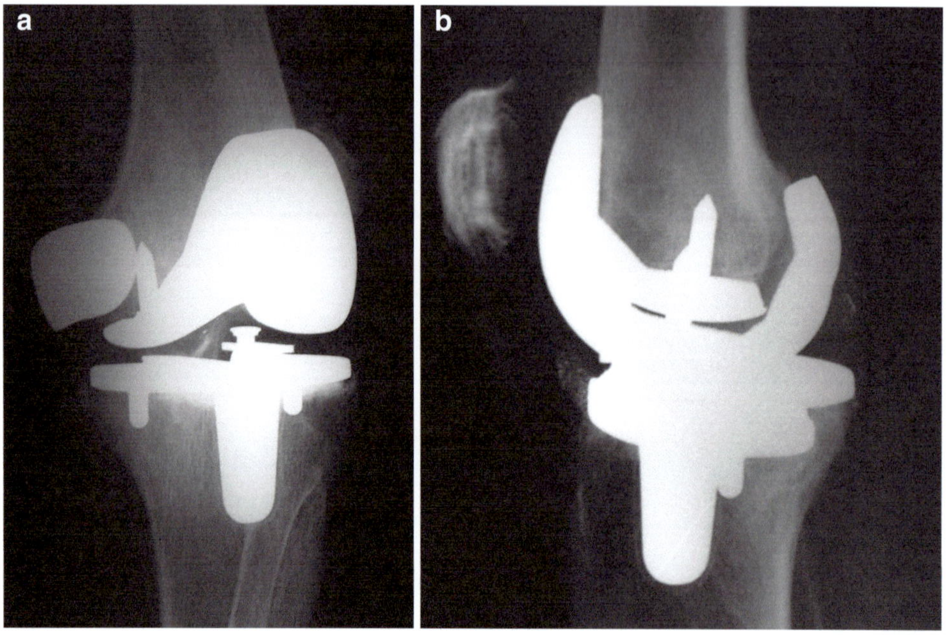

Fig. 3.35 Fracture of the posteromedial aspect of the femoral component seen in the AP (**a**) and lateral (**b**) views

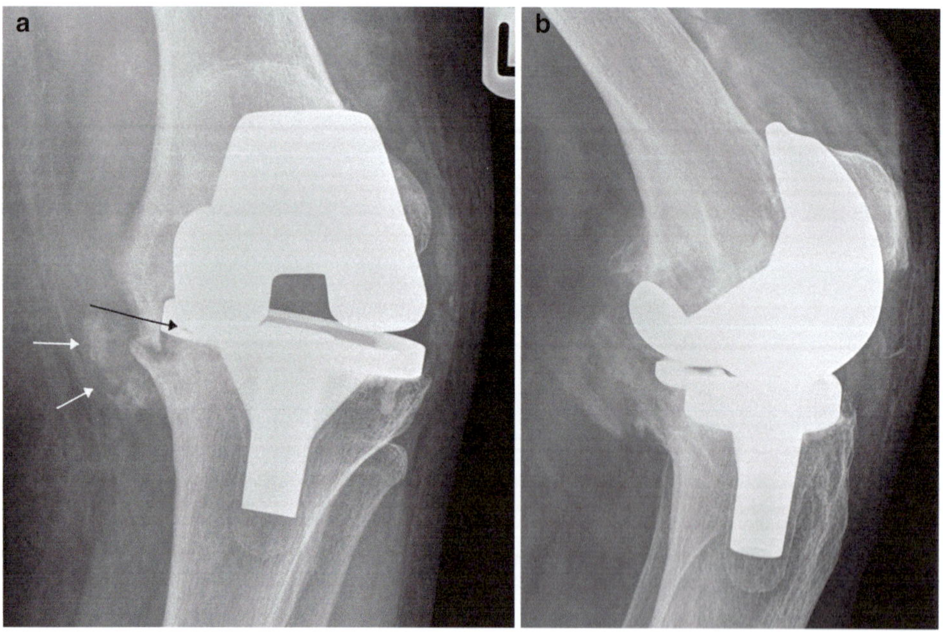

Fig. 3.36 Gross loosening of the implant with failure of the polyethylene insert. The femoral component has worn through the tibial tray as well (black arrows) seen in the AP (**a**) view, leading to metal debris (metallosis) in the joint (white arrows). Soft tissue shadows represent the metal debris in AP and lateral (**b**) view. (**c**) Retrieved implants from the patient in Fig. 3.35 showing the extent of damage to the polyethylene component and the tibial tray. In this implant system, the femoral component is made of cobalt-chrome alloy which is much harder than the titanium tibial component. Hence the tibial component has been eroded, with less damage to the femoral component. Postoperative radiographs of the same patient as Fig. 3.34 after revision to a hinged implant, AP (**d**) and lateral (**e**) view. The lack of integrity of the medial collateral ligament necessitated the use of a constrained prosthesis

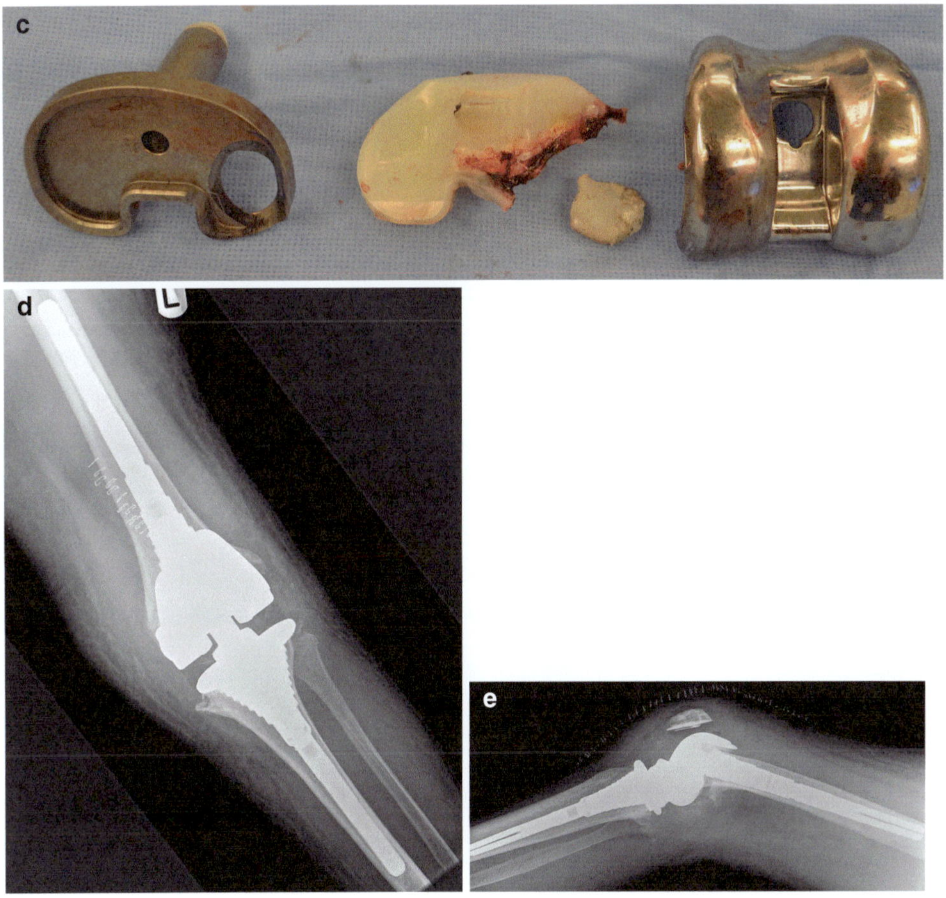

Fig. 3.36 (continued)

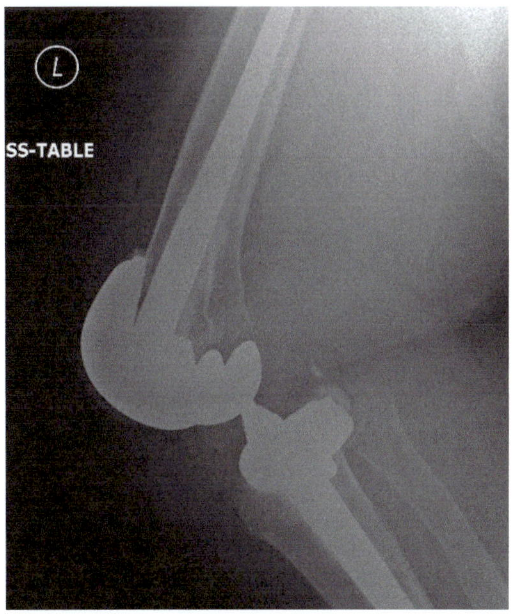

Fig. 3.37 Dislocation of the femoral cam over the post of the polyethylene insert. The femoral component is translated anteriorly in relation to the tibial component, with loss of congruity as seen in the lateral radiograph

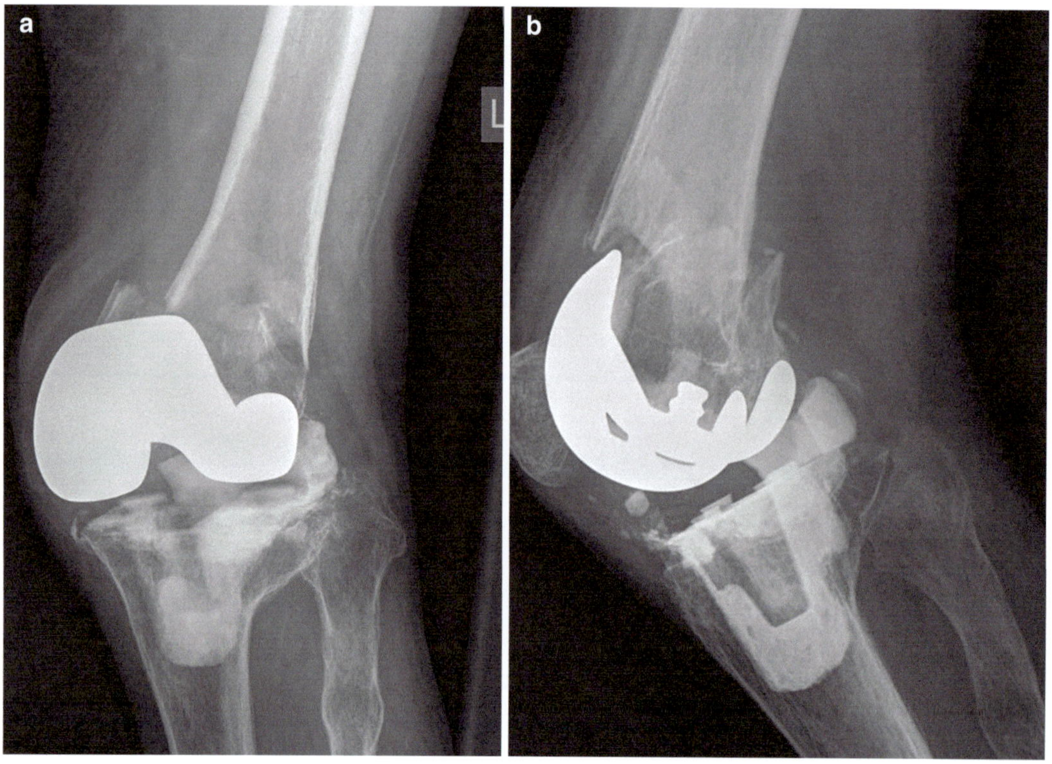

Fig. 3.38 Supracondylar periprosthetic fracture above a femoral component in AP (**a**) and lateral (**b**) view. The femoral component is loose. The tibial component is an all-polyethylene design. The extruded cement posteriorly is from the primary surgery. Lack of modularity of the tibial component restricts access to the posterior part of the knee after cementing. There is extensive osteopenia

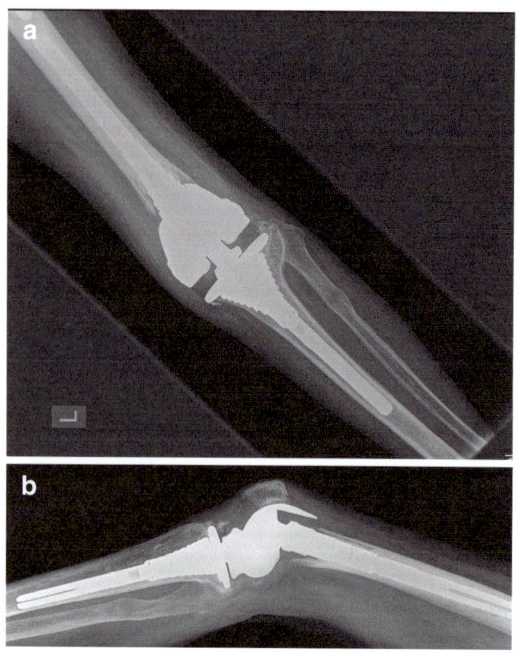

Fig. 3.39 Postoperative radiograph AP (**a**) and lateral (**b**) view following revision of the implant to a hinged prosthesis for the patient in Fig. 3.38. The distal femoral condyles have been removed. The implant is cemented. A distal femoral replacement prosthesis could have been considered in this situation, but the presence of a total hip replacement stem proximally imposed a limitation on the length of femur available for fixation

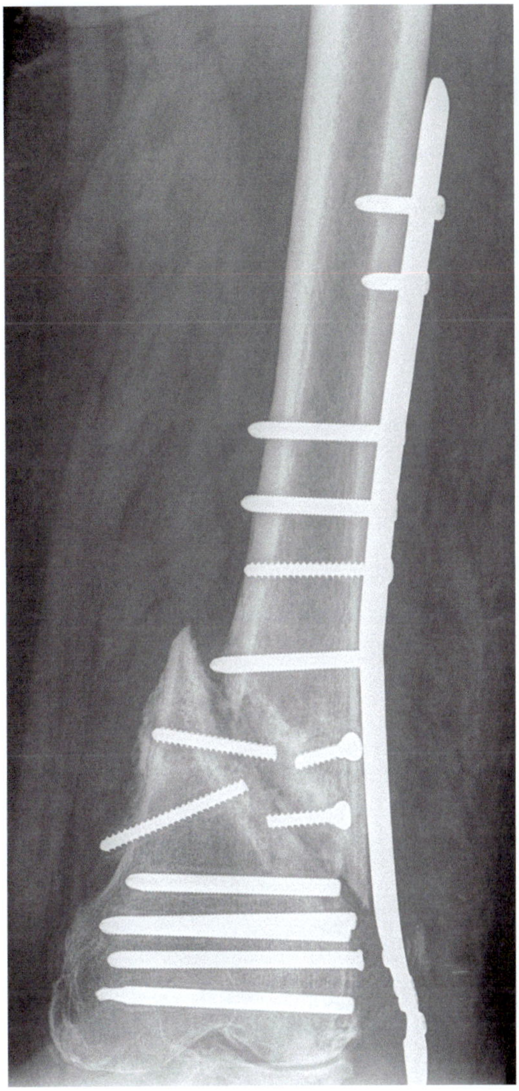

Fig. 3.40 Nonunion of a distal femoral fracture fixed with a distal femoral locking plate 3 years prior to presentation. The interfragmentary compression screws and all the screws in the distal fragment have failed

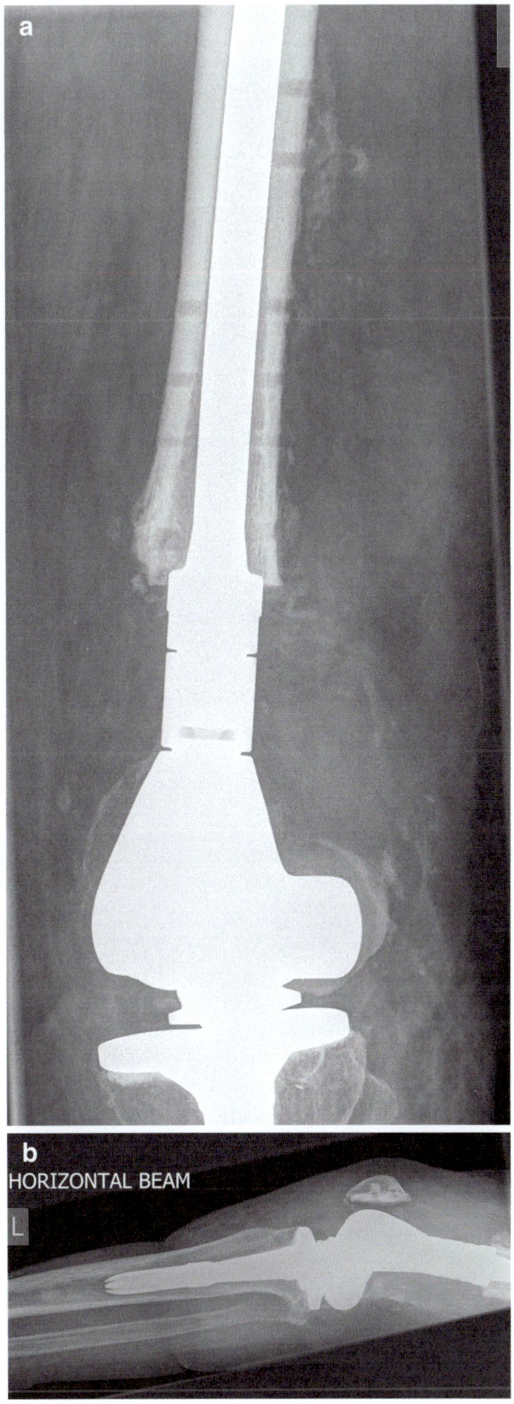

Fig. 3.41 Postoperative radiograph AP (**a**) and lateral (**b**) view of the patient from Fig. 3.40 showing removal of failed metalwork and reconstruction by a distal femoral replacement prosthesis

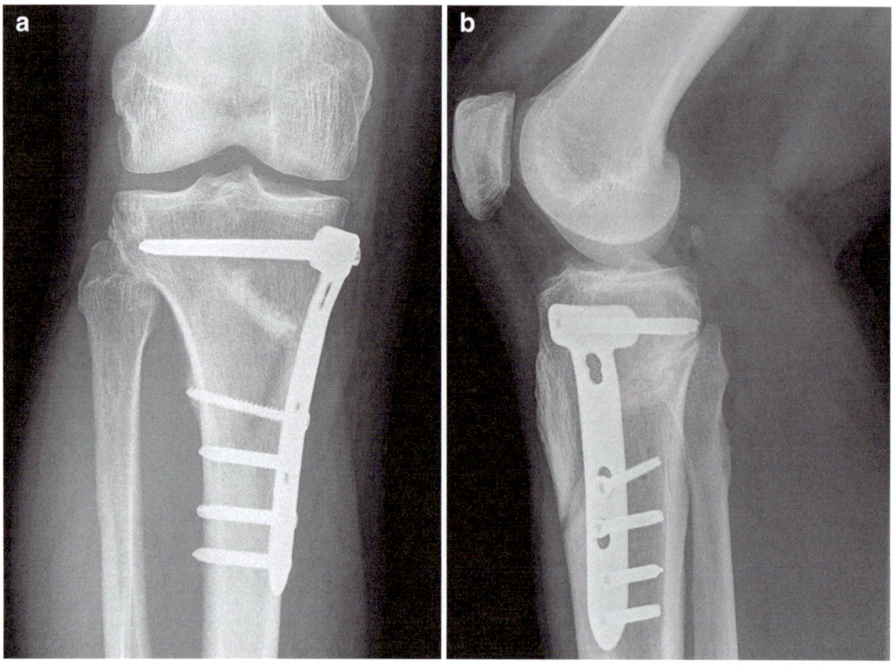

Fig. 3.42 AP (**a**) and lateral (**b**) radiograph following a high tibial osteotomy. This is an oblique medial opening wedge osteotomy stabilised with a locking plate

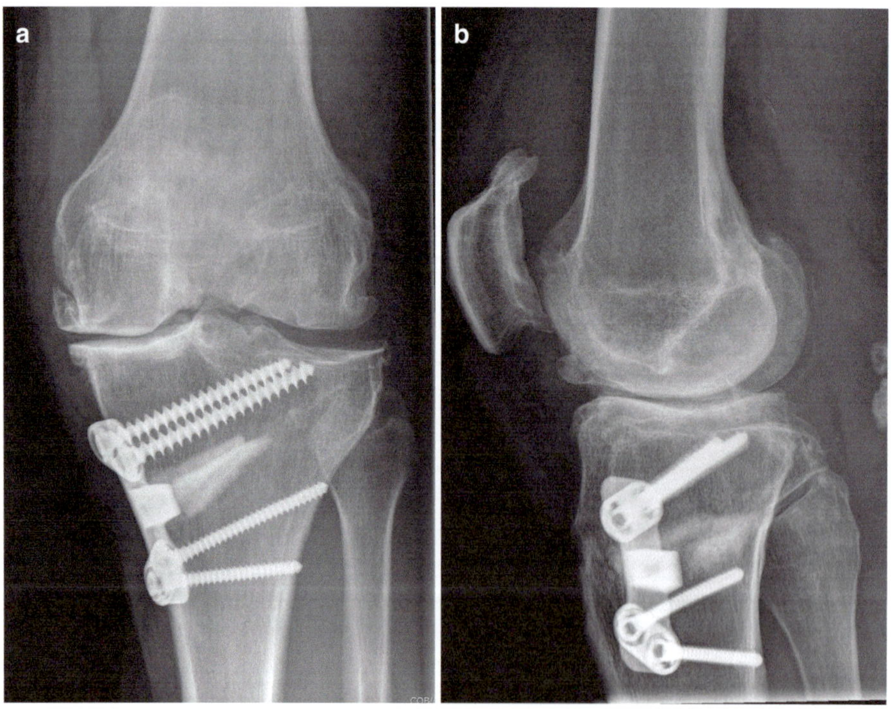

Fig. 3.43 An alternative implant for medial opening wedge high tibial osteotomy. This plate has a metal block seen in AP (**a**) and lateral (**b**) view, which helps to stabilise the osteotomy after a gap is created in the medial tibial cortex

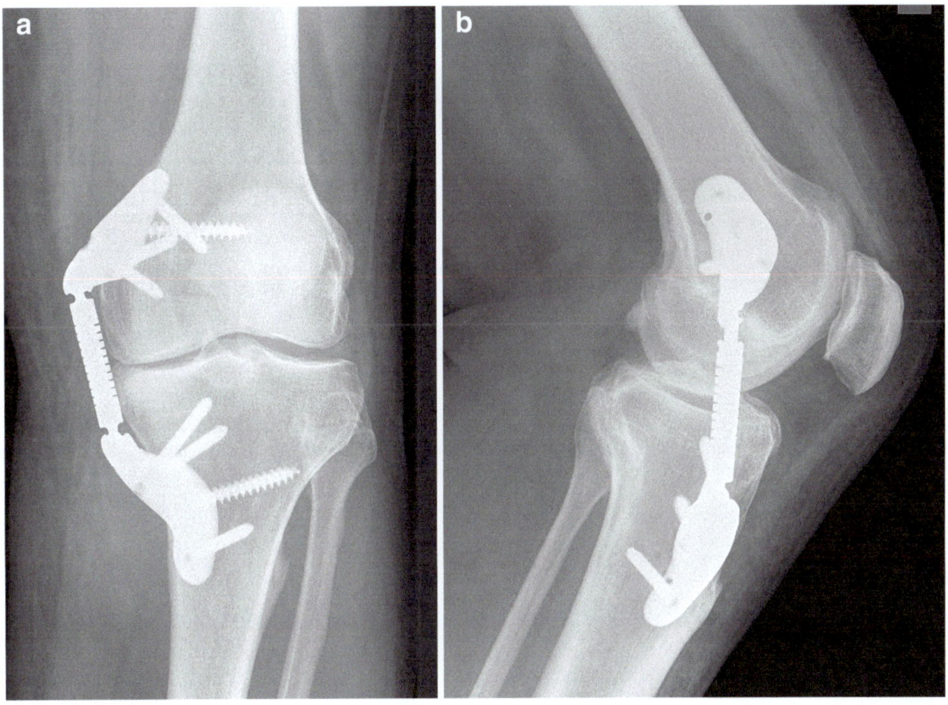

Fig. 3.44 The KineSpring device in AP (**a**) and lateral (**b**) view, designed to reduce the loading of the medial compartment of the knee

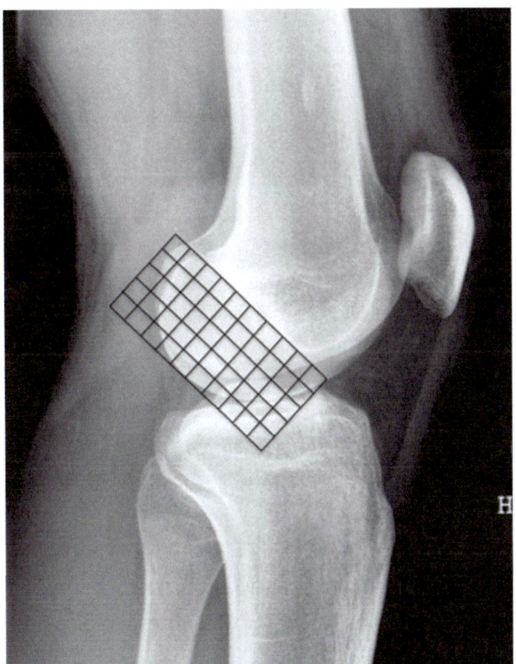

Fig. 3.45 The Bernard and Hertel grid projected on the lateral radiograph of the knee

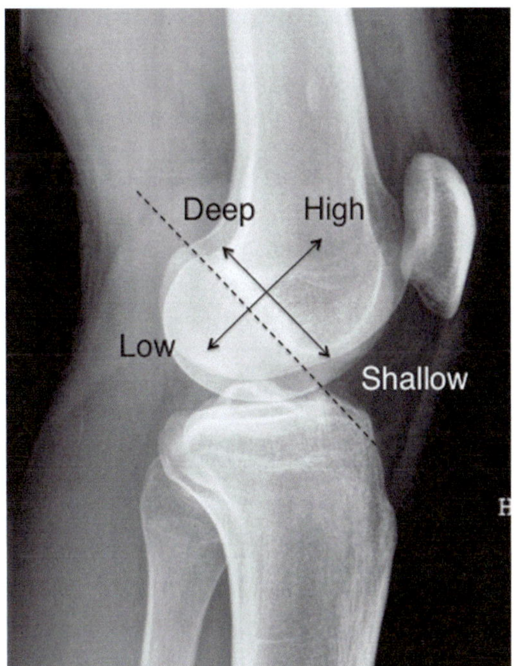

Fig. 3.46 Lines representing deep/shallow and high/low positioning of the femoral attachment of the ACL

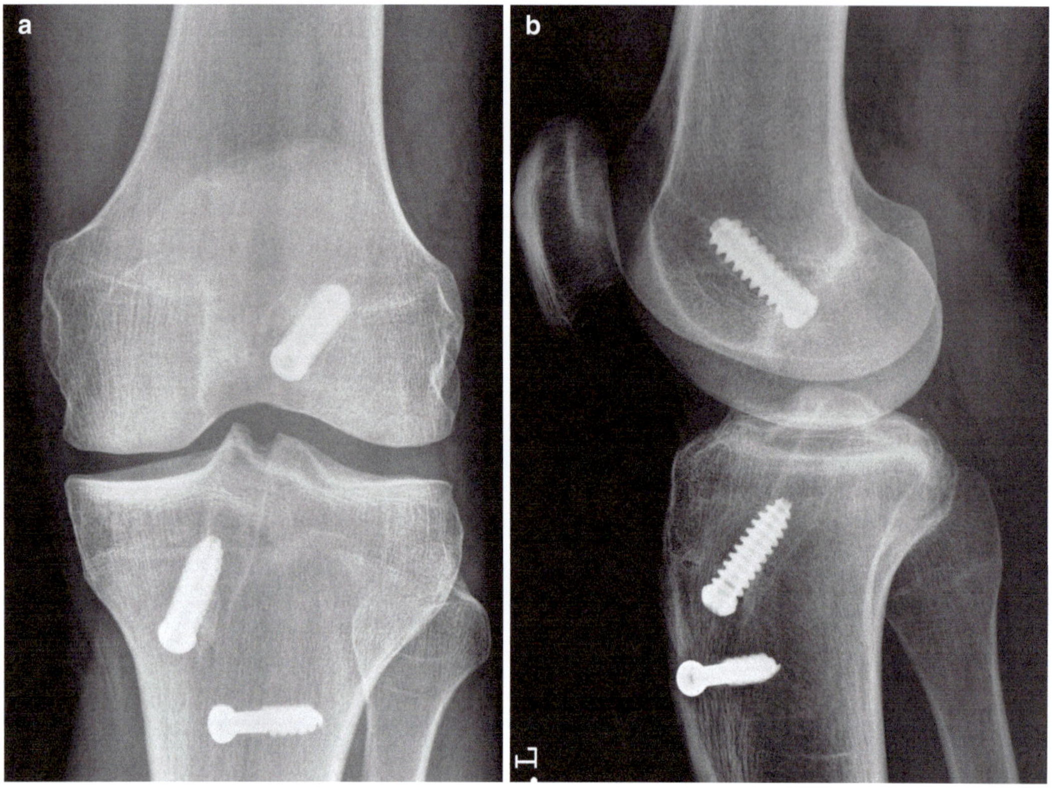

Fig. 3.47 AP (**a**) and lateral (**b**) view of the knee showing excessive shallow placement of the femoral tunnel in ACL reconstruction

posterior to a line drawn along the Blumensaat's line in the lateral view. In the AP view, for ACL reconstructions done through the trans-tibial technique, the tibial tunnel should be less than 72° from a line along the proximal tibial articular surface. More vertical tunnel placement may lead to graft impingement (Figs. 3.48 and 3.49).

Reconstruction of the posterior cruciate ligament (Fig. 3.50) is needed for moderate to severe instability following isolated injuries to the PCL or as part of management of multiligament injuries.

Realignment procedures to stabilise the patella may involve different strategies. Distal realignment is commonly through a tibial tubercle transfer, while proximally, reconstruction of the medial patellofemoral ligament is an option. In patients with a shallow trochlear groove, a trochleoplasty is performed to deepen the trochlear groove. This can be combined with other stabilisation procedures (Fig. 3.51).

Periprosthetic fractures around the knee are usually managed with either intramedullary fixation with an antegrade femoral nail (for more proximal fractures—Fig. 3.52) or plate fixation (for more distal fractures—Fig. 3.53).

With both techniques, it is important to try and achieve an overlap between the joint prosthesis and the fracture fixation device. This prevents the formation of a stress riser and decreases the risk of future fractures.

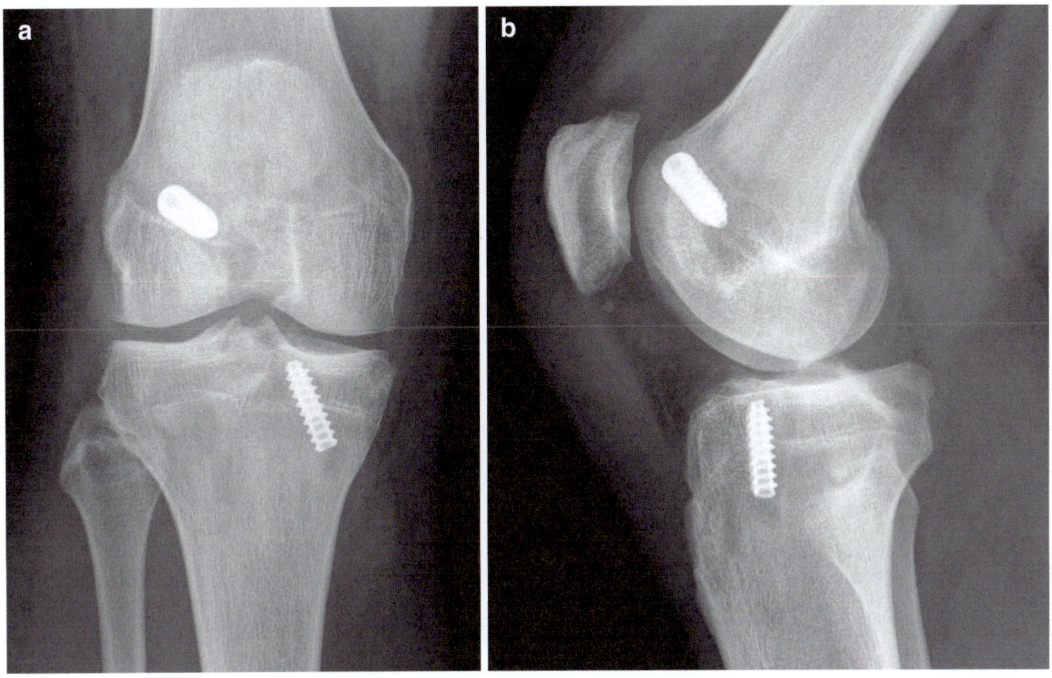

Fig. 3.48 Excessive medial (**a**) and anterior (**b**) placement of the tibial tunnel with shallow placement of the femoral tunnel. This position of the ACL graft will lead to impingement

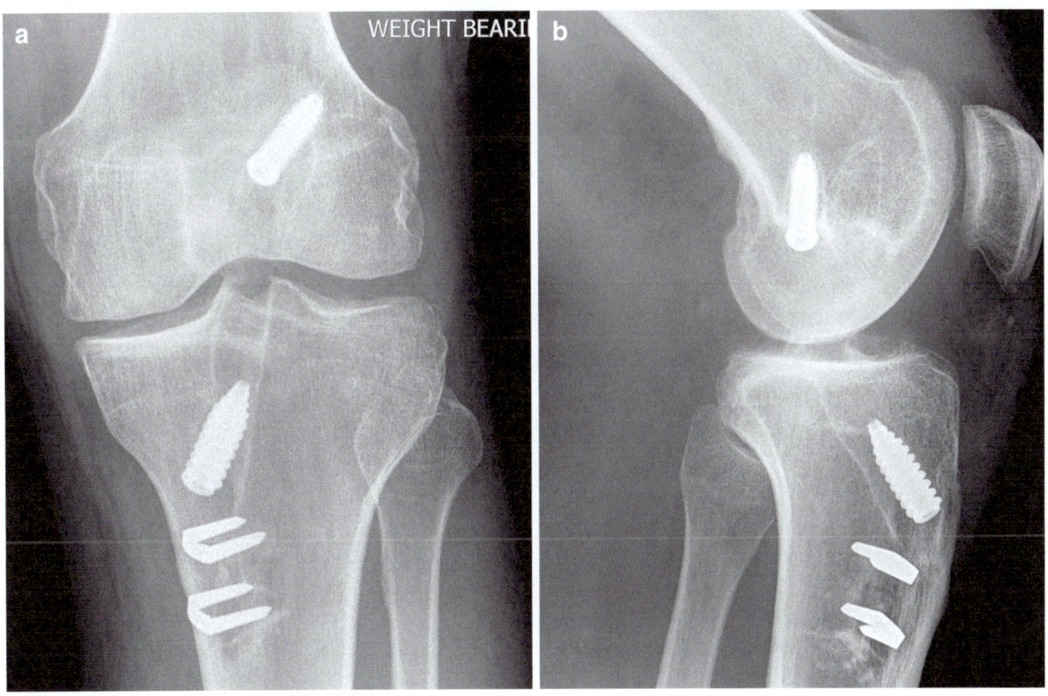

Fig. 3.49 Revision surgery for the patient in Fig. 3.47. The femoral and tibial tunnels have been repositioned

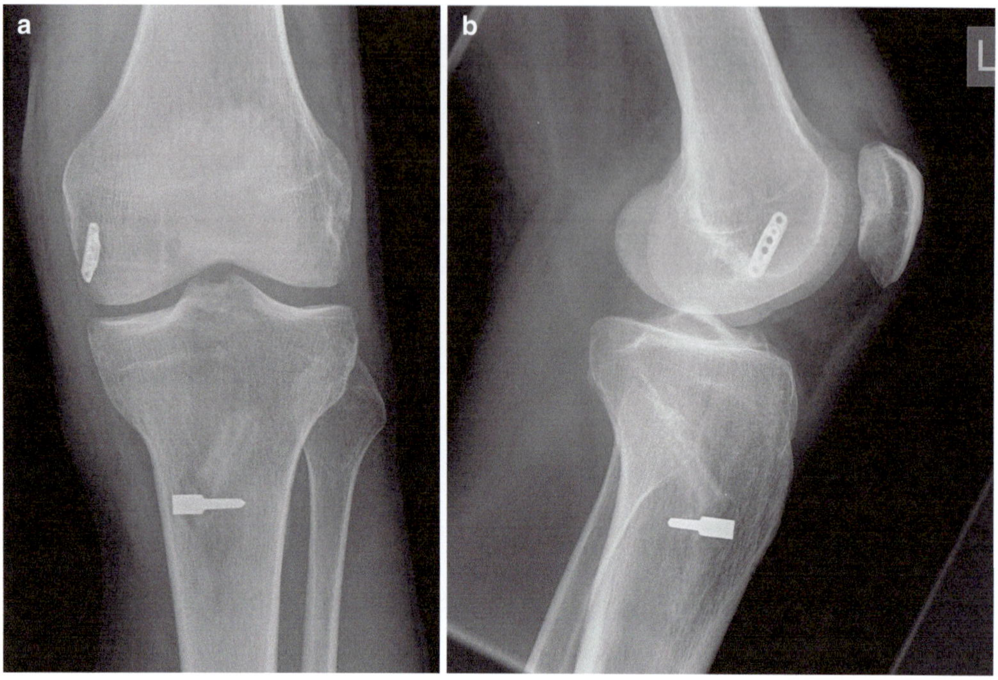

Fig. 3.50 PCL reconstruction using an ENDOBUTTON on the femur and a staple on the tibia to fix the graft in AP (**a**) and lateral (**b**) view

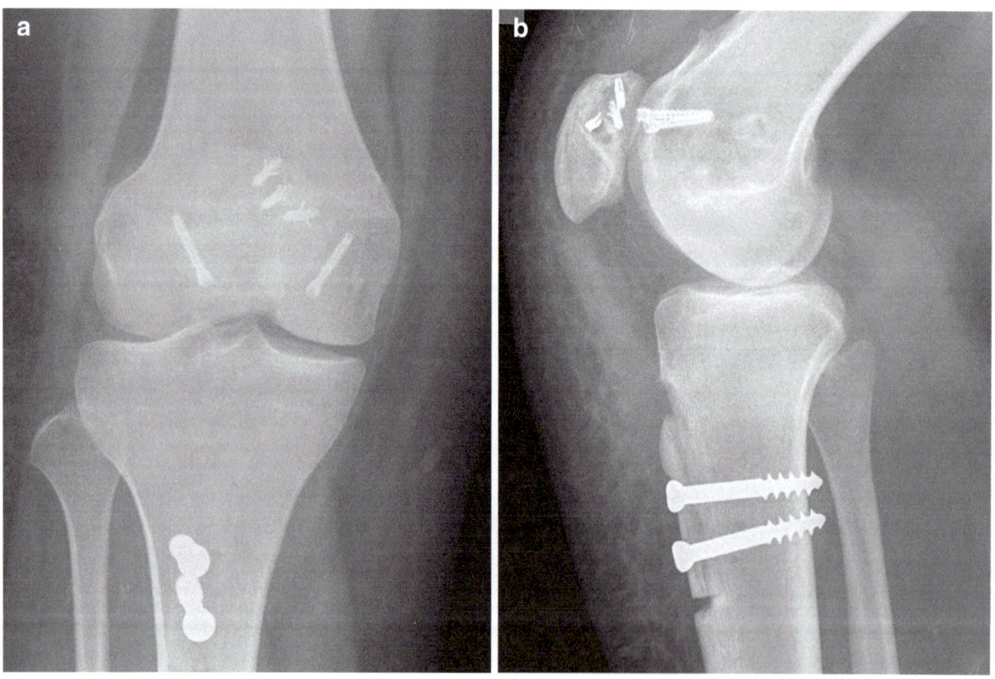

Fig. 3.51 A 17-year-old patient with recurrent patellar instability managed by trochleoplasty, medialisation of the tibial tubercle and reinforcement of the medial patellar retinaculum (**a**, **b**). The two headless screws in the trochlea help to fix the osteochondral flap of trochlear surface. Screws in the proximal tibia are used to stabilise the tibial tubercle. Anchors have been used for the medial repair in the medial margin of the patella

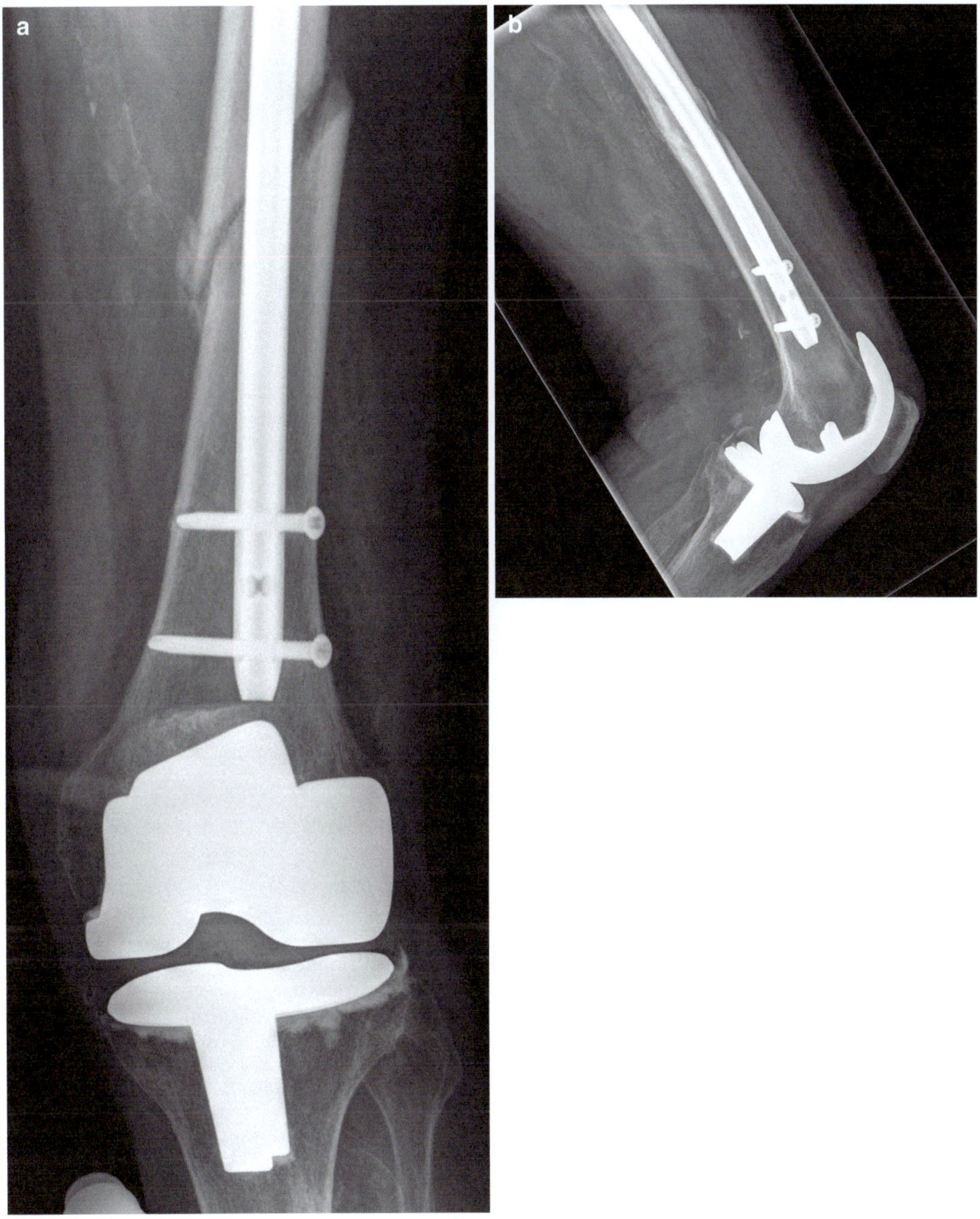

Fig. 3.52 Antegrade IM nail for fixation of a mid-shaft femoral fracture in a patient with a total knee replacement. The fracture is inadequately reduced in the AP view (**a**). In this case, there is no overlap between the implants (**b**), which could put the patient at risk of a further fracture at the site of the gap

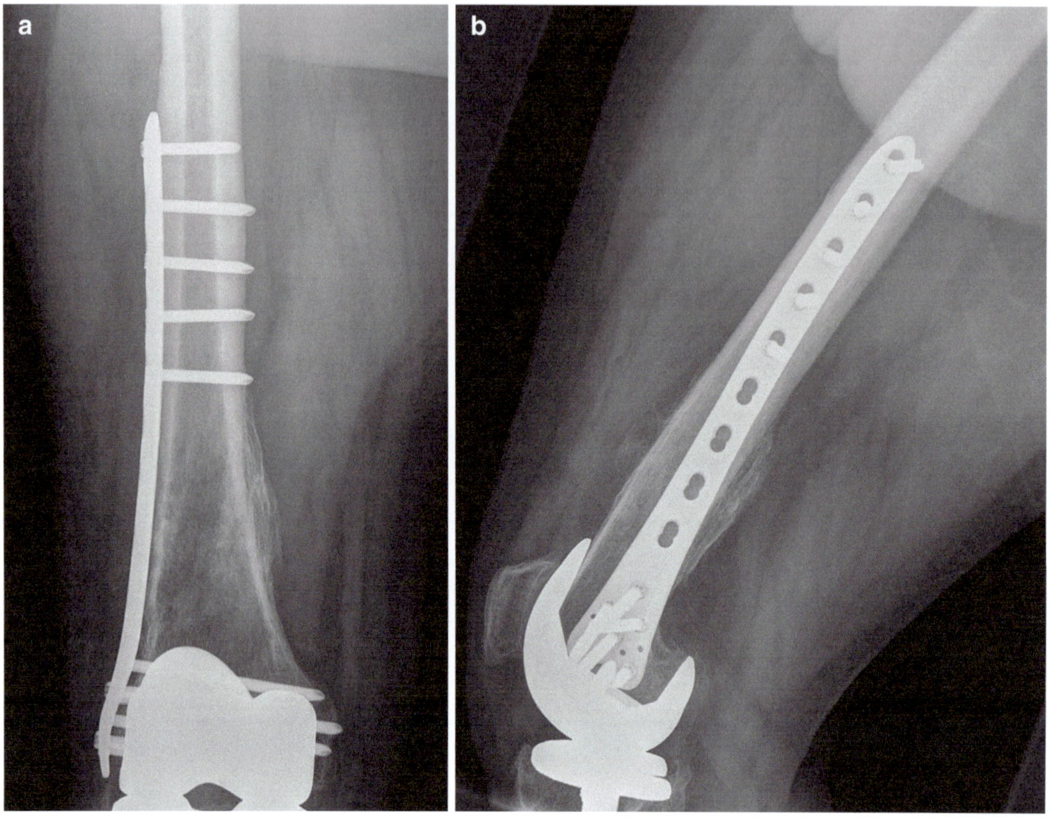

Fig. 3.53 Lateral plate fixation of a distal femoral shaft fracture in a patient with a knee replacement (**a**). The fracture has healed in an anatomic position. There are multiple screws passing from lateral to medial behind the anterior flange of the femoral component (**b**)

References

1. Ewald FC. The knee society total knee arthroplasty roentgenographic evaluation and scoring system. Clin Orthop Relat Res. 1989;248:9–12.
2. Schneider R, Hood RW, Ranawat CS. Radiographic evaluation of knee arthroplasty. Orthop Clin North Am. 1982;13:225–44.
3. Liebs TR, Kloos S-A, Herberg W, Ruther W, Hassenflug J. Bone Joint J. 2013;95(B):472–7.
4. Johal P, Hassaballa MA, Eldridge JD, Porteous AJ. The posterior condylar offset ratio. Knee. 2012;19(8):843–5.
5. Agarwal S, Azam A, Morgan-Jones R. The use of metal metaphyseal sleeves in revision total knee replacement. Bone Joint J. 2013;95:1640–4.
6. Bernard M, Hertel P, Hornung H, Cierpinski T. Femoral insertion of the ACL. Radiographic quadrant method. Am J Knee Surg. 1997;10:14–21.

4 Shoulder Implants

Timothy Matthews and Devdutt Neogi

The history of shoulder replacements goes back over 100 years. In 1893, Péan, a French surgeon, performed the first documented implantation of shoulder prosthesis. It was fashioned from platinum and rubber and inserted into a 37-year-old baker with tubercular arthritis. Unfortunately, it had to be removed after only 2 years, due to recurrence of the infection. Interestingly, one of the first X-ray machines to be developed helped detect an overwhelming reactive process in this patient.

In the 1950s, Neer [1] popularized shoulder replacements using a stemmed hemiarthroplasty for proximal humeral fractures. Since then, developments in design and techniques have resulted in a wide range of prostheses, with options for modularity, resurfacing arthroplasty and reverse arthroplasty.

Anatomic shoulder replacements are aimed at restoring the anatomy of the proximal humerus in conjunction with a glenoid surface replacement. The glenoid component usually has a keel or pegs for fixation. The humeral component can be stemmed, metaphyseal fit or resurfacing (Fig. 4.1a–c). The humeral component can also be used as a hemiarthroplasty, where the glenoid is not resurfaced.

Resurfacing shoulder arthroplasty is aimed at 'covering' the humeral head of the individual patient rather than attempting to reconstruct predetermined anatomical parameters, and this also can be used with or without a glenoid component.

Both glenoid and humeral components can be cemented in place or uncemented. In uncemented or cementless fixation, primary stability is achieved by a 'press fit' (accurate apposition of the implant against the prepared bone surface) of the prosthesis. Secondary stability is achieved by bone ingrowth or bone ongrowth.

Currently, a wide variety of glenoid component options are available, and these can be either 'all-polyethylene' (Fig. 4.1a, b) or metal-backed (Fig. 4.1c). The surface of metal-backed components allows for inset and augmented designs as well as provides a surface for bone ingrowth or ongrowth.

There is no consensus on which X-ray views should be performed postoperatively; however, anteroposterior (AP) views in internal and external rotation, together with axillary lateral views, are commonly reported as the standard method of radiographic evaluation in the current literature.

T. Matthews (✉) · D. Neogi
University Hospital of Wales, Cardiff, UK
e-mail: tjwmatthews@sky.com

S. Agarwal, G. J. Bansal (eds.), *Radiology of Orthopedic Implants*,
https://doi.org/10.1007/978-3-319-76009-4_4

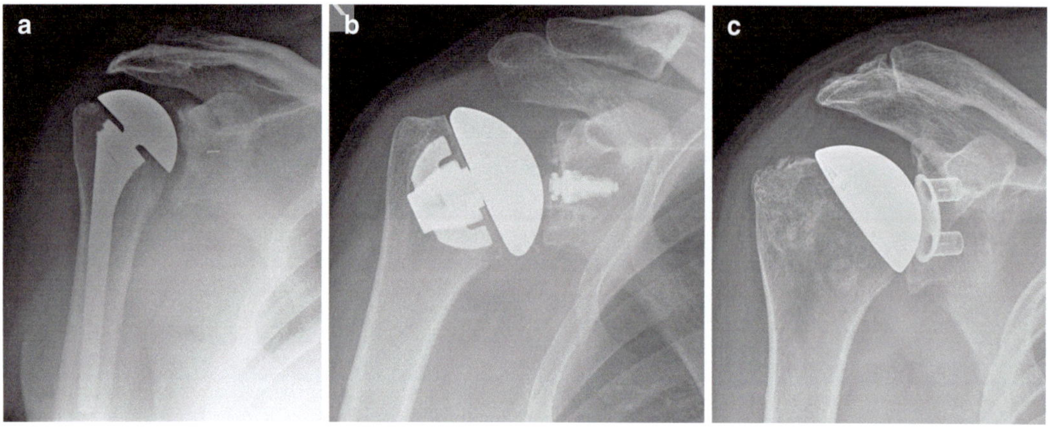

Fig. 4.1 Types of anatomic total shoulder replacements (TSR). (**a**) Stemmed TSR with all-polyethylene glenoid; (**b**) metaphyseal TSR with polyethylene glenoid with porous-coated central peg; (**c**) resurfacing TSR with metal-backed glenoid

AP Shoulder Radiograph

Features to note on the humeral component:

1. Head-neck angle
2. Humeral head height
3. Glenohumeral offset, medial and lateral
4. Cephalotuberosity index
5. Articular surface thickness
6. Restoration of diameter of curvature of the articular surface of the humeral head
7. Periprosthetic fracture
8. Cementation of humeral component (if cemented stem is used)
9. Humeral stem placement (for stemmed humeral implants)

Features to note on the glenoid component:

1. Implant seating
2. Cementation
3. Periprosthetic fracture
4. Height

Axillary View

Features to note on the humeral component, both stemmed and resurfacing:

1. Humeral head version
2. Articular surface thickness
3. Restoration of diameter of curvature of the articular surface of the humeral head

Features to note on the glenoid component:

1. Implant seating
2. Cementation
3. Periprosthetic fracture

On Long-Term Follow-Up Radiographs

1. Evidence of loosening of the humeral or glenoid components
2. Wear of the glenoid—evidenced by eccentric articulation of the humeral head
3. Superior humeral migration—evidence of rotator cuff tendon failure
4. Periprosthetic fracture
5. Stress shielding

Head-Neck Angle

The head-neck or inclination angle is the angle between the proximal metaphyseal (intramedullary) axis and a line perpendicular to the plane of the articular margin (Fig. 4.2). A cadaveric study [2] showed a range of 123–136° with the mean at approximately 130°. Anatomical replacements

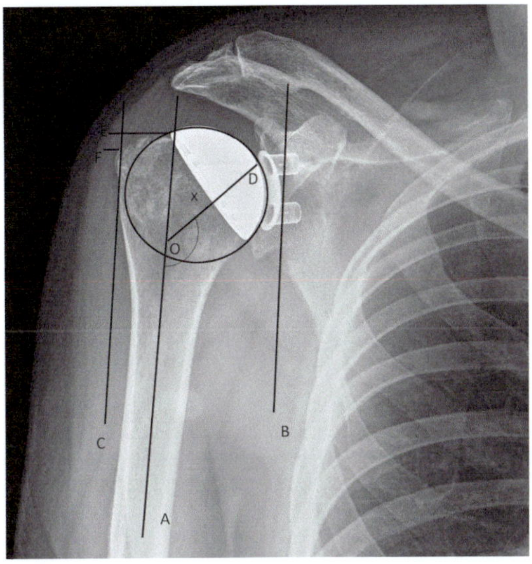

Fig. 4.2 Bony landmarks around the shoulder on the AP radiograph. Line A, humeral shaft axis; angle AOD, humeral neck-shaft angle; Line B, vertical line from the glenoid; Line C, vertical line from the lateral point on the proximal humerus; distance between Line B and Line C, lateral humeral offset; Point X, the centre of rotation of the humeral head; perpendicular distance between Point X and Line A, medial humeral offset; distance between X and humeral surface, radius of curvature of the humeral head; distance between Line E and Line F, cephalotuberosity index

aim to recreate this angle accurately within their design, but resurfacing humeral components rely on surgical technique for accuracy (Fig. 4.3a, b). Biomechanical and cadaveric studies have considered this angle to be important when preventing against impingement from malposition. However, there are no clinical studies to corroborate this view [3, 4].

Humeral Head Retroversion

Humeral head retroversion is defined as the angle between a line perpendicular to the articular margin plane of the implant and the transepicondylar axis or the tangent elbow axes.

This may be appreciated on the axillary view (Fig. 4.4) but is difficult to calculate accurately as most commonly acquired shoulder images do not include the elbow. Calculation is possible from standard AP radiographs with the forearm held in 35° of external rotation using a simple mathematical formula based upon the humeral head appearing as an ellipse. Anatomically, the retroversion is markedly variable, not only between individuals but also between the right and left shoulder of

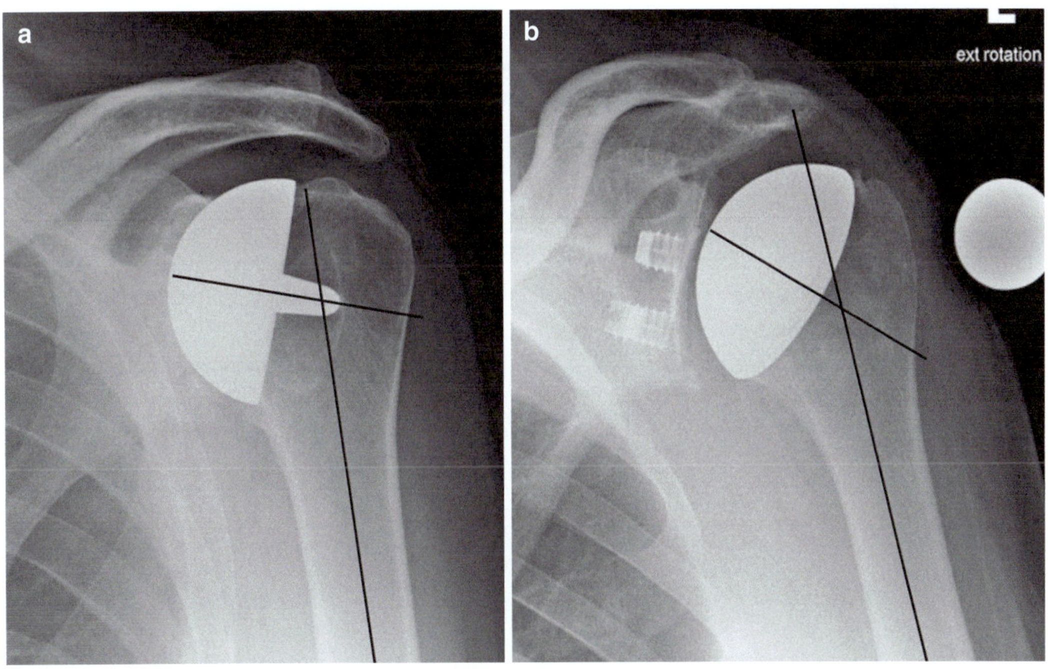

Fig. 4.3 Humeral component in varus alignment (**a**) and humeral component in normal alignment (**b**)

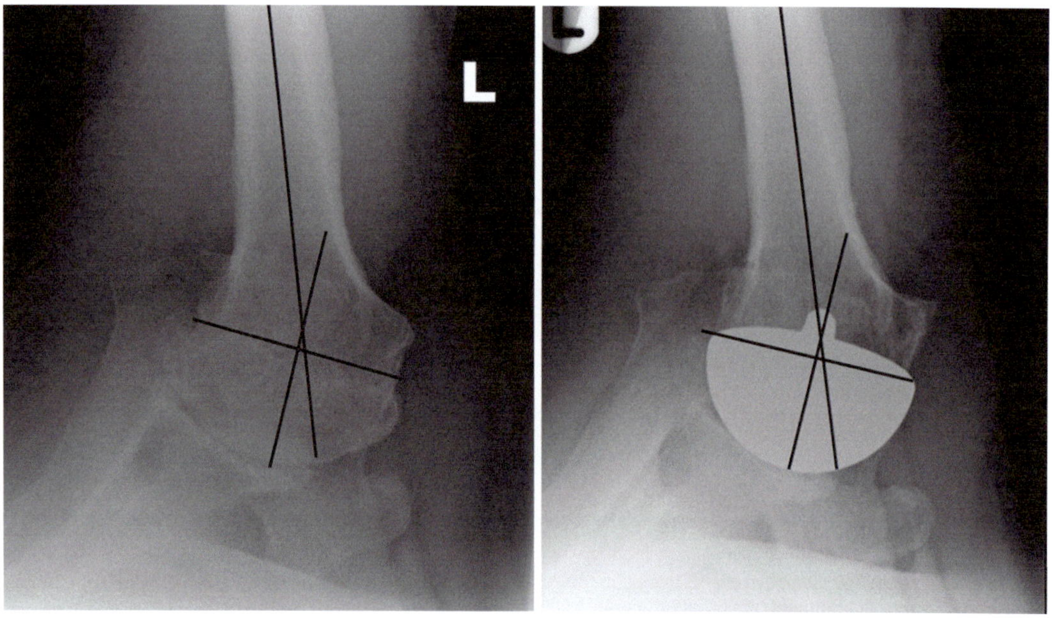

Fig. 4.4 Axillary view depicting humeral head version in comparison with preoperative radiograph. The lines indicate the axis of the humeral shaft and the alignment of the humeral component, which matches the normal anatomy

the same individual. Clinical and cadaveric studies have recommended retroversion of implants to be between 20 and 40° but may be closer to 30–40° to account for more anteriorly positioned stems. Malposition may be associated with instability, altered joint kinematics and pain [5–7].

Lateral Humeral Offset

The distance between the base of the coracoid process and most lateral part of the greater tuberosity on the plain radiograph [8, 9] is the lateral humeral offset (LHO) (Fig. 4.2). The LHO correlates both with the deltoid and rotator cuff moment arm and the humeral head size [10]. Restoration of LHO is thought to improve shoulder function and stability and to decrease glenoid wear [8].

Medial Humeral Offset

The medial humeral offset (Fig. 4.2) has been defined by the distance of the centre of the humeral head from the central axis of the humeral canal. Irrespective of the method used, measurements before and after surgery can be made and the offset difference calculated. Significant increases in offset have been considered to represent 'overstuffing of the joint' and may be responsible for poorer outcomes [11]. This is more commonly seen in resurfacing humeral head arthroplasty, as insufficient quantities of the cartilage and subchondral bone may be reamed to make space for the metal 'cap'. Cadaveric studies have demonstrated that increase in medial offset by more than 4 mm may lead to impingement.

Radius of Curvature

Restoring a radius of curvature close to normal is essential (Fig. 4.2) because an excessive increase does not increase lateral humeral offset but may induce overstuffing of the joint (Fig. 4.5) [12].

Cephalotuberosity Index

The distance between the superior most point on the humeral head and the greater tuberosity is the

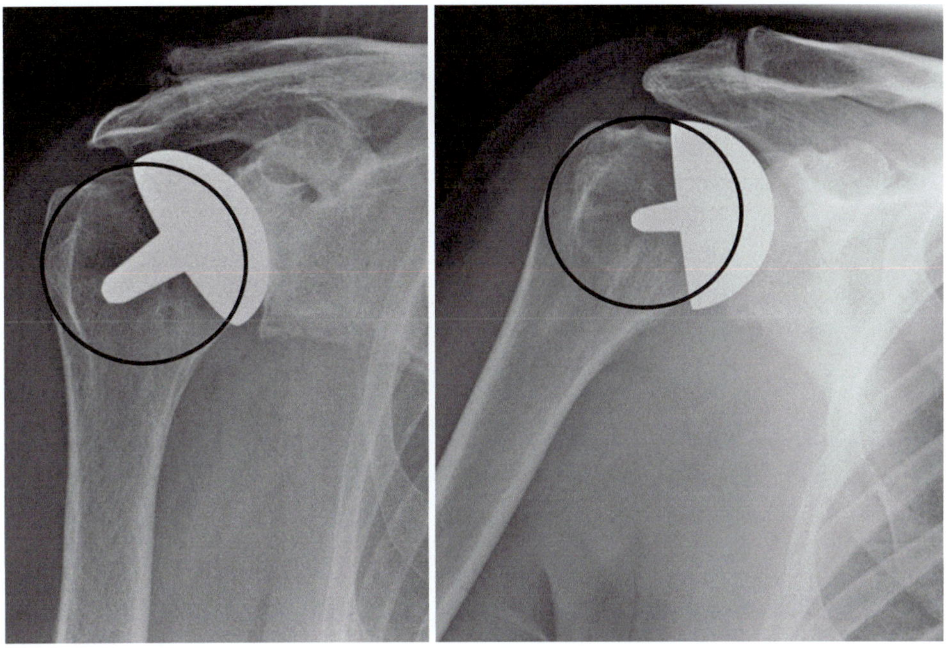

Fig. 4.5 'Overstuffing' of the shoulder joint. Insufficient removal of the bone results in a prosthesis, which extends beyond the curvature of the humeral head

cephalotuberosity index (Fig. 4.2). It has been reported to be 8 ± 3.2 mm in the normal glenohumeral joint [10, 13]. Accurate positioning of the resurfacing implant relative to the top of the greater tuberosity is important. If the prosthesis is placed inferiorly, it may lead to impingement of the greater tuberosity under the acromion (Fig. 4.6). Placing it superiorly will lead to overstuffing of the cuff tendons with limited range of motion. An increase of the humeral height of 5 mm or greater will lead to a decrease of 20–30° of range of motion [14].

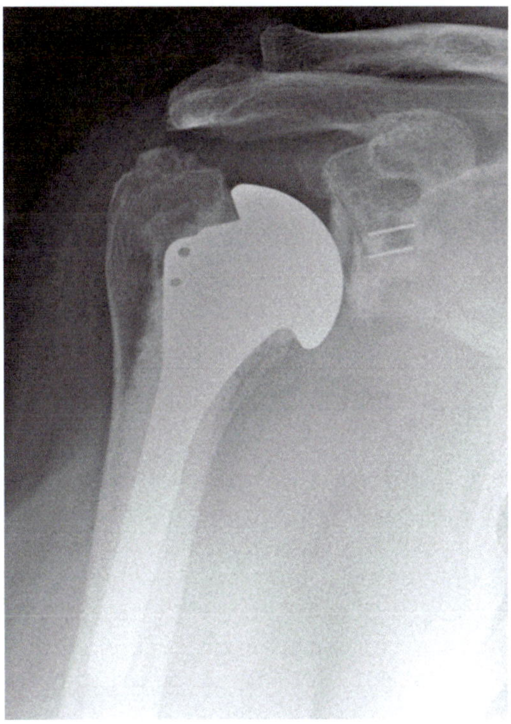

Fig. 4.6 Inferior humeral component placement leading to impingement at greater tuberosity with restriction of shoulder abduction

Loosening

Radiographic assessment of glenoid loosening was developed [15] to evaluate the integrity of the bone-cement interface in keeled all-polyethylene glenoid components (Fig. 4.7). These were graded according to the presence of radiolucent lines.

This classification was modified [16] so that cemented pegged all-polyethylene components could be similarly evaluated (Fig. 4.8), and a

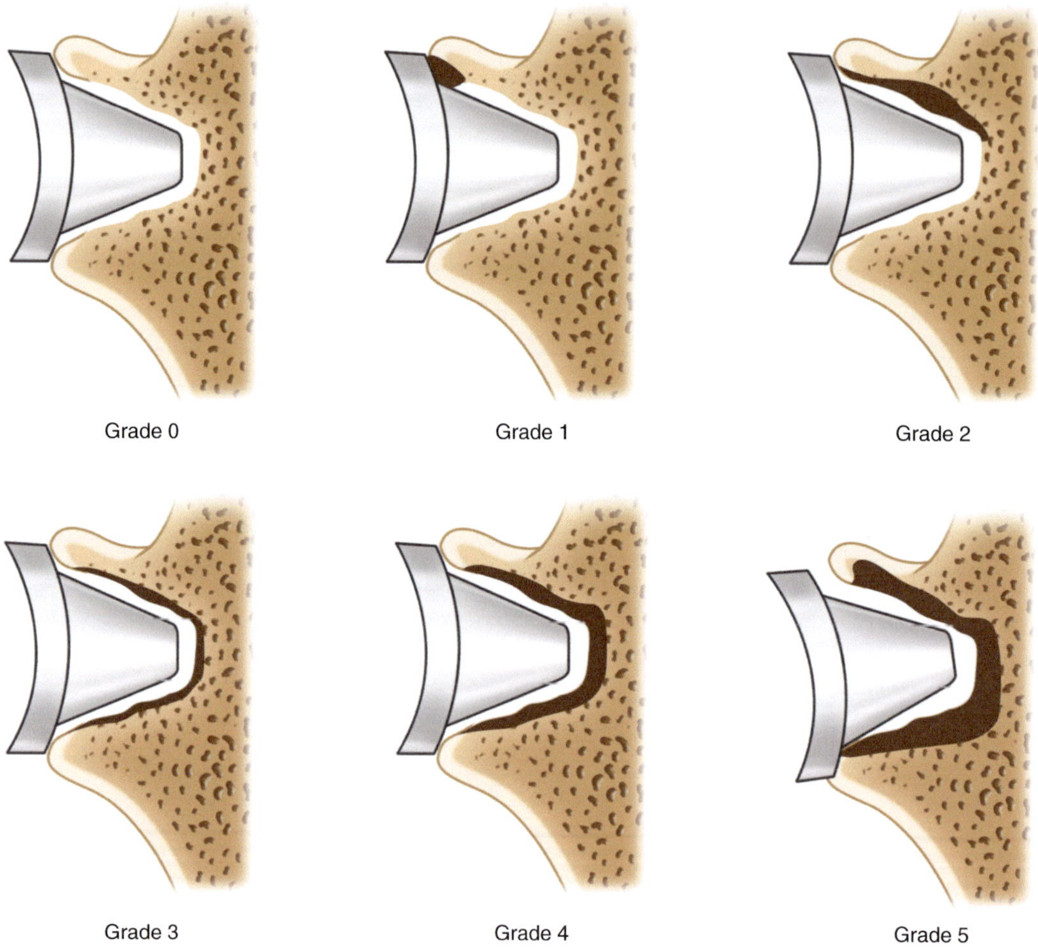

Fig. 4.7 Grading system used to depict radiolucencies around keeled components (reproduced with permission) [15]

grading scale was developed for completeness of glenoid component 'seating' as this reflected the amount of host subchondral bone directly in contact with the back of the glenoid component (Fig. 4.9).

Loosening in bone ingrowth components can be described [17] in five zones around the glenoid (Fig. 4.10) and eight zones around the humeral stem (Fig. 4.11). Loosening in cemented humeral components (Fig. 4.12) has also been described [18] using eight zones (Fig. 4.11).

A humeral component is considered radiographically 'at risk' for clinical loosening when a radiolucent line 2 mm or greater in width was present in three or more zones or tilt or subsidence was identified on sequential radiographs [18]. Malposition of the glenoid implant has a direct effect on the clinical and radiological outcomes [19]. In a three-dimensional orientation, implanting the glenoid component in neutral rotation, neutral to slightly retroverted and neutral to 20° of superior inclination is recommended.

Computer modelling using normal CT shoulders suggests that positioning the glenoid component more inferiorly might reduce the risk of a 'rocking horse phenomenon' [20] by reducing shear forces.

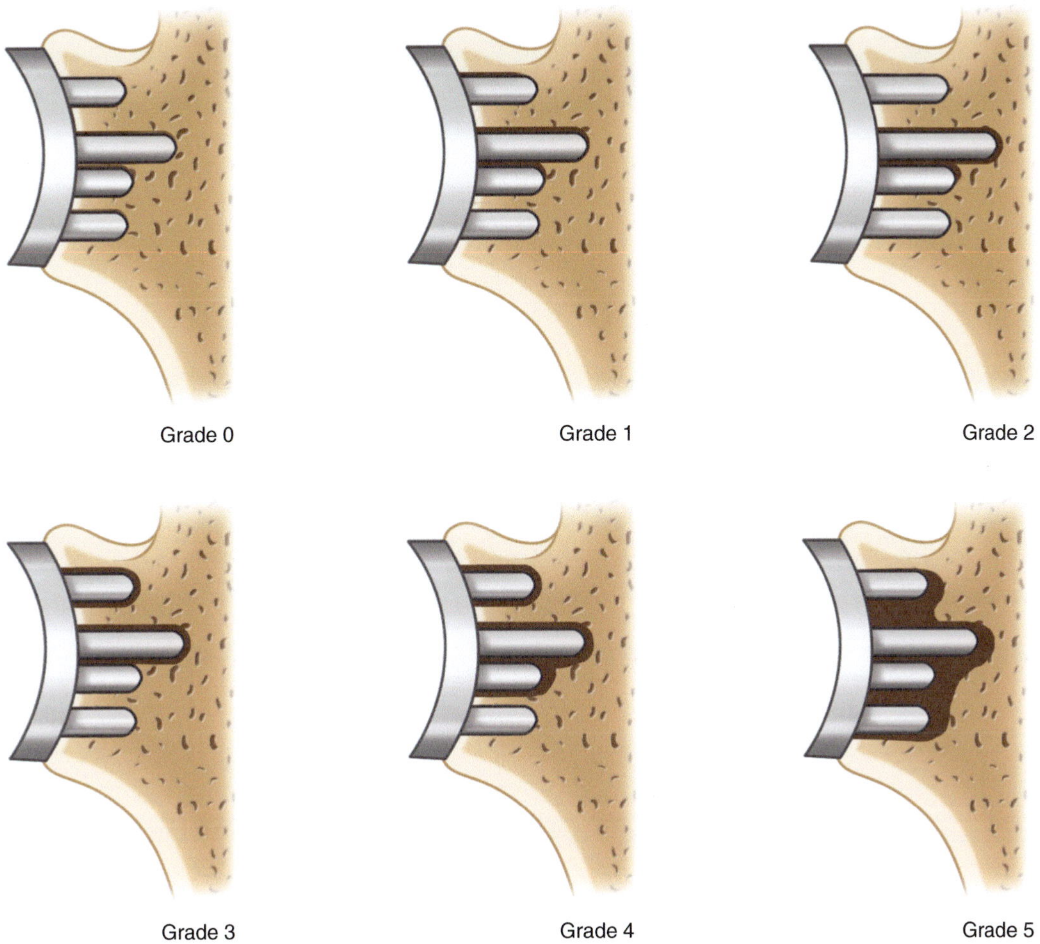

Fig. 4.8 Illustration depicting grading system used to depict radiolucencies around pegged components (reproduced with permission) [16]

Reverse Shoulder Replacement

Significant shoulder arthritis in the presence of large irreparable rotator cuff deficiency historically has proved a challenge to the surgeon. In the past attempts were made to address this problem by designing a constrained or semiconstrained arthroplasty which could replace the joint but also restore the biomechanical imbalance caused by the loss of the rotator cuff.

In the 1980s, Paul Grammont designed the reverse shoulder arthroplasty, which was based upon the use of a large hemisphere glenoid component with no neck and a small humeral cup with a head-neck angle of 155°.

This design medialized the centre of rotation, placing it at the surface of the glenoid, thus minimizing torque forces and prosthesis loosening. By creating a fixed centre of rotation, the humeral head was prevented from migrating superiorly, and the length of the deltoid muscle fibres could be restored. This provided a stable arthroplasty and placed the deltoid at a biomechanical advantage for movement.

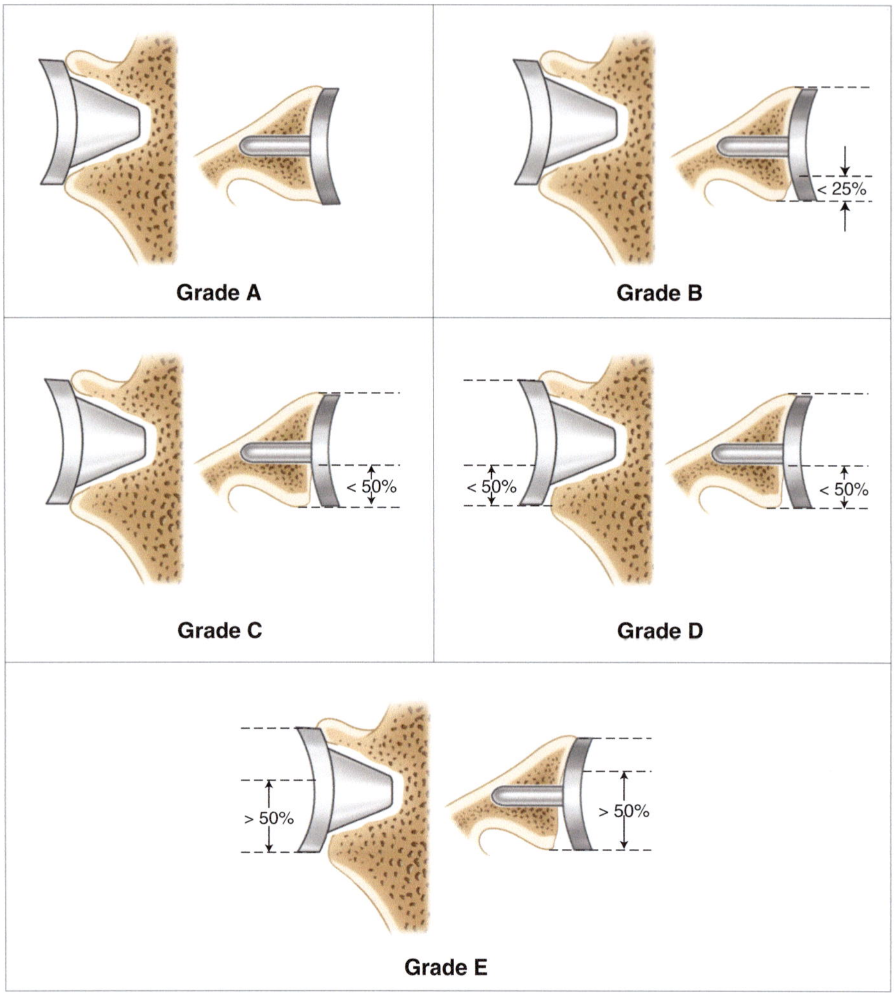

Fig. 4.9 Illustration depicting the grading system used to assess the completeness of glenoid component seating on the host bone. Representative anteroposterior and axillary views are depicted for each grade (reproduced with permission) [16]

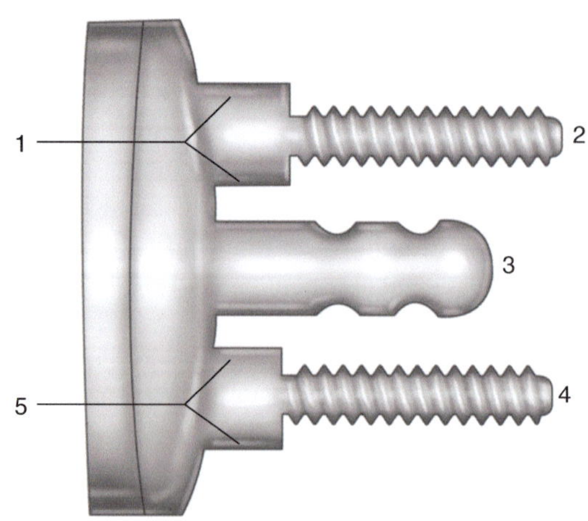

Fig. 4.10 Glenoid component interface is divided into five radiographic zones (reproduced with permission) [17]

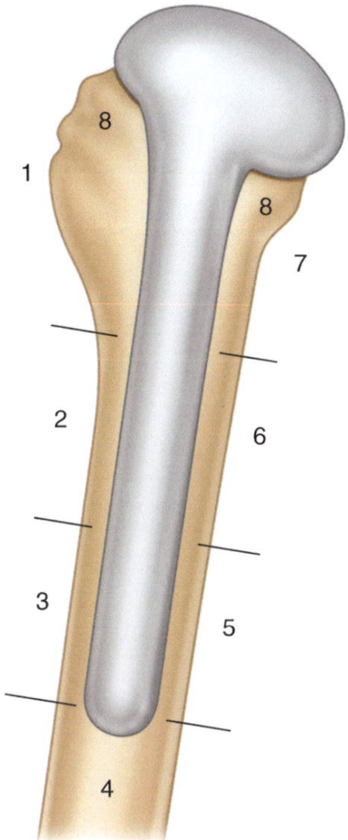

Fig. 4.11 Humeral component interface is divided into eight radiographic zones (reproduced with permission) [17]

Reverse prosthesis is also becoming increasingly popular in the unreconstructable three- or four-part proximal humeral fractures in the elderly, particularly in the light of poor results from hemiarthroplasty. Grammont's design has now evolved into an uncemented humeral stem, with an uncemented glenoid component augmented by screws. The majority of contemporary components are fixed in this way, although cemented humeral components are also common, particularly in the trauma setting. There are also short humeral components that rely on metaphyseal fixation without the need for a stem. There is an increasing vogue for 'platform' systems, which build upon a universal stem and then are added to a humeral body. The aim of these is to allow accurate reconstruction of the anatomy but also provide more straightforward revision options should the need arise.

There is a lack of consensus on X-ray views which should be performed postoperatively. However, AP views in internal and external rotation, together with axillary lateral views, are commonly reported as the standard method of radiographic evaluation in the most recent published series.

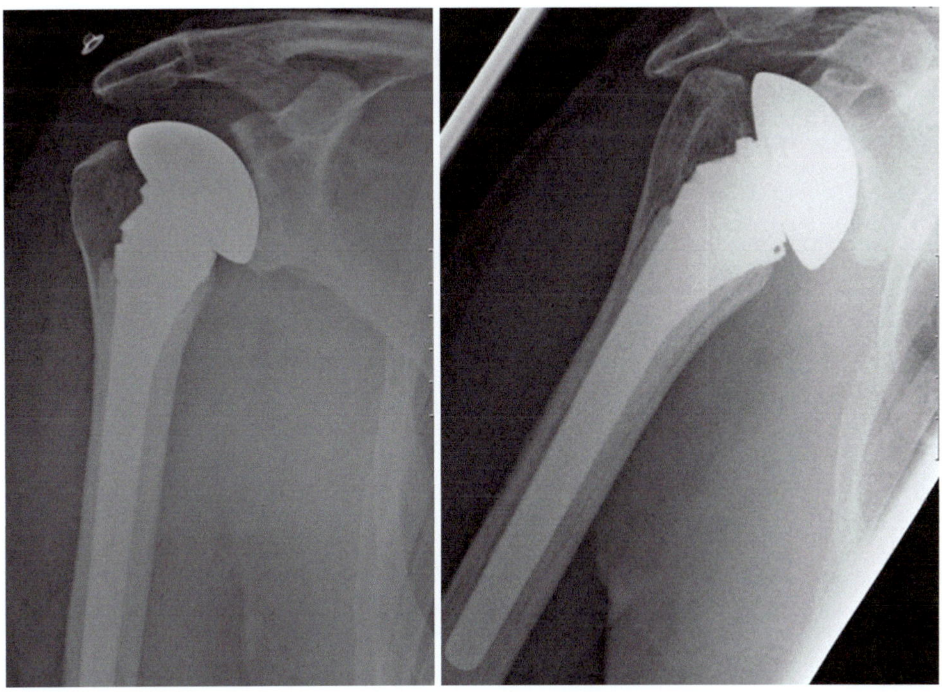

Fig. 4.12 Sequential radiographs demonstrating humeral component loosening

Postoperative AP radiographs should make note of:

1. The head-neck angle of the humeral stem
2. Cementation of humeral and glenoid components (if cemented stem is used)
3. Periprosthetic fracture
4. Glenosphere height and size
5. Position of glenoid base plate screws
6. Seating of glenoid base plate
7. Integrity of the acromion
8. Evidence of scapular notching
9. Dislocation

Axillary views can provide some idea into the version of the humeral component particularly if they include the epicondylar axis of the elbow as a point of reference.

Head-Neck Angle

The head-neck angle is set by the prosthesis design and is usually between 135 and 155° (Fig. 4.13). Prosthesis design, where the humeral neck angle is lower, reduces humeral contact with the scapula neck and can potentially reduce the incidence of scapula notching [21] but may have implications with reduced movement and instability.

Scapular Notching

Scapular notching was a commonly reported complication in the early reports and raised significant concerns that it was associated with poorer outcomes and potentially catastrophic failure [22]. Nerot-Sirveaux score [23] established a method (Table 4.1) for

Table 4.1 The Nerot-Sirveaux score

0	No defect
1	Defect affecting only lateral pillar
2	Defect in contact with inferior screw
3	Defect extends beyond inferior screw
4	Defect extends to base plate

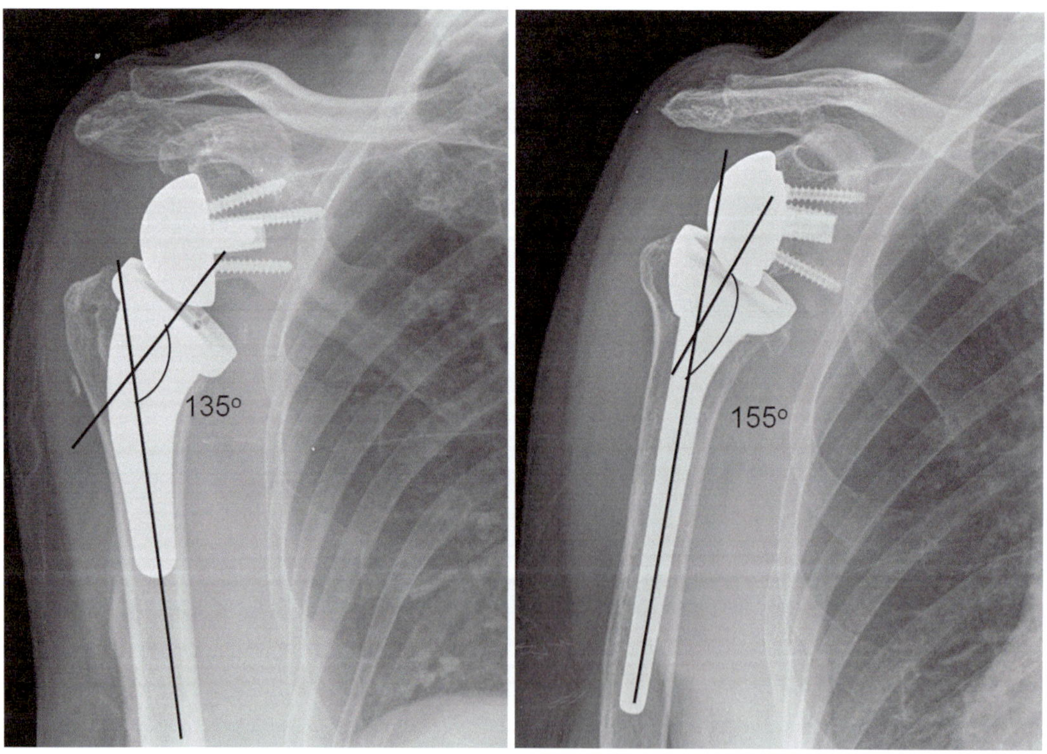

Fig. 4.13 Illustration showing different neck-shaft angles of the humeral component

describing the extent of postoperative scapular neck erosion on plain radiographs (Figs. 4.14 and 4.15).

Factors associated with notching are glenosphere position and humeral neck-shaft angle. Inferior placement, inferior eccentricity or even overhang of the glenoid component is associated with less common occurrence of scapular notching [24].

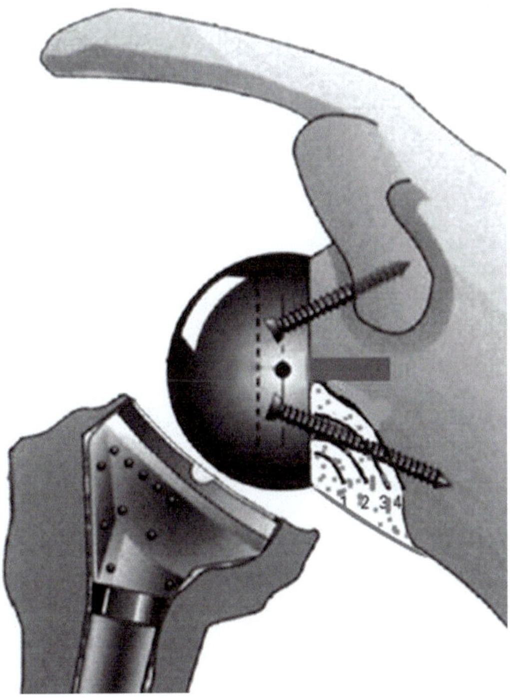

Fig. 4.14 Sirveaux grading for scapular notching on a schematic diagram

Humeral Component Version

Early series recommended retroversion of the humeral component to facilitate maximum rotation without having a detrimental effect on stability.

Placing the humeral component in 0–20° of retroversion allows maximum internal rotation with the arm at the side, a movement that is required for daily activities. This limits external rotation with the arm at the side but has no effect on external rotation with the arm elevated. Biomechanically this provides sufficient teres minor length and moment arm, as well as causes minimum impingement [25, 26].

There is however some evidence to suggest that retroversion of the humeral component can predispose to abnormal anterior instability, recommending that the component should be placed in a neutral version [27].

Dislocation

The incidence is reported to be between 0 and 8% and depends on indication for surgery, surgical technique and patient-related factors [28]. Many patients are unaware that their prosthesis is dislocated, and thus, it behoves the surgeon to obtain radiographs throughout the acute postoperative period, even in patients who are clinically doing well (Fig. 4.16). In addition, a 10° inferior tilt of the glenoid is associated with a reduced risk of dislocation when compared to neutral tilt. It does

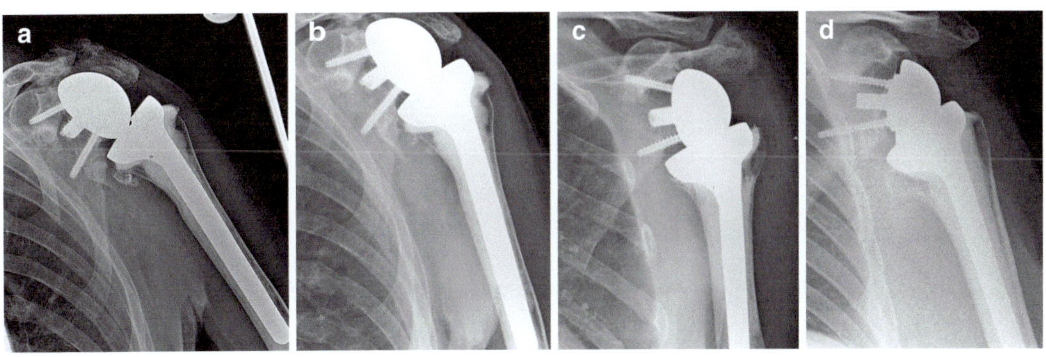

Fig. 4.15 Scapular notching from grade 1 to 4 as demonstrated on radiographs

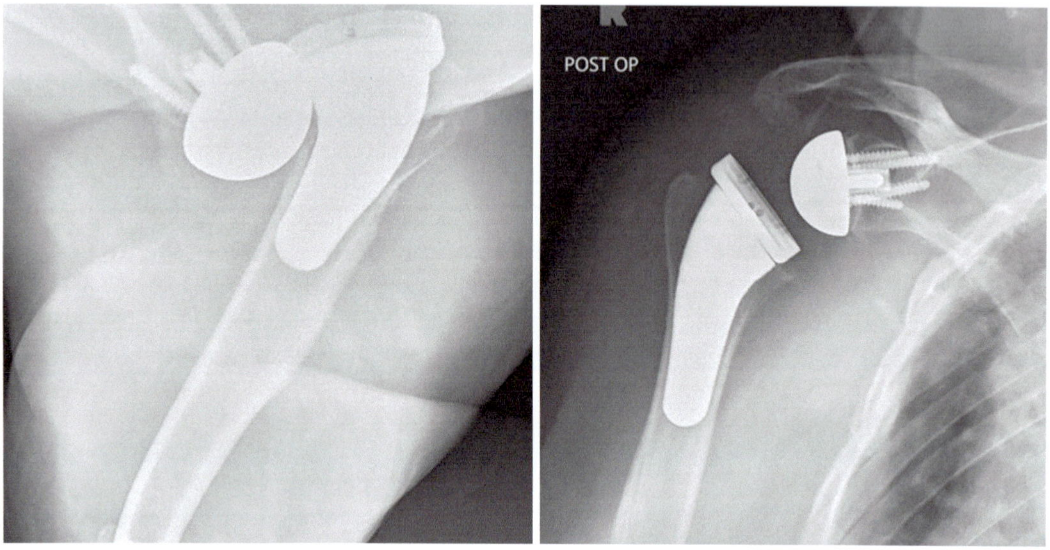

Fig. 4.16 Dislocated reverse shoulder prosthesis

not however reduce the incidence or severity of radiographic scapular notching [29].

Acromial Fractures

Stress fractures to the acromion (Fig. 4.17) are seen in over 10% of reverse shoulders at 5 months post surgery. The occurrence of an acromial fracture does not necessarily translate into clinical relevance.

Excision of tumours of the humerus requires reconstruction with extensive prosthesis (Fig. 4.18).

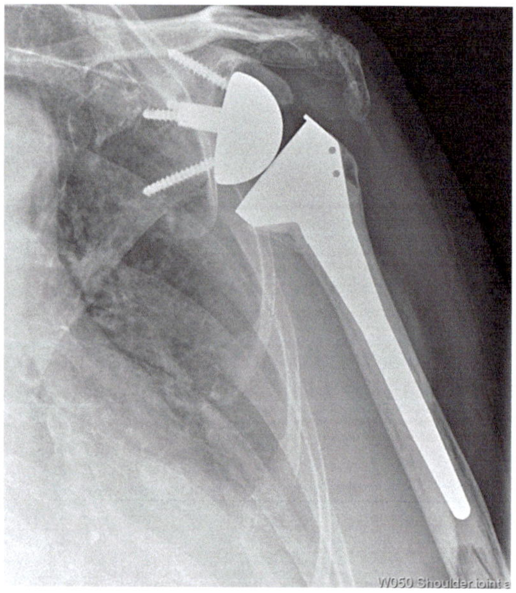

Fig. 4.17 Acromial stress fracture

Elbow Implants

Prior to 1947, resection and interposition arthroplasties were the primary surgical procedures for the treatment of severe posttraumatic deformity, trauma and rheumatoid arthritis of the elbow. Since 1947 surgeons began performing partial elbow arthroplasty of the distal part of the humerus and proximal part of the ulna, but the results were unfavourable. In the 1970s, the first simple hinged prosthesis was inserted with the use of methyl methacrylate fixation. This improved the stability of the construct, but loosening rates were high. Over the years, there have been significant improvements in designs and materials [30].

Currently the indications for total elbow arthroplasty (TEA) have expanded from inflammatory arthropathy to include unreconstructable

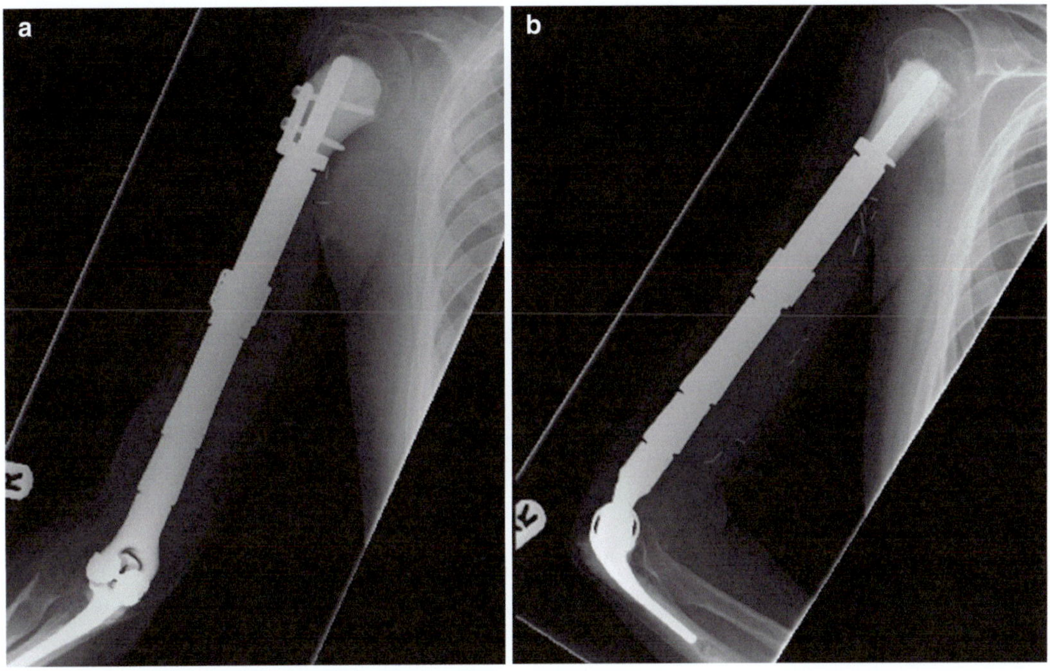

Fig. 4.18 Replacement of the humeral shaft and elbow joint using a prosthesis after resection for tumour AP (**a**) and lateral (**b**) view. There is limited bone in the proximal humerus and fixation using an intramedullary stem, and extramedullary plate has been used. Distally, the elbow joint has been replaced with a hinge design

fractures and primary osteoarthritis. Nevertheless TEA is still generally considered mainly for patients with low physical demands, and the reported survival is not as good as hip or knee replacements.

The modern elbow replacements can be broadly divided into linked, unlinked and linkable. The mechanism of linkage is the main distinguishing feature between the subtypes. The linkage refers to the physical connection of the humeral and ulnar components at the time of surgery, in order to avoid subluxation or dislocation [30].

The early linked implants allowed purely flexion and extension. These were associated with high failure rates secondary to the transmission of high stresses to the implant-cement-bone interface. The modern linked implants are semi-constrained, with the linking mechanism behaving as a 'sloppy hinge' allowing flexion and extension with some valgus-varus movement. They are designed to transmit less stress to the implant-cement-bone interface. These changes replicate more accurately with helical motion of elbow movement and have generally resulted in more reliable long-term results [31, 32].

Examples of the linked total elbow prostheses include the Coonrad-Morrey, Discovery, GSB III, Norway, Pritchard Mk II and Pritchard-Walker.

The unlinked implants are not mechanically linked. Therefore, the maintenance of prosthesis congruency depends on the adequate position of each component, the ligamentous integrity and the dynamic stabilizing effect of the musculature.

Examples of the unlinked implants include the Capitellocondylar, iBP, Kudo, Sorbie and Souter-Strathclyde [31].

The Acclaim and Latitude prostheses are newly designed implants that are linkable systems. In these, the surgeon can choose to either link or unlink the implant depending on the intra-operative assessment of the stability.

Postoperative Radiological Assessment

Immediate postoperative radiographs include AP and lateral views.

They are used to assess:

1. Alignment of the implanted stems (humeral and ulnar) in relation to the long axis of the bone
2. Normal articulation between the humeral and ulnar components, with no evidence of subluxation or dislocation
3. No evidence of periprosthetic fractures
4. Cementation

Long-term follow-up radiographs should be scrutinized for any features of:

1. Loosening
2. Instability
3. Infection
4. Periprosthetic fracture

Loosening is graded from grade 0 to grade 4 (Table 4.2) as described by Morrey [32]. Radiolucency around pegged and keeled glenoid components are classified in Tables 4.3 and 4.4.

Subluxation or dislocation is unlikely in linked prosthesis; however, wear of the polyethylene bushings can be identified and is a precursor for implant failure.

Disengagement of the linking pin will also result in elbow instability.

Polyethylene bushing wear can be evaluated based on the description by Ramsey et al. [33], which is based on a true AP radiograph of the prosthesis. A line is drawn parallel to the yoke of the humeral component, and another line is drawn parallel to the medial or lateral surface of the ulnar component. Normally the prosthesis has about 7° of varus-valgus and axial rotational laxity. An angle of intersection of more than 7° between these two lines is indicative of excessive tolerance of the bushings due to wear or plastic deformation (Fig. 4.19).

The presence of periosteal new bone formation, periprosthetic bone resorption, soft tissue or periprosthetic gas and periprosthetic loosening may indicate infection.

Periprosthetic fractures are classified (Fig. 4.20) based on the location of the fracture based on the Mayo classification [34] (Table 4.5) and also consider the bone quality and the stability of the component. It applies to both humeral and ulnar fractures.

Table 4.2 Classification of loosening of elbow prosthesis

Type 0, a radiolucent line which is <1 mm thick and involves <50% of the interface
Type 1, a radiolucent line which is 1 mm thick and involves <50% of the interface
Type 2, a radiolucent line which is >1 mm thick and involves >50% of the interface
Type 3, a radiolucent line which is >2 mm thick and involves the whole interface
Type 4, gross loosening

Table 4.3 Grading scale for radiolucencies around keeled glenoid components [16]

Grade	Finding
0	No radiolucency
1	Radiolucency at superior and/or inferior flange
2	Incomplete radiolucency at keel
3	Complete radiolucency (≤2 mm wide) around keel
4	Complete radiolucency (>2 mm wide) around keel
5	Gross loosening

Table 4.4 Grading scale for radiolucencies around pegged glenoid components [16]

Grade	Finding
0	No radiolucency
1	Incomplete radiolucency around one or two pegs
2	Complete radiolucency (<2 mm wide) around one peg only, with or without incomplete radiolucency around one other peg
3	Complete radiolucency (<2 mm wide) around two or more pegs
4	Complete radiolucency (>2 mm wide) around two or more pegs
5	Gross loosening

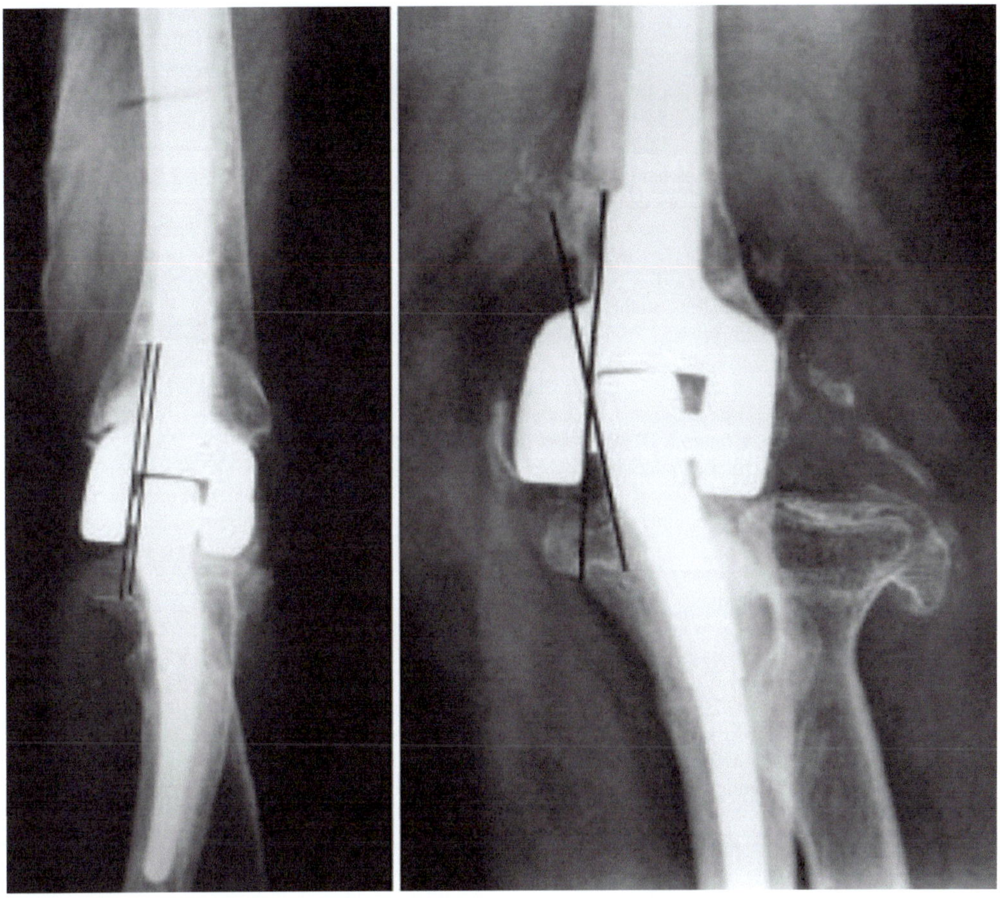

Fig. 4.19 On a true anteroposterior radiograph, a qualitative determination of wear of the bushings may be estimated by observing the angular relationship between the ulnar component and the humeral yoke. A normally aligned implant (**a**) and image showing wear of the bushings (**b**) (reproduced with permission)

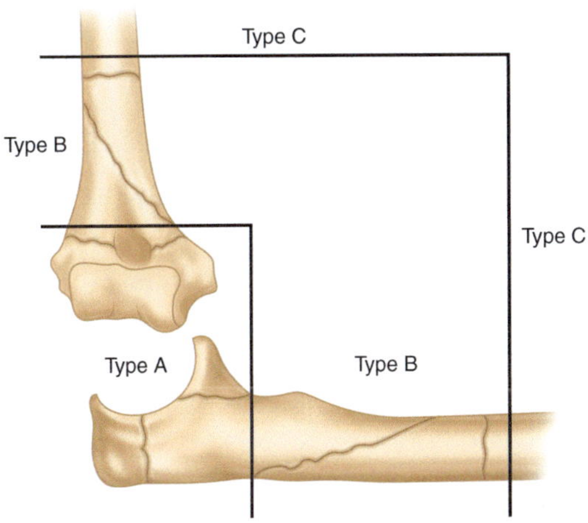

Fig. 4.20 Periprosthetic fractures of the humerus and ulna can be classified according to the region of the bone involved (reproduced with permission) [34]

Table 4.5 Elbow periprosthetic fracture classification

1. Based on anatomical region
(a) Periarticular (humerus + condyle, epicondyle) (ulna + olecranon, coronoid)
(b) Shaft around or at tip of stem
(c) Shaft beyond tip of stem
2. Based on status of stem and bone stock
(a) Well-fixed, adequate bone quality
(b) Loose, adequate bone quality
(c) Severe bone loss or osteolysis

References

1. Neer CS II. Prosthetic replacement of the humeral head: indications and operative technique. Surg Clin North Am. 1963;43:1581–97.
2. Boileau P, Walch G. The three dimensional geometry of the proximal humerus. Implications for surgical technique and prosthetic design. J Bone Joint Surg Br. 1997;79(5):857–65.
3. Favre P, Moor B, Snedeker JG, Gerber C. Influence of component positioning on impingement in conventional total shoulder arthroplasty. Clin Biomech (Bristol, Avon). 2008;23(2):175–83. Epub 2007 Nov 5.
4. Williams GR Jr, Wong KL, Pepe MD, Tan V, Silverberg D, Ramsey ML, Karduna A, Iannotti JP. The effect of articular malposition after total shoulder arthroplasty on glenohumeral translations, range of motion, and subacromial impingement. J Shoulder Elbow Surg. 2001;10(5):399–409.
5. Neer CS 2nd, Watson KC, Stanton FJ. Recent experience in total shoulder replacement. J Bone Joint Surg Am. 1982;64(3):319–37.
6. Ovesen J, Nielsen S. Prosthesis position in shoulder arthroplasty. A cadaver study of the humeral component. Acta Orthop Scand. 1985;56(4):330–1.
7. Frich LH, Møller BN. Retroversion of the humeral prosthesis in shoulder arthroplasty. Measurements of angle from standard radiographs. J Arthroplasty. 1989;4(3):277–80.
8. Takase K, Yamamoto K, Imakiire A, Burkhead WZ Jr. The radiographic study in the relationship of the glenohumeral joint. J Orthop Res. 2004;22(2):298–305.
9. Kadum B, Sayed-Noor AS, Perisynakis N, Baea S, Sjödén GO. Radiologic assessment of glenohumeral relationship: reliability and reproducibility of lateral humeral offset. Surg Radiol Anat. 2015;37(4):363–8.
10. Iannotti JP, Gabriel JP, Schneck SL, Evans BG, Misra S. The normal glenohumeral relationships. An anatomical study of one hundred and forty shoulders. J Bone Joint Surg Am. 1992;74(4):491–500.
11. Mechlenburg I, Amstrup A, Klebe T, Jacobsen SS, Teichert G, Stilling M. The Copeland resurfacing humeral head implant does not restore humeral head anatomy. A retrospective study. Arch Orthop Trauma Surg. 2013;133(5):615–9.
12. de Leest O, Rozing PM, Rozendaal LA, van der Helm FC. Influence of glenohumeral prosthesis geometry and placement on shoulder muscle forces. Clin Orthop Relat Res. 1996;330:222–33.
13. Nyffeler RW, Sheikh R, Jacob HAC, Gerber C. Influence of humeral prosthesis height on biomechanics of glenohumeral abduction. An in vitro study. J Bone Joint Surg Am. 2004;86:575–80.
14. Harryman DT, Sidles JA, Harris SL, Lippitt SB, Matsen FA. The effect of articular conformity and the size of the humeral head component on laxity and motion after glenohumeral arthroplasty: a study in cadavera. J Bone Joint Surg Am. 1995;77:555–63.
15. Franklin JL, Barrett WP, Jackins SE, Matsen FA III. Glenoid loosening in total shoulder arthroplasty. Association with rotator cuff deficiency. J Arthroplasty. 1988;3:39–46.
16. Lazarus MD, Jensen KL, Southworth C, Matsen FA III. The radiographic evaluation of keeled and pegged glenoid component insertion. J Bone Joint Surg Am. 2002;84-A(7):1174–82.
17. Sperling JW, Cofield RH, O'Driscoll SW, Torchia ME, Rowland CM. Radiographic assessment of ingrowth total shoulder arthroplasty. J Shoulder Elbow Surg. 2000;9(6):507–13.
18. Sanchez-Sotelo J, O'Driscoll SW, Torchia ME, Cofield RH, Rowland CM. Radiographic assessment of cemented humeral components in shoulder arthroplasty. J Shoulder Elbow Surg. 2001;10(6):526–31.
19. Gregory TM, Sankey A, Augereau B, Vandenbussche E, Amis A, Emery R, Hansen U. Accuracy of glenoid component placement in total shoulder arthroplasty and its effect on clinical and radiological outcome in a retrospective, longitudinal, Monocentric Open Study. PLoS One. 2013;8(10):e75791.
20. Karelse A, Van Tongel A, Verstraeten T, Poncet D Jr, De Wilde LF. Rocking-horse phenomenon of the glenoid component: the importance of inclination. J Shoulder Elbow Surg. 2015. pii: S1058-2746(14)00684-3.
21. de Wilde LF, Poncet D, Middernacht B, Ekelund A. Prosthetic overhang is the most effective way to prevent scapular conflict in a reverse total shoulder prosthesis. Acta Orthop. 2010;81(6):719–26.
22. Ek ET, Neukom L, Catanzaro S, Gerber C. Reverse total shoulder arthroplasty for massive irreparable rotator cuff tears in patients younger than 65 years old: results after five to fifteen years. J Shoulder Elbow Surg. 2013;22(9):1199–208.
23. Lévigne C, Boileau P, Favard L, Garaud P, Molé D, Sirveaux F, Walch G. Scapular notching in reverse shoulder arthroplasty. J Shoulder Elbow Surg. 2008;17(6):925–35.
24. De Biase CF, Ziveri G, Delcogliano M, de Caro F, Gumina S, Borroni M, Castagna A, Postacchini R. The use of an eccentric glenosphere compared with a concentric glenosphere in reverse total shoulder arthroplasty: two-year minimum follow-up results. Int Orthop. 2013;37(10):1949–55.
25. Gulotta LV, Choi D, Marinello P, Knutson Z, Lipman J, Wright T, Cordasco FA, Craig EV, Warren RF. Humeral component retroversion in reverse total shoulder arthroplasty: a biomechanical study. J Shoulder Elbow Surg. 2012;21(9):1121–7.
26. Berton A, Gulotta LV, Petrillo S, Florio P, Longo UG, Denaro V, Kontaxis A. The effect of humeral version on teres minor muscle moment arm, length, and impingement in reverse shoulder arthroplasty during activities of daily living. J Shoulder Elbow Surg. 2015;24(4):578–86.
27. Favre P, Sussmann PS, Gerber C. The effect of component positioning on intrinsic stability of the

reverse shoulder arthroplasty. J Shoulder Elbow Surg. 2010;19(4):550–6.
28. Chalmers PN, Rahman Z, Romeo AA, Nicholson GP. Early dislocation after reverse total shoulder arthroplasty. J Shoulder Elbow Surg. 2014;23(5):737–44.
29. Edwards TB, Trappey GJ, Riley C, O'Connor DP, Elkousy HA, Gartsman GM. Inferior tilt of the glenoid component does not decrease scapular notching in reverse shoulder arthroplasty: results of a prospective randomized study. J Shoulder Elbow Surg. 2012;21(5):641–6.
30. Cross MB, Sherman SL, Kepler CK, Neviaser AS, Weiland AJ. The evolution of elbow arthroplasty: innovative solutions to complex clinical problems. J Bone Joint Surg Am. 2010;92(Suppl 2):98–104. https://doi.org/10.2106/JBJS.J.00777.
31. Sanchez-Sotelo J. Total elbow arthroplasty. Open Orthop J. 2011;5:115–23. https://doi.org/10.2174/1874325001105010115.
32. Schneeberger AG, Adams R, Morrey BF. Semiconstrained total elbow replacement for the treatment of post-traumatic osteoarthrosis. J Bone Joint Surg Am. 1997;79:1211–22.
33. Ramsey ML, Adams RA, Morrey BF. Instability of the elbow treated with semiconstrained total elbow arthroplasty. J Bone Joint Surg Am. 1999;81(1):38–47.
34. O'Driscoll SW, Morrey BF. Periprosthetic fractures about the elbow. Orthop Clin North Am. 1999;30(2):319–25.

Foot and Ankle Implants

5

Anthony Perera, Monier Hossain, and Faiz Khan

An increasing variety of specialised implants are used in foot and ankle surgery. Fixation devices used can be either internal fixation devices—plates, screws, staples, wires or intramedullary nails—or external fixation devices, fine wire fixators or ring fixators.

Plates are a common method of internal fixation. A commonly used plate is the one-third tubular plate. This is often used as a neutralisation plate in fibular fracture fixation. The plate is thin and malleable and often contoured at the time of the operation to lateral fibular cortex (Fig. 5.1).

New locking compression plates are recognisable by their combination holes that allow screw insertion in both locking and non-locking modes and are larger than conventional plate holes. Locking compression plates are used in tibial plafond fixation (Fig. 5.2) where compression across the fracture site may not be achievable due to comminution.

Screws are widely used and are of different types. They can be fully or partially threaded. Cortical and cancellous screws are the commonest in use. Cortical screws tend to have finer threads, and cancellous screws have deeper threads with longer distance between threads (Fig. 5.1).

Locking screws have additional threads in the screw head that lock within the reciprocal threads in the hole of the plate. Locking screw threads are shallower compared to conventional non-locking screws, and they also have a sharper, self-drilling, self-tapping tip. Another useful clue is that conventional screws are used for bicortical fixation, whereas locking screws can be used for unicortical fixation. However, although initial fixation principles recommended unicortical fixation with locking screws, bicortical fixation is more commonly used generally.

Headless compression screws (Fig. 5.3) are also widely used in forefoot elective surgery. The lack of a head allows the screw to be buried in the bone and produce compression through differential pitch.

A. Perera (✉) · F. Khan
University Hospital of Wales, Cardiff, UK

M. Hossain
Wirral University Teaching Hospital, Wirral, UK
e-mail: nunierh@doctors.org.uk

S. Agarwal, G. J. Bansal (eds.), *Radiology of Orthopedic Implants*,
https://doi.org/10.1007/978-3-319-76009-4_5

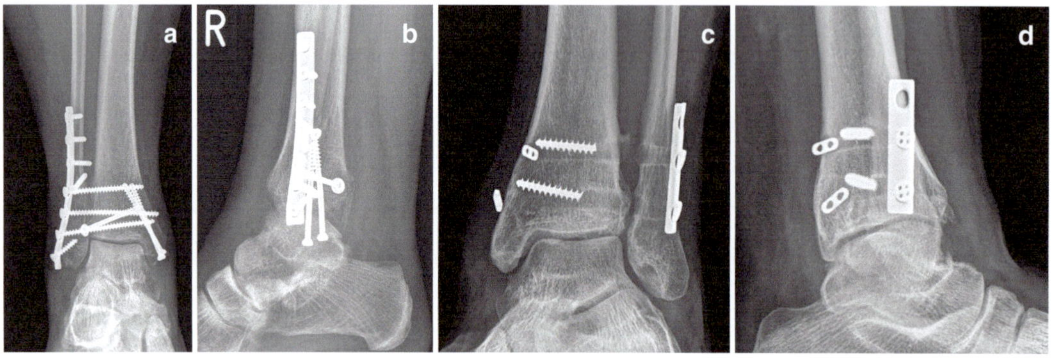

Fig. 5.1 AP (**a**) and lateral (**b**) view after fixation of an ankle fracture. The fibular fracture has been stabilised with a one-third tubular plate along with a lag screw. The medial malleolus and the anterolateral fragment from the distal tibia have been fixed with partially threaded cancellous screws to achieve compression. Three screws from the fibular plate extend into the distal tibia for additional fixation in view of osteopenia, as well as to stabilise the syndesmosis. The fibulo-tibial screws are fully threaded cancellous for optimum fixation. The proximal three screws in the fibular plate are cortical screws with shorter distance between threads compared to cancellous screws. AP (**c**) and lateral (**d**) view of the ankle showing an example of syndesmosis stabilisation using two screws from the fibula to the tibia. The screws have broken, and the lateral half of the screws has been retrieved. The syndesmosis has been stabilised using two tight rope anchors. The tight rope has a metal button at either end connected by a suture. In view of the relatively large hole on the fibular cortex, a three-hole one-third tubular plate was used to provide a stable surface for positioning the button of the tight rope

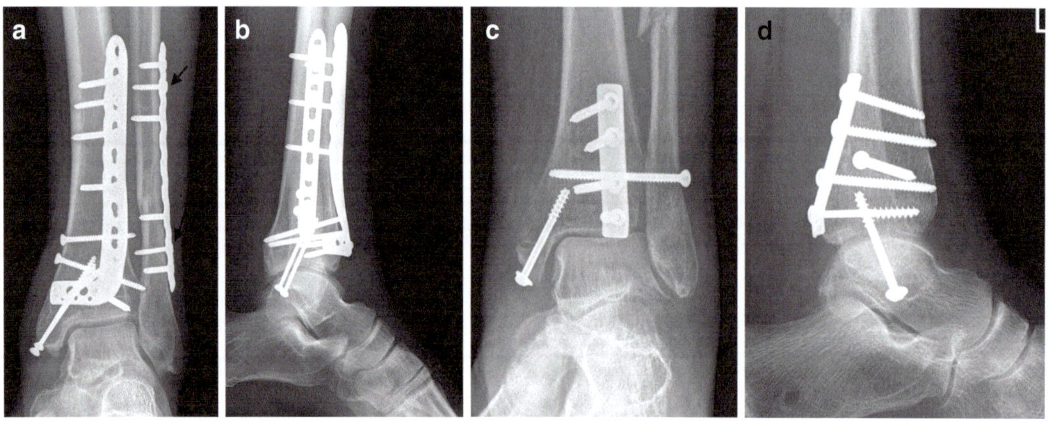

Fig. 5.2 AP (**a**) and lateral (**b**) views of the ankle after fixation of a Pilon fracture. The fibula has been stabilised with a locking plate. There are two cortical screws in the fibula (solid black arrows), and the remaining four screws are locking. The distance between threads in locking screws is shorter than cortical screws. The tibial fracture has a locking plate contoured to match the shape of the bone. There are two additional fully threaded cortical screws for the medial cortical fragment and two partially threaded cancellous screws for the medial malleolus. Stabilisation of an ankle fracture through the posterior approach—AP (**c**) and lateral (**d**) view. The one-third tubular plate has been used as a buttress plate to stabilise the posterior distal tibial fracture. There is a single screw for the medial malleolus and a single screw to stabilise the syndesmosis

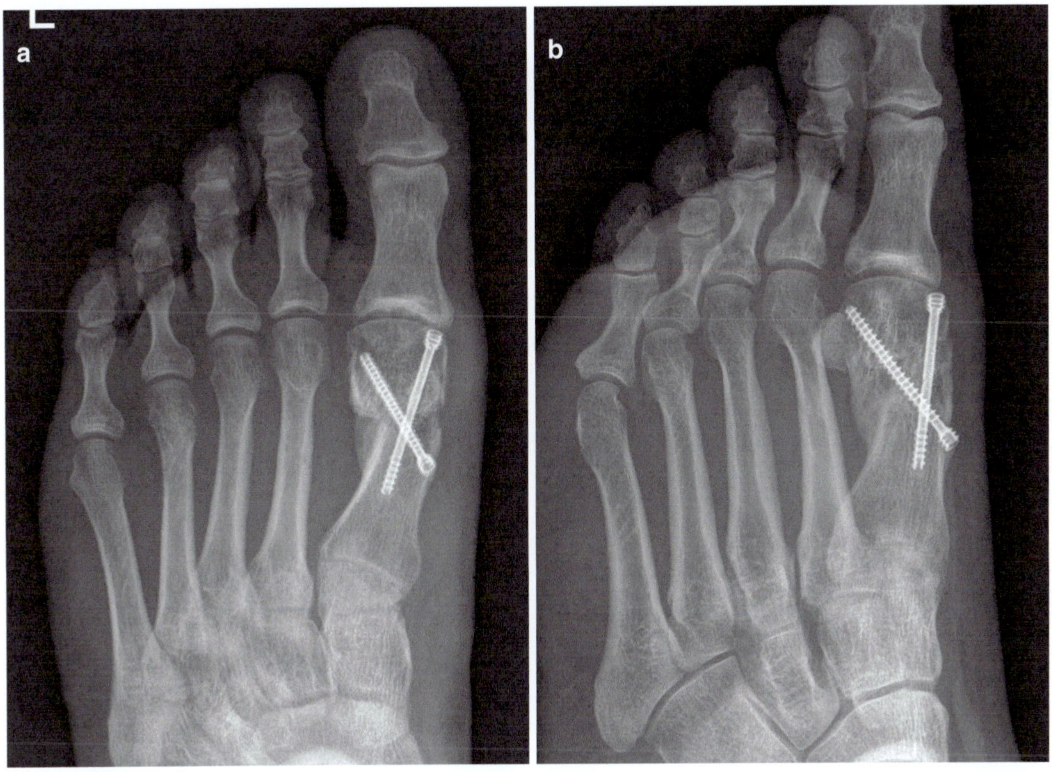

Fig. 5.3 AP (**a**) and oblique (**b**) view of hallux valgus correction using headless screws. The screws have two separate sets of threads with a different pitch, and this produces compression as the screw is tightened

Staples are used frequently in foot and ankle elective surgery to achieve compression, for instance, in arthrodesis or following osteotomy (Fig. 5.4). A common use is following hallux valgus correction where the proximal phalanx of the great toe is angulated to achieve better correction. This staple is positioned near the MTP joint and may inadvertently penetrate the articular surface.

Wires are used for lesser toe corrective surgery. As these are smooth, they have a tendency to migrate, and it is not uncommon to see wires in soft tissue in post-operative images. An intramedullary nail may be used for tibiotalocalcaneal (TTC) arthrodesis (Fig. 5.5). There are two different designs in use: straight entry nail and valgus entry nail. Valgus entry nail has a distal lateral bend to allow a valgus hindfoot positioning.

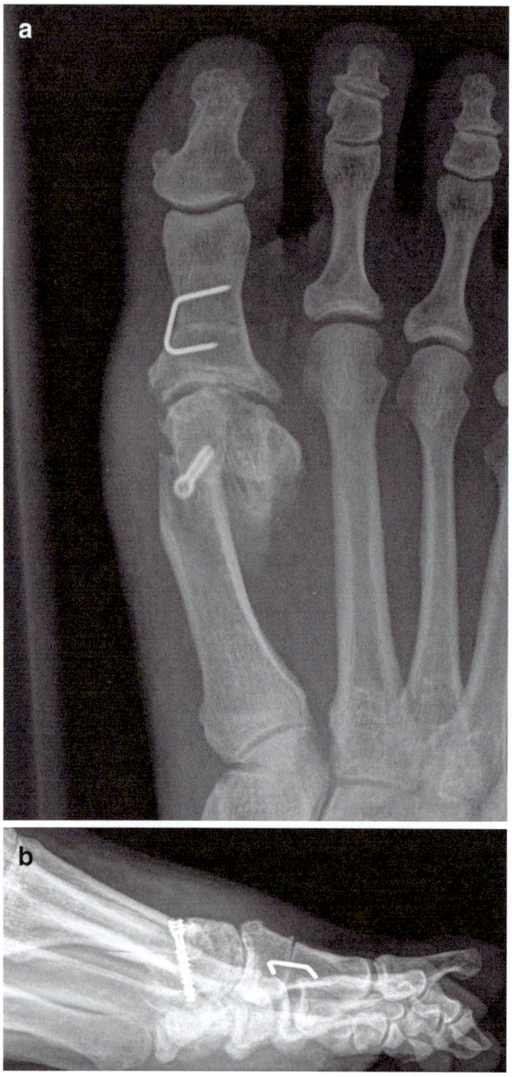

Fig. 5.4 AP (**a**) and lateral (**b**) view of the forefoot illustrating the use of a staple to stabilise the corrective osteotomy of the proximal phalanx great toe

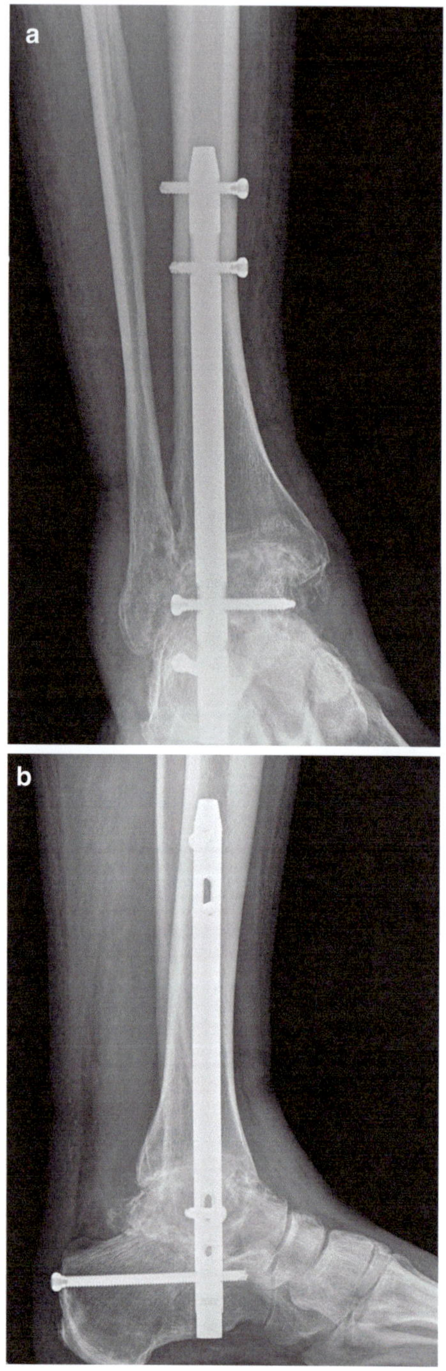

Fig. 5.5 AP (**a**) and lateral (**b**) views of the ankle following a hindfoot nail. The nail stabilises the subtalar and the tibiotalar joints. This is an example of a straight nail

Implants Used for Managing Injuries

For ankle fractures, adequate radiological assessment requires a standing AP, lateral and mortise view. Table 5.1 gives an indication for acceptable reduction criteria [1] following ankle fractures.

Lisfranc fractures are usually fixed with a combination of screws (Fig. 5.6) for the first and second tarsometatarsal joints (TMTJ). Additional fixation with wires may be needed for the third, fourth and fifth TMTJ. Weight-bearing AP, lateral and oblique views are useful for assessment of Lisfranc injuries. In case of subtle injuries, it may

Table 5.1 Radiographic markers of ankle malunion

Consider reconstruction if:	
Medial malunion/instability	
Medial clear space	>4 mm or >superior space
Talar tilt	>5 degrees
Syndesmosis	
Fibula overlap	<10 mm
Tibiofibular clear space	<5 mm
Talar shift	>1 mm
External rotation stress test	Compare with the opposite side
CT scan of syndesmosis	Incongruency
Fibula length	
Talocrural angle	Average = 83 ± 40 but compare with the opposite side
Fibula shortening	>2 mm
Fibula rotation	
CT fibula torsional angle	>150
Distal tibial malunion	
Tibial plafond angle	>100

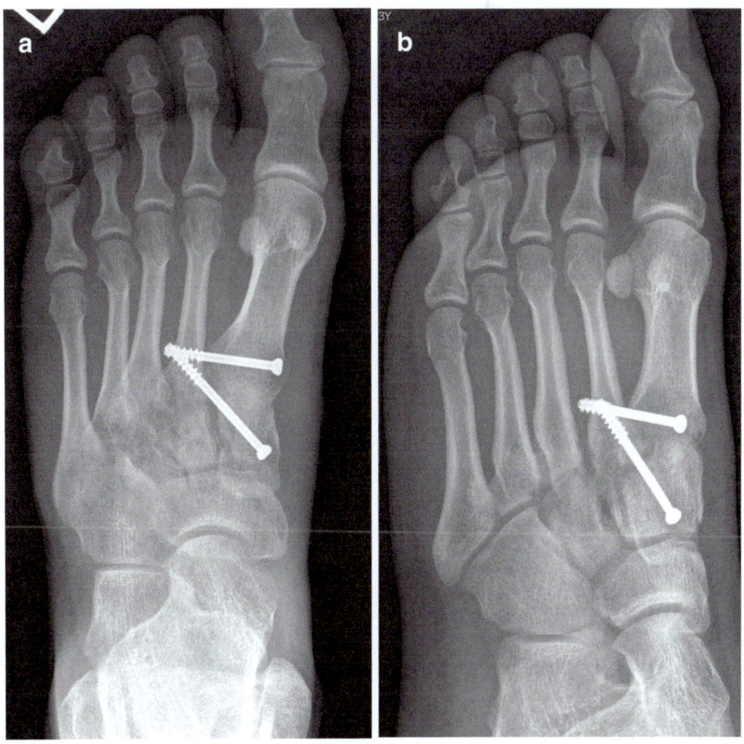

Fig. 5.6 AP (**a**) and oblique (**b**) view of the midfoot showing stabilisation of a Lisfranc injury of the first ray using two partially threaded cancellous screws

be useful to obtain a CT scan or comparison views of the contralateral foot.

A number of collinear lines are helpful to assess adequacy of reduction:

1. Medial border of the base of the second metatarsal should be in line with the medial border of the intermediate cuneiform (best seen in AP view).
2. Medial border of the third metatarsal should be in line with the medial border of the lateral cuneiform (best seen in oblique view).
3. Medial border of the fourth metatarsal should be in line with medial border of cuboid (best seen in the oblique view).
4. The fourth metatarsal styloid process should project beyond the lateral margin of the cuboid (best seen in the oblique view).
5. Flattening of the longitudinal arch is evident in the lateral view. This is best assessed by the talo-first metatarsal angle. Normal range is 0 ± 50°.

Navicular fractures are usually fixed with screws (Fig. 5.7). If the lateral navicular fragment is small, the screw may extend into the cuboid. Both the naviculocuneiform and talonavicular joint should be congruent following fixation.

For Chopart joint fracture/dislocation, both AP and lateral views of the foot are useful. On the AP view, the proximal edges of the cuneiforms must line up with the distal edge of the navicular. The calcaneocuboid joint space should not exceed 2 mm, and there should be no overlap between any of the opposing sides of the Chopart joints. On the lateral view, Chopart's joint should be outlined as a smooth S shape, also called the cyma line, which is formed by the talonavicular and the calcaneocuboid joints.

Talar neck fractures are usually fixed with two screws. However, a medial contoured plate (Fig. 5.8) may be used especially if there is medial neck comminution. Canale view gives optimal observation of the talar neck. Following fixation, it is important to assess whether there is any persistent medial neck comminution and varus angulation. Hawkins sign is best seen in the mortise X-ray 6–8 weeks after injury. The presence of subchondral radiolucency under the talar dome indicates resorption of subchondral bone and intact vascularity.

Calcaneal fracture is fixed with screws or locking plates (Fig. 5.9). Adequate radiological assessment requires a lateral view of the foot and ankle, dorsoplantar and oblique view of the foot

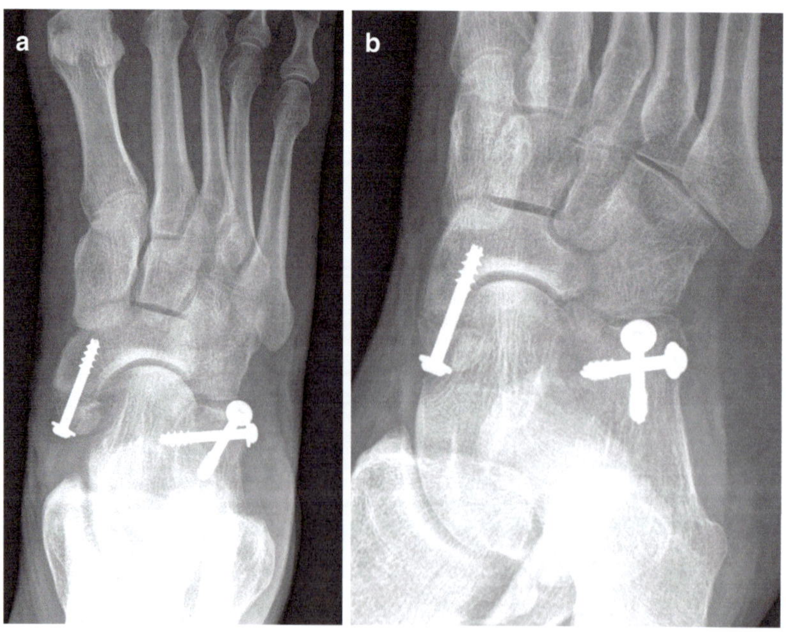

Fig. 5.7 AP (**a**) and oblique (**b**) view of the midfoot. Fixation of the navicular and the calcaneum for Chopart fracture dislocation of the foot. The partially threaded screw in the navicular helps achieve compression as it is tightened

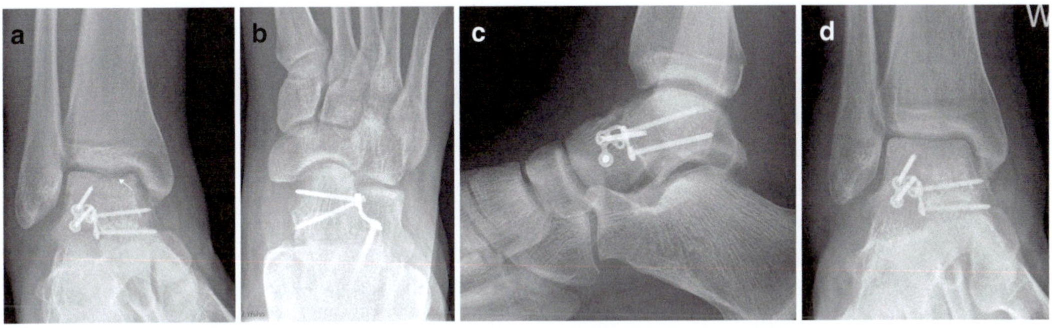

Fig. 5.8 Talar neck fixation using an anterolateral plate (**a–c**). On the initial AP view of the ankle (**a**), there is a radiolucency under the talar dome (arrow). This is the Hawkins sign signifying maintenance of blood supply to the talus. Lateral and oblique views (**b**, **c**) show the metalwork on the talar neck. On follow-up radiographs (**d**), the radiolucency has disappeared, and the talar bone architecture is maintained

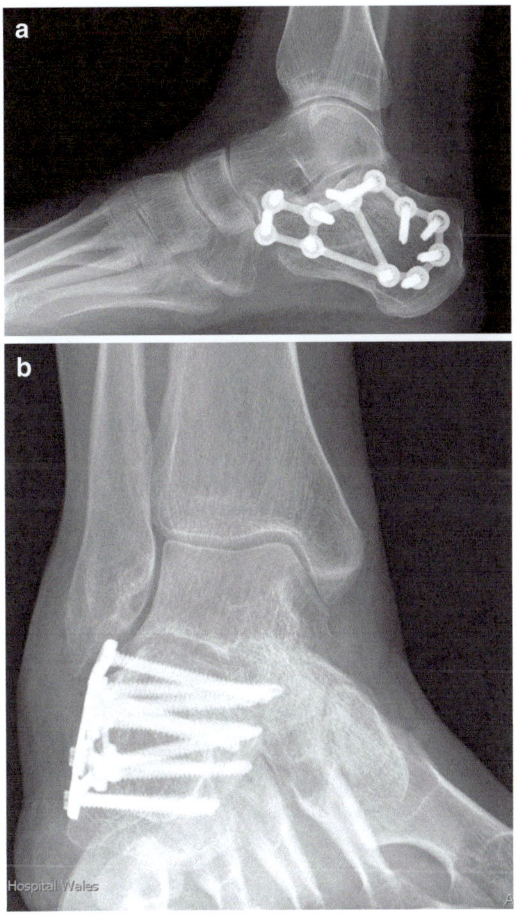

Fig. 5.9 Fixation of the calcaneum using a lateral plate—lateral (**a**) and AP (**b**) view. The plate provides multiple screw options to stabilise the fragments. Restoration of the subtalar congruity is evident on these radiographs

and axial Harris view. The lateral view is useful for assessing the position of the middle and posterior facet and the calcaneal height.

Calcaneal height is indicated by the Bohler angle. Normal range is 20–40°. Flattening represents collapse of the posterior facet, and double density is indicative of subtalar joint incongruity. Normal Gissane angle range is 130–145°. An increase of this angle is indicative of collapse of the posterior facet. Double density sign is present when injury only involves the lateral portion of the posterior facet. Both Bohler's angle and Gissane angles are normal when double density sign is present.

Axial view is useful for assessing varus angulation and lateral wall displacement. Broden's view is useful for assessing the articular surface of the posterior facet. A step of more than 2 mm is considered significant. CT scan is very useful for assessing calcaneal fracture morphology. Coronal scan is especially important to assess heel width, subfibular impingement and comminution and displacement of the subtalar joint and the posterior facet.

Radiological Assessment of Hallux Valgus Deformity

A number of radiological measurements have been described for assessment of hallux valgus angle. Although the measurements are well described and widely in use, the interobserver reliability is low, and their accuracy can be affected by the position of the foot and the great toe and their weight-bearing status [2–4]. These measurements should therefore be performed with weight-bearing AP and lateral views of the foot taken in identical positions.

Radiological assessment is based on various angles. The hallux valgus angle is formed between two lines bisecting the first metatarsal shaft and the proximal phalanx. Normal value is less than 15 degrees. Intermetatarsal angle is formed between two lines bisecting the first and the second metatarsal shafts. Normal value is less than 9°. The distal metatarsal articular angle (DMAA) is formed between two lines, one bisecting the first metatarsal shaft and the other drawn perpendicular to the distal articular surface of the first metatarsal head. Normal value is less than 10 degrees. The interphalangeal angle is formed between two lines bisecting the base and the shaft of the proximal phalanx. Normal value is less than 10 degrees.

As hallux valgus deformity progresses, there is progressive subluxation of the metatarsal head compared to the sesamoid position. Hardy and Clapham had originally devised a scoring system to measure the severity of metatarsal head subluxation. This is graded from 1 to 7 by measuring the tibial sesamoid position compared to a line drawn bisecting the first metatarsal shaft. This scoring system was subsequently simplified by the American Orthopaedic Foot and Ankle Society. The new grading system has a score from 0 to 3. Grade 0 is no lateral displacement of the tibial sesamoid compared to the mid-metatarsal shaft. Grade 1 is less than 50% lateral subluxation, grade 2 is less than 100% subluxation, and grade 3 is 100% subluxation (Fig. 5.10).

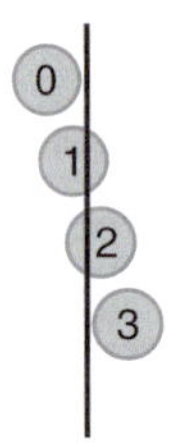

Fig. 5.10 Scoring system for position of tibial sesamoid in relation to the axis of the first metatarsal

For determination of first metatarsophalangeal (MTP) joint subluxation, two lines are drawn connecting the medial and lateral articular margin of the first metatarsal and the proximal phalanx. The first MTP joint is considered congruent if the lines are parallel. If the lines are not parallel, the joint is deviated or subluxed.

The relative length of the first metatarsal compared to the second is assessed. A number of different techniques have been described. A simple technique is to draw the axis of the second metatarsal and parallel lines perpendicular to this line from the distal end of the metatarsals (Fig. 5.11). Most of the surgical techniques described for hallux valgus correction involve a degree of first metatarsal shortening, and this measurement is especially important in individuals who experience transfer metatarsalgia following surgery. A difference in length ±2 mm of the first metatarsal compared to the second is normal. However, first metatarsal should not be

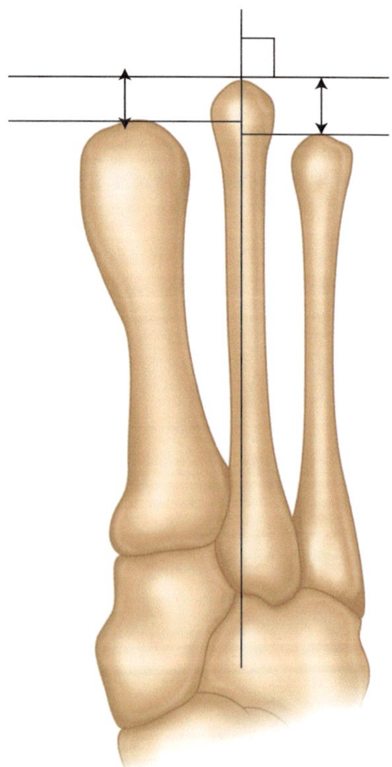

Fig. 5.11 Determination of the relative length of the first metatarsal

longer than the second following surgery, and up to 4 mm shortening is acceptable. Some reports have claimed that a relative first metatarsal length of less than 82.5% of the second metatarsal may cause symptoms [5, 6].

Weight-bearing sesamoid view is not routinely performed preoperatively but is useful for assessment of recurrent hallux valgus to determine the position of the sesamoids in relation to the sesamoid facets of the first metatarsal.

Radiological Assessment of Flatfoot Deformity

Adult-acquired flatfoot results in loss of medial longitudinal arch, peritalar subluxation and planovalgus deformity. A number of radiological markers are available to assess this deformity. Deformity is mainly noted in the talonavicular (TN) joint, but the naviculocuneiform (NC) and the first tarsometatarsal (TMT) joint may also be affected.

Weight-bearing AP and lateral views of the foot and the ankle are required. In addition some specific views have also been described for assessment of flatfoot deformity.

With increasing flatfoot deformity, the navicular subluxes laterally and the talus become increasingly uncovered. The talonavicular coverage angle can be quantified on the dorsoplantar view. This angle is formed by two lines drawn perpendicular to the articular surfaces of the talus and the navicular. An angle greater than 7° indicates lateral subluxation of the navicular.

The talo-first metatarsal angle is formed by the long axis of the talus and the first metatarsal on the weight-bearing lateral view. Normally, the axis of the two bones should be collinear. An angle which is convex downwards and greater than 4° is suggestive of pes planus (Figs. 5.12 and 5.13). Angle of greater than 15° is considered as moderate deformity, and angle greater than 30° is severe pes planus.

The anterior talocalcaneal angle is formed by the long axis of the talus and the calcaneus. This is increased due to talocalcaneal divergence in planovalgus deformity.

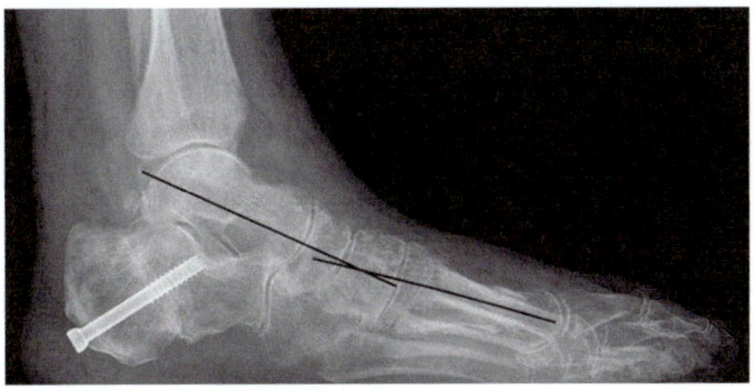

Fig. 5.12 The talo—first metatarsal angle on the weight-bearing lateral view of the foot

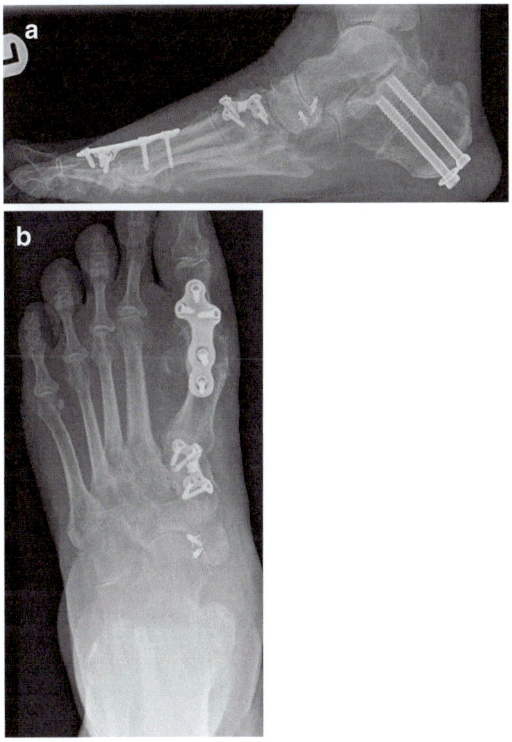

Fig. 5.13 Reconstruction of flatfoot deformity with a medialising calcaneal osteotomy, repair of medial ligaments, medial cuneiform osteotomy and fusion of the metatarso-phalangeal joint. Lateral (**a**) view and AP (**b**) view demonstrated

Arunakul et al. [7] have described the relationship of the talar head in respect to the foot tripod formed by the heel centre and the medial and lateral borders of the foot. They termed this the "tripod index" and stated that this measurement is a summation of fore, mid- and hindfoot deformities in multiple planes and demonstrated the effect of overall foot alignment on the subtalar joint. Tripod index has been validated for assessment of both flatfoot and cavovarus deformity. On a weight-bearing AP radiograph of the foot, the centre of calcaneus, talar head, lateral edge of the fifth metatarsal head and the medial edge of the medial sesamoid are marked. The tripod is formed by two lines joining the centre of calcaneus with the fifth metatarsal and the medial sesamoid. The index is positive if the line joining the centre of talar head and calcaneus is outside of the tripod. The more positive the tripod index, the more medial the talar head and the more severe the flatfoot deformity.

AP view of the ankle is important in long-standing cases to rule out talar tilt and degenerative changes of the ankle. The standing ankle height can be measured in the AP view from the talar dome to the calcaneal tubercle. Standing ankle height is reduced in unilateral planovalgus deformity. Severe planovalgus deformity may give rise to stress fracture of the fibula 5–10 cm above the tip of the lateral malleolus, and this can be detected on the AP view of the ankle.

Calcaneal pitch is the angle formed by a line drawn parallel to the floor and another drawn connecting the inferior point of the calcaneocuboid joint and the antero-inferior margin of the calcaneal tuberosity. Normal values are between 17 and 32°, with an angle less than 10° considered abnormal. Calcaneal pitch is reduced in flatfoot deformity. A reduction in the distance between the medial cuneiform and the fifth metatarsal is also indicative of loss of arch height. This is best compared with the opposite side.

Radiological Assessment of Ankle Joint Replacements

Ankle joint replacements are relatively recent and less common compared to hip and knee replacements. The first generation of constrained, cemented implants was introduced in the early 1970s. They were not very successful, nor widely adopted. These implants incorrectly considered an ankle joint to be a single axis hinge joint. Subsequent development of uncemented implants has produced better clinical results. The polyethylene insert can be mobile or fixed with the mobile design being more commonly used currently (Figs. 5.14, 5.15 and 5.16).

The radiographic assessment of ankle replacement requires standing anteroposterior and lateral views. Serial images over a period of time are more relevant and useful. In some situations, CT scans are needed to evaluate problems.

Post-operative radiological assessment can be divided into two separate aspects—component position and complications.

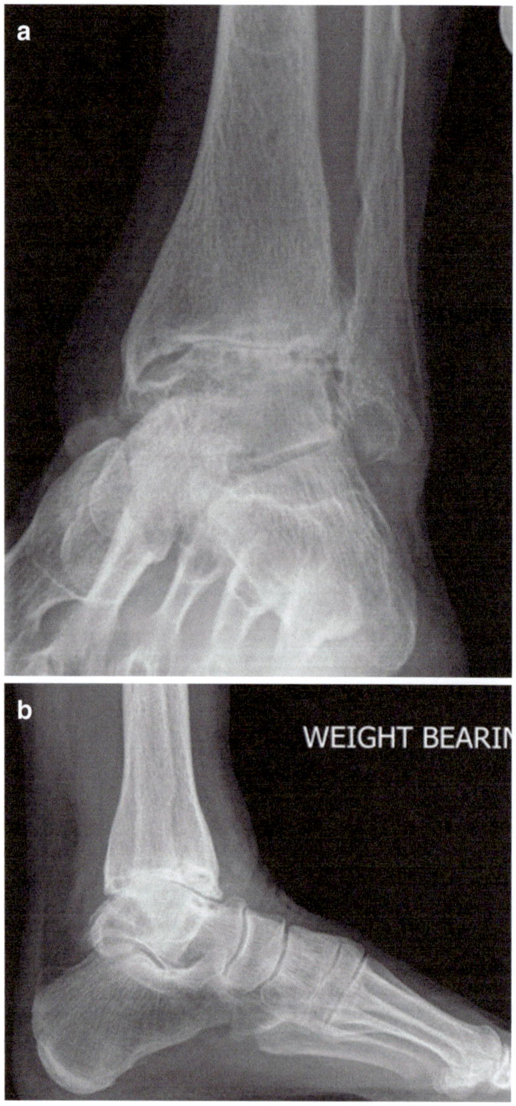

Fig. 5.14 Weight-bearing AP (**a**) and lateral (**b**) views of the ankle with osteoarthritis. Loss of joint space, osteophytes and cysts are seen in both views

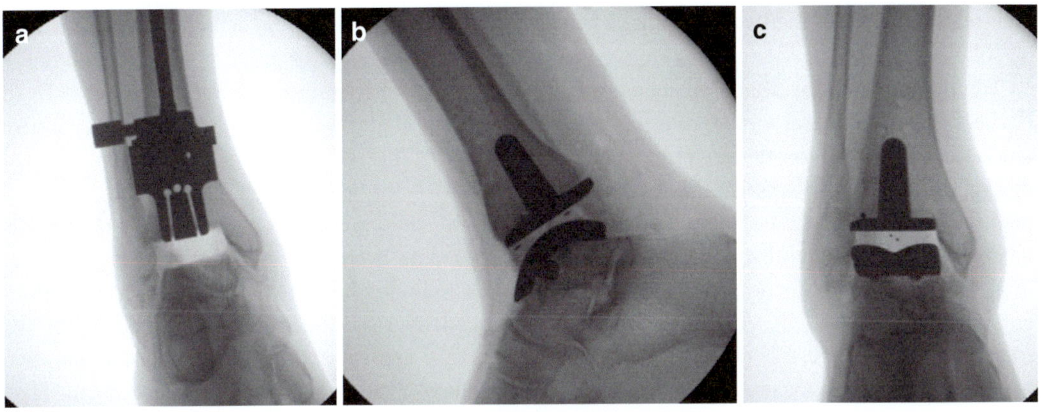

Fig. 5.15 Intraoperative image intensifier films with alignment jig and implants

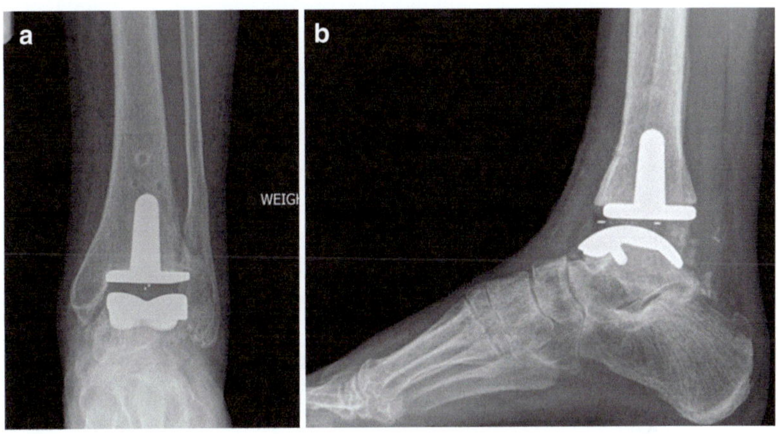

Fig. 5.16 Post-operative AP (**a**) and lateral (**b**) views following TAR

The tibial and the talar components are assessed for varus, valgus, flexion or extension alignment. Other features to note include component overhang, relative angle between the tibia and talus, quality of cementing in case of cemented implants, any retained cement, component migration and osseointegration. Possible complications which should be checked for include periprosthetic fracture, stress fracture of the medial malleolus, loosening, osteolysis, component subsidence, cavitation, spacer migration or fracture and heterotopic bone formation.

Various radiological measurements have been described. The alpha angle defines the position of the tibial component in the anteroposterior view and is formed by the intersection of two lines: one line is drawn in the long axis of the tibia, and the other line is drawn parallel to the flat plate of the tibial component [8]. This angle should normally be 90°.

The beta angle defines the tibial component position in the lateral view and is formed by the intersection of the same lines drawn in the AP view. This angle should also ideally be 90°.

Gamma angle is used to describe the position of the talar component in the lateral view and is formed by the intersection of two lines, one drawn along the long axis of the talar component and the other line drawn through the middle of the talar neck. Normal range of gamma angle is between 11 and 33°. This measurement may not be precise if there is a deformity of the hindfoot.

Displacement of the talar component relative to the tibial component can be assessed by drawing lines through the centre of both components. The relative position of the two lines is the tibial–

talar relationship. Normally, the two lines should be collinear.

Tibial component overhang or undercoverage is checked in the lateral view by noting the distance between the most anterior and posterior margin of the tibial component. Medial impingement is measured in the AP view and is the distance between the lateral margin of the medial malleolus and the tibial component. A change in angular measurement of either component by more than 5° is suggestive of component migration or subsidence. A change in talar component position of more than 5 mm in the lateral view also suggests possible migration.

Radiolucency at the bone–implant interface in the early post-operative radiograph may be the result of surgical technique. However, radiolucent lines at the bone–implant interface that are progressive or more than 2 mm wide are considered significant and are suggestive of osteolysis.

In order to better localise abnormalities and to facilitate communication, a number of different zonal systems similar to Gruen zones for assessment of hip arthroplasty have been described. However, in view of the different designs of implants, there is no universally accepted zonal classification system.

Researchers reporting mobility ankle outcome described 15 zones for assessment of radiolucencies: ten zones for tibial component (five in AP view and five in lateral view) and five zones for talar component (two in AP and three in lateral view) [9, 10]. Tibial component interface for the agility prosthesis [11] was divided into six zones in the AP view and three zones in the lateral view. However, assessment of radiolucency around ankle arthroplasty may be difficult for a number of reasons. Periprosthetic osteolysis may not be evident until a significant proportion of the bone is lost because it happens mainly around the cancellous bone of the distal tibia and proximal talus. Additionally, even if osteolysis is present, it may be obscured by the metallic overhang of tibial or talar components. CT scan is often a more accurate assessment tool for this [12].

The presence of radiolucency around the entire length of a zone or of more than 2 mm width at any point indicates possible lack of osseointegration.

Some of the current ankle replacement systems like the agility ankle system incorporate a design feature to allow concomitant arthrodesis of the tibiofibular joint. In assessing post-operative imaging, it is important to assess whether the syndesmosis fusion has taken place or not.

An anteroposterior and a lateral X-ray view is needed to ascertain adequate implant position. The radiographic appearance after TAR is influenced by the intraoperative positioning of the implant and the type of implant used. The two primary components are tibial and talar. They may be cemented particularly in the earlier generations but are predominantly uncemented in the current generation of implants. They are made from metal alloys and are thus visualised on radiographs, but some earlier implants particularly tibial were made from polyethylene and therefore are not well visualised.

The polyethylene insert may be an independent third component or incorporated into the tibial component. This is an important distinction to make, as the mobile insert may present as a dislocation. Mobile inserts usually have radio-opaque markers that allow its position to be determined. These may be in the form of metal dots or a metal bar along the longitudinal axis of the polyethylene spacer (Fig. 5.17).

The bioactive coating on the implant may present as a linear radiolucency at the bone–implant interface, particularly in the immediate post-operative views until osseointegration takes place. Heterotopic ossification may also be seen after TAR.

There are multiple important radiological findings in relation to TAR outcomes. The most common complications are mechanical and include loosening, dislocation and disintegration. Post-operative X-rays may show a fracture of the lateral or the medial malleolus. This can occur during preparation of the joint surfaces or during insertion of the implant and may not be seen on image intensifier films in theatre. The position of the implants plays a significant role in the long-term outcomes of TAR as it significantly affects the loading of the joint. The orientation of the tibial implant should be at a right angle to the long axis of the tibia on the AP and lateral views. The posi-

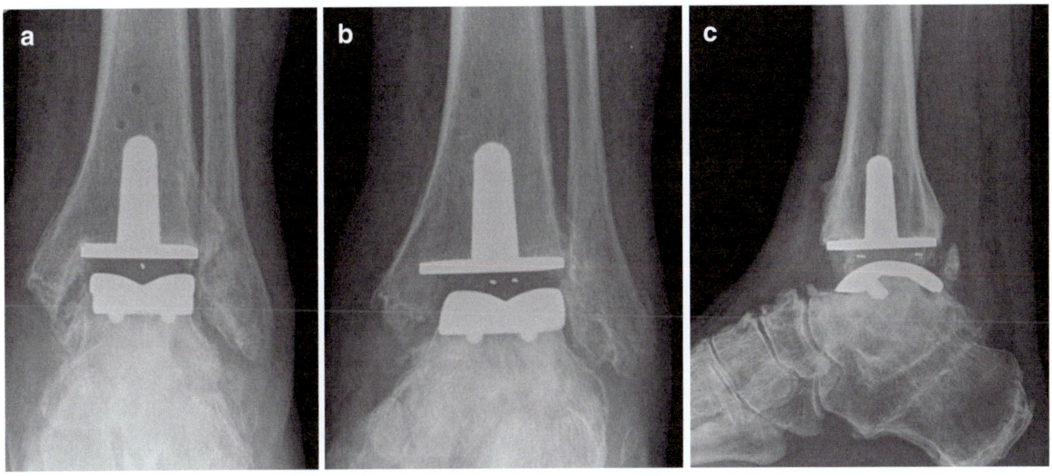

Fig. 5.17 (**a–c**) AP views post-TAR with the metal markers in the polyethylene spacer. They are placed along the long axis of the spacer. On a true AP view (**a**), they appear as one dot, and the dots are besides each other on an oblique AP view (**b**). On the lateral view (**c**), they appear as two linear markers along an imaginary longitudinal line in the spacer

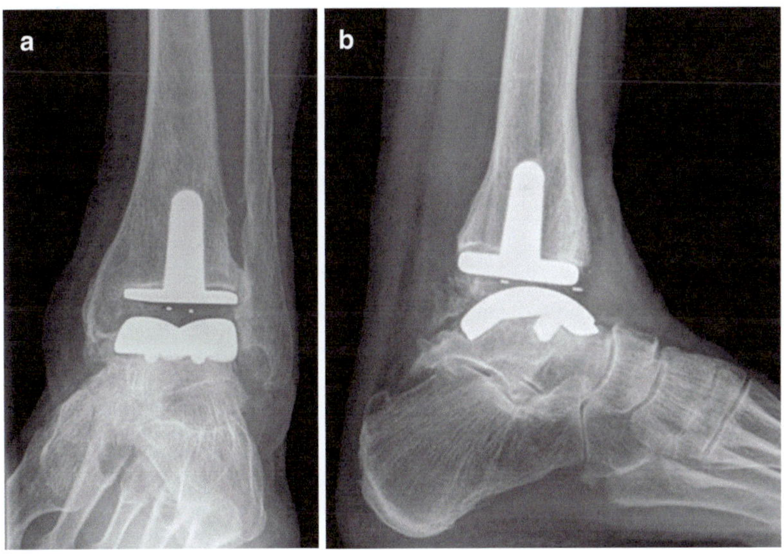

Fig. 5.18 AP (**a**) and lateral (**b**) weight-bearing views 3 years post-TAR with complaints of pain. Lucent areas are seen in both views at the bone–implant interface

tion of the talar component should correspond to the native talus and not be anterior or posterior. The metal dots or bar in the insert should be central and aligned with the tibial and talar implants. Narrowing of the spacer due to wear can take place over time, and this may be even or uneven depending on ankle loading (Fig. 5.18). This is best assessed on serial weight-bearing images.

Loosening of the implants can occur over time and can be septic or aseptic. The presence of radiolucent lines at the bone–implant interface and development of periarticular cysts indicate loosening. It is best appreciated in serial X-rays which would show progression of the lines and enlargement of cysts. A radiolucent line of 2 mm or a progressive increase in size of a line which is already present is highly suspicious of loosening, as is subsidence of over 5 mm of the talar implant as seen on the lateral view. Change in the position of the implant on serial radiographs is an absolute sign of loosening.

In the absence of radiological abnormality, determination of source of pain after ankle replacement can be difficult. The pathology may be in the ankle or in the subtalar and other adjacent joints. In order to identify the source of pain, selective local anaesthetic injections are done under ultrasound guidance into the suspected joints of the foot or the ankle joint. The ultrasound guidance technique is also very useful if joint sepsis is suspected. It is used for aspiration of the joint to obtain samples for culture.

The use of SPECT scan to localise the site of the pathology after TAR is being shown to be of statistical significance. In the presence of a metal implant, a plain X-ray may not view the joint adequately. A CT scan will have a certain degree of scatter due to the metal in the implants and thus may not show the underlying pathology. SPECT scans combine a CT scan with the use of a radioisotope. Hence, its use is an important tool to localise the site of the pathology.

With more widespread use of ankle replacements, the radiological features and their understanding continue to evolve.

References

1. Perera A, Myerson M. Surgical techniques for the reconstruction of malunited ankle fractures. Foot Ankle Clin. 2008;13:737–51.
2. Coughlin MJ, Freund E. The reliability of angular measurements in hallux valgus deformities. Foot Ankle Int. 2001;22:369–79.
3. Vittetoe DA, Saltzman CL, Krieg JC, Brown TD. Validity and reliability of the first distal metatarsal articular angle. Foot Ankle Int. 1994;15:541–7.
4. Fuhrmann RA, Layher F, Wetzel WD. Radiographic changes in forefoot geometry with weight-bearing. Foot Ankle Int. 2003;24:326–31.
5. Carr CR, Boyd BM. Correctional osteotomy for metatarsus primus varus and hallux valgus. J Bone Joint Surg Am. 1968;50(7):1353–67.
6. Schemitsch E, Horne G. Wilson's osteotomy for the treatment of hallux valgus. Clin Orthop Relat Res. 1989;240:221–5.
7. Arunakul M, Amendola A, Gao Y, et al. Tripod index: a new radiographic parameter assessing foot alignment. Foot Ankle Int. 2013;34:1411–20.
8. Bestic JM, Peterson JJ, DeOrio JK, Bancroft LW, Berquist TH, Kransdorf MJ. Postoperative evaluation of the total ankle arthroplasty. AJR Am J Roentgenol. 2008;190(4):1112–23.
9. Muir D, Aoina J, Hong T, Mason R. The outcome of the Mobility total ankle replacement at a mean of four years: can poor outcomes be predicted from pre- and post-operative analysis? Bone Joint J. 2013;95-B(10):1366–71.
10. Wood PL, Karski MT, Watmough P. Total ankle replacement: the results of 100 mobility total ankle replacements. J Bone Joint Surg Br. 2010;92(7):958–62.
11. Kopp FJ, Patel MM, Deland JT, O'Malley MJ. Total ankle arthroplasty with the agility prosthesis: clinical and radiographic evaluation. Foot Ankle Int. 2006;27(2):97–103.
12. Hanna RS, Haddad SL, Lazarus ML. Evaluation of periprosthetic lucency after total ankle arthroplasty: helical CT versus conventional radiography. Foot Ankle Int. 2007;28(8):921–6.

Spinal Implants

6

Sashin Ahuja, Kiran Lingutla, and Abdul Gaffar Dudhniwala

Spinal surgery, like other disciplines of orthopaedics, has experienced an immense expansion in range of implants. The era of instrumentation in spinal surgery began in 1970s with the development of Harrington rods by Paul Harrington. It provided distraction rods as well as compression hooks. Currently, the common indications for spinal instrumentation are to stabilise unstable segments, correct spinal deformities, achieve bony union/fusion, promote soft tissue healing, reduce need for external immobilisation and allow early mobilisation.

Anterior Cervical Fusion Cages

Anterior cervical interbody fusion is the gold standard in the treatment of symptomatic degenerative and traumatic conditions of the cervical spine. Various materials are used to manufacture these cages. The most common materials used are polyetheretherketone (PEEK), titanium, carbon fibre, trabecular metal and more recently allograft-machined cages.

Cages can be used as stand-alone devices with or without integrated screw mechanism or in combination with a plate (Fig. 6.1). The level of the operation should be confirmed on both the AP and lateral views. On AP view, the position of the cage in the interbody space is checked along with adequacy of fixation methods.

On lateral view, sagittal position of the cages is checked. The full metal cage implant or the metal markers on the radiolucent PEEK cages are helpful to assess the position of the cage with respect to the anterior and posterior vertebral lines. Other features to note are restoration of intervertebral height, restoration of foraminal height, adequacy of cervical lordosis, facet joint integrity and congruity and any soft tissue swelling.

On long-term follow-up, osseous integration may be evident with a bony bridge across fusion segments. Any subsidence of the implant is noted, along with any lucency around cages or the screws and implant failures, e.g. screw fracture. The subsidence of the cage can lead to segmental kyphosis. The adjacent disc spaces are checked and compared to previous X-rays for degenerative changes or progression with loss of disc height and osteophyte formation.

Anterior Cervical Plates

Various types of plates are available for use in the cervical spine. They can be static/rigid plates, dynamic plates and buttress plates. Static plates are used in trauma management scenarios

S. Ahuja (✉) · K. Lingutla · A. G. Dudhniwala
University Hospital of Wales, Cardiff, UK

S. Agarwal, G. J. Bansal (eds.), *Radiology of Orthopedic Implants*,
https://doi.org/10.1007/978-3-319-76009-4_6

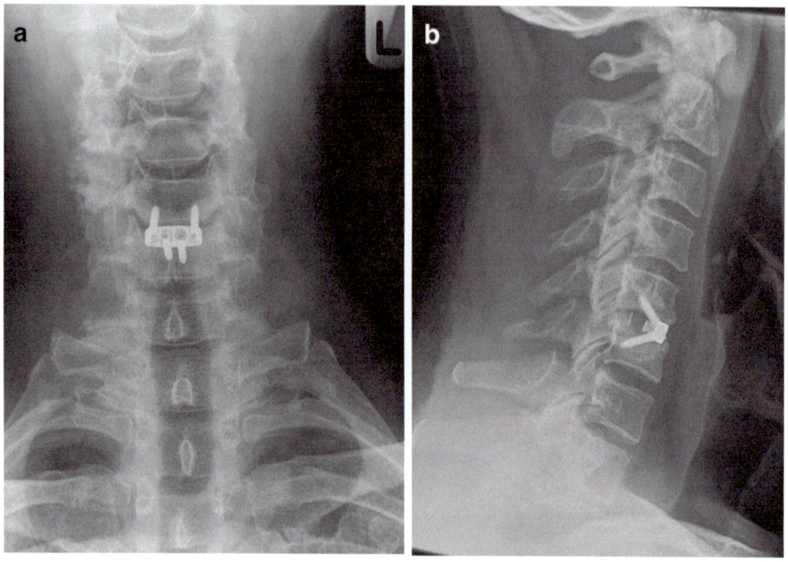

Fig. 6.1 Anterior cervical fusion cage (stand alone). AP (**a**) and lateral (**b**) view

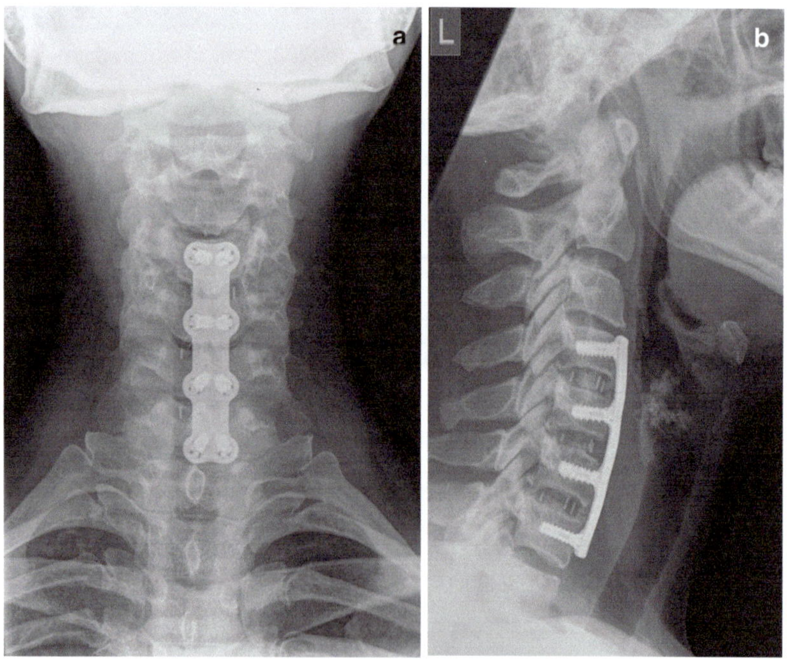

Fig. 6.2 (**a**, **b**) Multilevel anterior cervical fusion with radiolucent PEEK cages and a plate. AP (**a**) and lateral (**b**) view

whereas dynamic plates are used in degenerative fusion procedures.

On both AP and lateral views, the level of the operation is confirmed (Fig. 6.2). On the AP view, adequate positioning of the plate and screws to the vertebral body/bodies is checked. On lateral view, the positioning of the plate on either side of the disc space is checked. The screws should not extend beyond the posterior vertebral body (bicortical screws extend up to the posterior vertebral body). The screws should be in the vertebral body and not breaching the endplate into the disc space. Proximity of the superior or inferior ends of the plate to the adjacent endplates has been shown to accelerate adjacent segment degeneration and osteophytes formation. The plate should be sitting snug to the vertebral bodies and shouldn't be prominent. If the plate sits off the vertebral bodies (which can occur if the anterior osteophytes haven't been excised adequately) it can potentially cause problems with swallowing. Pre vertebral soft tissue and maintenance of cervical lordosis is noted.

Supra-adjacent disc space degenerative changes, evidence of fusion at the operated levels, i.e. bony bridging, and any lucency around metal work suggesting pseudarthrosis are checked on long-term follow-up.

Cervical Disc Replacement

Replacement of the cervical disc is used as motion preservation technique at the affected spinal segment. It is hypothesised that motion preservation reduces the incidence of adjacent segment degeneration. Numerous devices with various bearing surfaces and endplate fixation methods are used (Fig. 6.3). Most of the disc replacements are metallic although some of these can be made of PEEK. If the cervical disc replacement is made of PEEK the metal markers on the device are utilised to assess positioning on the AP and lateral X-rays of the cervical spine.

On both AP and lateral views, the level of the operation is confirmed.

On AP view, the midline positioning of implant is assessed. A keel, if present, helps in this assessment. This view also helps ascertain central location of the entire device in the disc space. The spinous process could also be used as a guide to assess this, but is not always reliable due to rotation. The contact area of the disc replacement implant with vertebral body is assessed by disc congruity with the vertebral endplate.

On lateral view, anterior and posterior margin of the disc replacement are checked to assess adequate placement of the implant. The disc replacement should be congruent with the vertebral endplates. Position of the disc replacement device can be judged, i.e. neutral, flexed or extended. Restoration of intervertebral height, adequacy of endplate fixation, congruency of the facet joints and any soft tissue swelling are noted.

On long-term follow-up, the implant position and alignment is checked. Subsidence of the implant into the vertebral body leading to segmental kyphosis as discussed above. Lucency around the device may be evident suggesting loosening of the implant. Bridging osteophytes or heterotropic ossification may be present across the replaced level. Segment integrity is checked and flexion-extension radiographs are helpful to demonstrate preservation of motion at the replaced level.

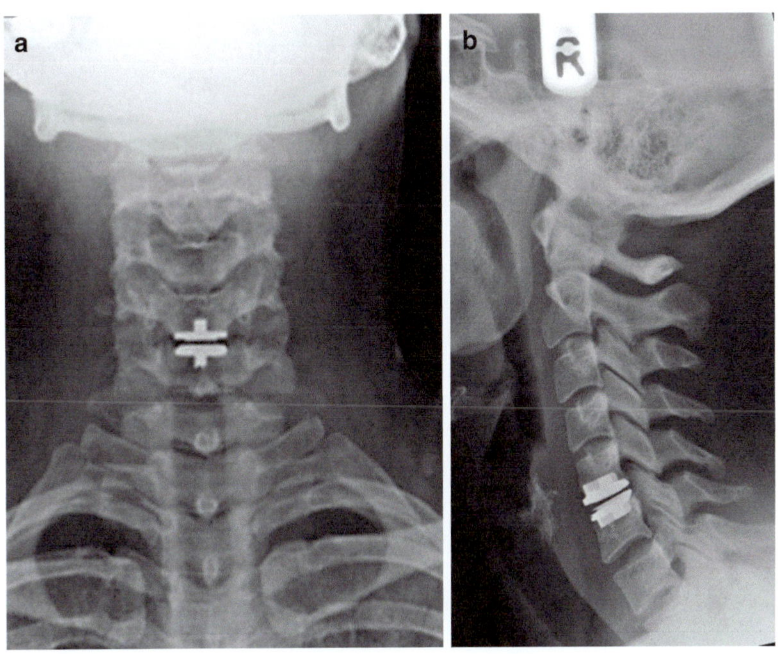

Fig. 6.3 AP (**a**) and lateral (**b**) view—cervical disc replacement

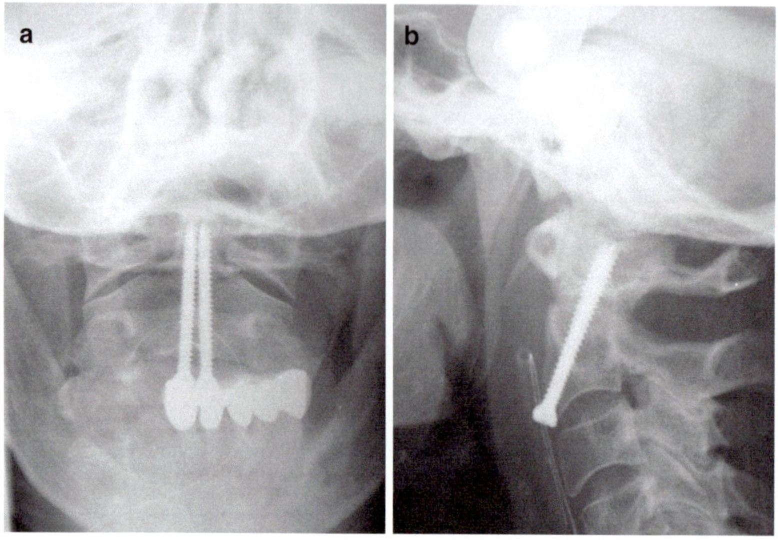

Fig. 6.4 Odontoid process screws. Open mouth (**a**) view and lateral view (**b**). The screws should be within the outline of the odontoid process

Odontoid Process (C2) Screws

One or two screws are used for the fixation of C2 odontoid process fractures, and these are directed retrograde from the antero-inferior part of the body of C2 to the tip of the odontoid (Fig. 6.4).

Two views are obtained to assess the metalwork. In the 'open mouth view', the level of operation is confirmed. If one screw is used, the position should be central, and if two screws have been used, the screws should be parallel and contained in the odontoid peg. The length of screw should be adequate.

In the lateral view, appropriate direction and length of the screws is checked and well as satisfactory reduction and compression at the fracture site. If a cancellous screw is utilised then the threaded portion of the screw should be past the fracture line and in the tip of the odontoid peg.

Posterior Cervical Spine Fixation

Posterior cervical spine fixation can be achieved with screws placed in the occiput, C1 articular (lateral) mass, C2 (pedicle/pars/translaminar) and lateral mass screws for subaxial spine (C3–C7), which are more commonly used compared to pedicular screws (Fig. 6.5). These screws are used in conjunction with appropriate rods, wires or plate.

For the subaxial spine (C3–C7) lateral mass screws, on AP view, the level of operation is confirmed. The lateral mass screws project upwards and outwards as compared to the pedicle screws, which are medially directed. There should be adequate length of the rod, i.e. above and below the caps. The rods are sometimes connected with cross connectors, which increase the stability of the construct.

On lateral view, the level of operation is confirmed. Lateral mass screws are directed cranially and parallel to the cervical facet joints, whereas pedicle screws are directed into the vertebral body. The screws should not encroach into the cranial facet joint. The rod length and contour are assessed along with the alignment of the spine, i.e. cervical lordosis.

Posterior fixation for C1 and C2 can be achieved with wires or screws. The posterior wires for stabilisation can be done by Gallie or Brooks technique. Gallie technique involves an iliac crest bone graft held between C1 and C2 with a wire from under the arch of C1 to the spinous process of C2. The Brooks technique uses two bone grafts between the arch of C1 and the lamina of C2 held with two separate sublaminar wires. Various modifications of these two techniques have also been described.

Transarticular C1–C2 screw stabilisation was described by Magerl (Fig. 6.6). Posterior screws are directed cranially and medially from the inferior articular edge of C2 traversing the C1–C2

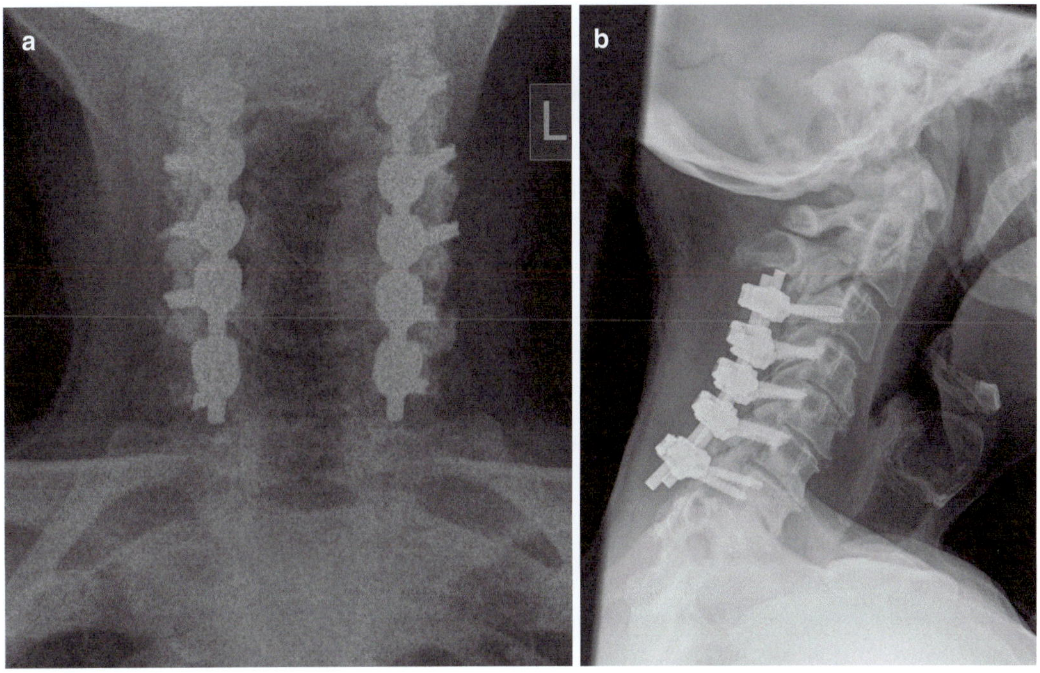

Fig. 6.5 Cervical lateral mass screw fixation. AP (**a**) and lateral (**b**) view

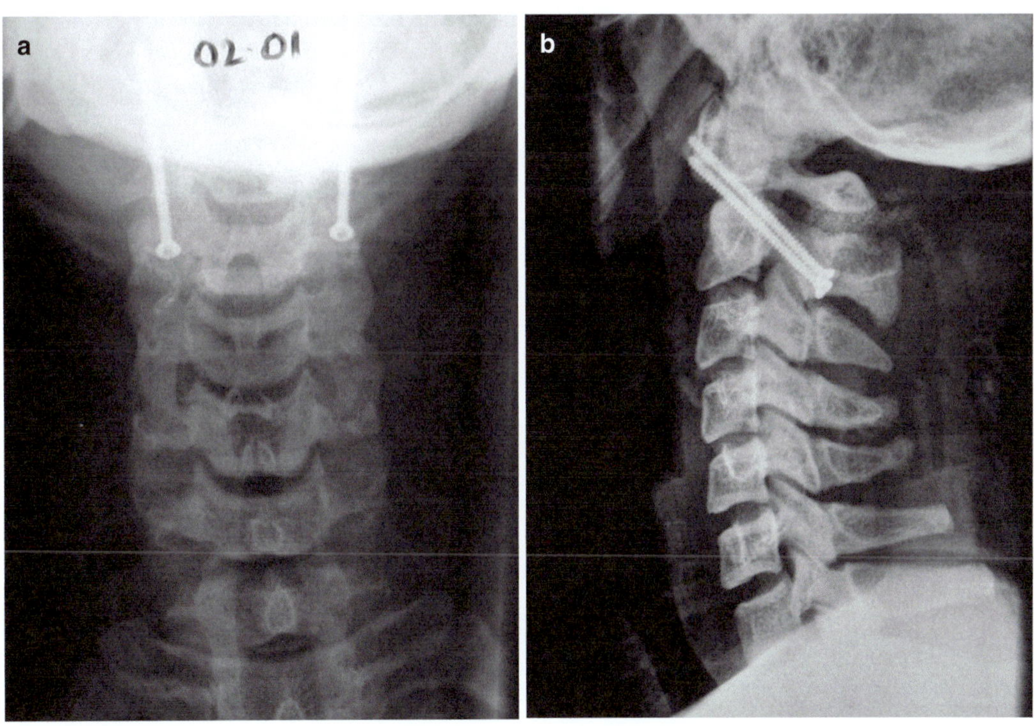

Fig. 6.6 Transarticular C1–C2 screw stabilisation. The screws traverse the facet joint between C1 and C2. AP (**a**) and lateral (**b**) views

facet joint to the lateral mass of C1. These are augmented with posterior bone graft.

On the AP view, the level of operation is confirmed. The screws project upwards and outwards from the base of C2 to the C1 lateral mass crossing the C1–C2 articulation and should be of adequate length. The placement of the bone graft posteriorly between C1 and C2 is checked.

On the lateral view, the level of operation is confirmed. The screws should be directed cranially from inferior articular edge of C2 up to the anterior arch of C1 but should not breach it. The length of screws should be adequate.

C1 Lateral Mass and C2 Pedicular/Pars Screw Fixation

C1 lateral mass screws are directed medially and cephalad starting from a point above the C1–C2 articulation at the junction of lateral mass with the arch of C1 and the centre of lateral mass in medial-lateral plane. The C1 screw is usually a shaft screw which is a cancellous screw with a long smooth shaft and threads at the distal end. This it to avoid irritation of the greater occipital i.e. C2 nerve as it come out between C1 and C2 i.e. in contact with the smooth part of the screw. These are connected to C2 (pedicle/pars) screw with rods (Fig. 6.7).

The level of operation is confirmed on both views. On the AP view, the C1 lateral mass, C2 pedicle/pars screws project upwards and inwards. The C2 pedicle screw enters the lateral part of C2 body; hence, their anterior ends are more medially placed as compared to the C2 pars screws. C2 laminar screws are almost transversely placed with the right laminar screw starting from the left side and vice versa. Adequate rod length, i.e. above and below the caps, is checked.

On the lateral view, the screws are directed cephalad from their starting point and should be contained within the vertebra. The screws should not encroach into the cranial facet joint and the C2 nerve foramen. The rod length and contour is assessed along with the alignment of the atlanto-axial joint.

Occipito-Cervical Fixation

Occipito-cervical fusion is used in the management of cranio-cervical junction instability. Fixation is achieved commonly by a combination of occipital plates, screws, rods and lateral mass screws for cervical spine (Fig. 6.8).

Radiological assessment for the cervical part of fixation is the same as for the lateral mass screws of subaxial spine. For the occipital part of fixation, AP view shows central placement of the plate and helps assess alignment of cranio-cervical junction. The lateral view confirms the level of operation and assesses alignment of cranio-cervical junction. The length of occipital screws should be adequate and not breach the inner table of the cranium. Occipital plate should be seated in close contact with the occiput.

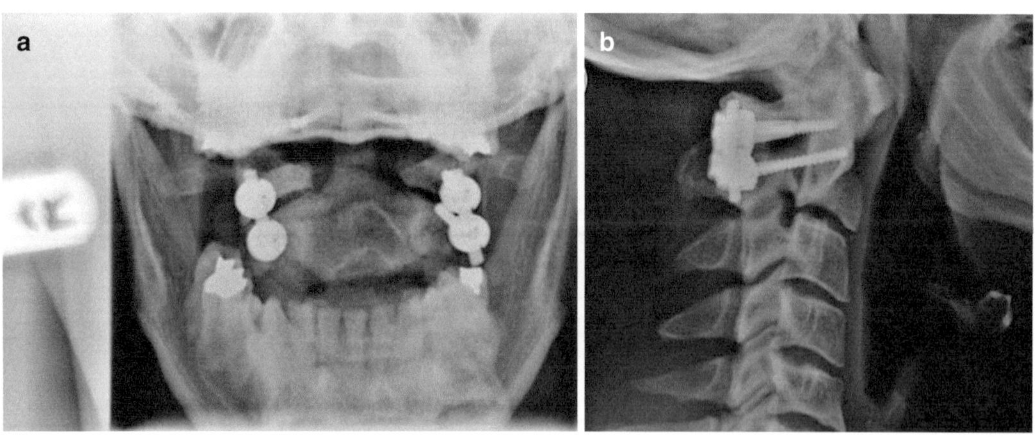

Fig. 6.7 C1–C2 posterior stabilisation with C1 lateral mass and C2 pedicle screws. Open mouth AP (**a**) and lateral view (**b**)

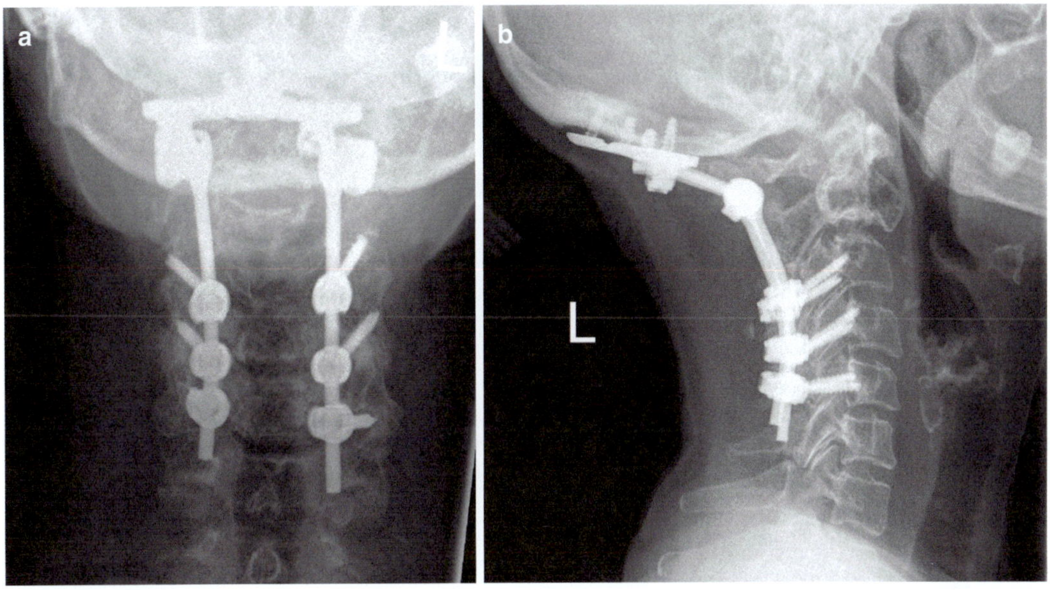

Fig. 6.8 Occipito-cervical fixation AP (**a**) and lateral (**b**) view

Cervical Corpectomy Cages

The radiological assessment for cervical corpectomy cages (Fig. 6.9) is similar to intervertebral cages. In addition, the AP view helps to see midline placement of the cage and the positioning of the cage within the confines of the cephalad and caudal vertebral bodies. The lateral view shows positioning of the cage within the confines of cephalad and caudal vertebral bodies, restoration of the segmental height and lordosis, prevertebral soft tissue alignment and implant bone interface to ensure no subsidence into vertebral body. On long-term follow-up, the maintenance of alignment is checked along with evidence of fusion. These cages could be metallic i.e. made of titanium or PEEK cages which are radiolucent but they have metal markers to assess the proximal and the distal ends and anterior and posterior ends of the endplate of the corpectomy cage.

Anterior Spinal Instrumentation

Anterior spinal instrumentation can be either extracolumnar or intracolumnar. Extracolumnar implies vertebral body screws connected to a plate or rod. Intracolumnar instrumentation (Fig. 6.10) resides within the contour of the vertebral body. Implant options are bone, metal or synthetic materials. Metal options are titanium mesh cages, expandable mesh cages and stackable modular cages.

The level of the operation is confirmed on both views. On the AP view, screws should be cited in the vertebral body in the safe zone. These screws can also be bicortical. The plate is placed on the lateral aspect to increase stability of the construct. The interbody corpectomy cage should be in the midline and well anchored to the endplates.

On the lateral view, the interbody cages should be positioned anterior to spinal canal. The screw should be positioned within the confines of vertebral body. Normal spinal curvature should be restored.

Pedicle Screw Stabilisation for the Thoracolumbar Spine

Pedicle screw stabilisation of the thoracolumbar spine is commonly utilised during decompression and fusion procedures for degenerative conditions, to stabilise the unstable segments following trauma (Fig. 6.11), pathological fractures and metastatic cord compression (Fig. 6.12). Pedicle screw systems are also employed in the procedures for the correction of a spinal deformity—scoliosis or kyphosis (Fig. 6.13).

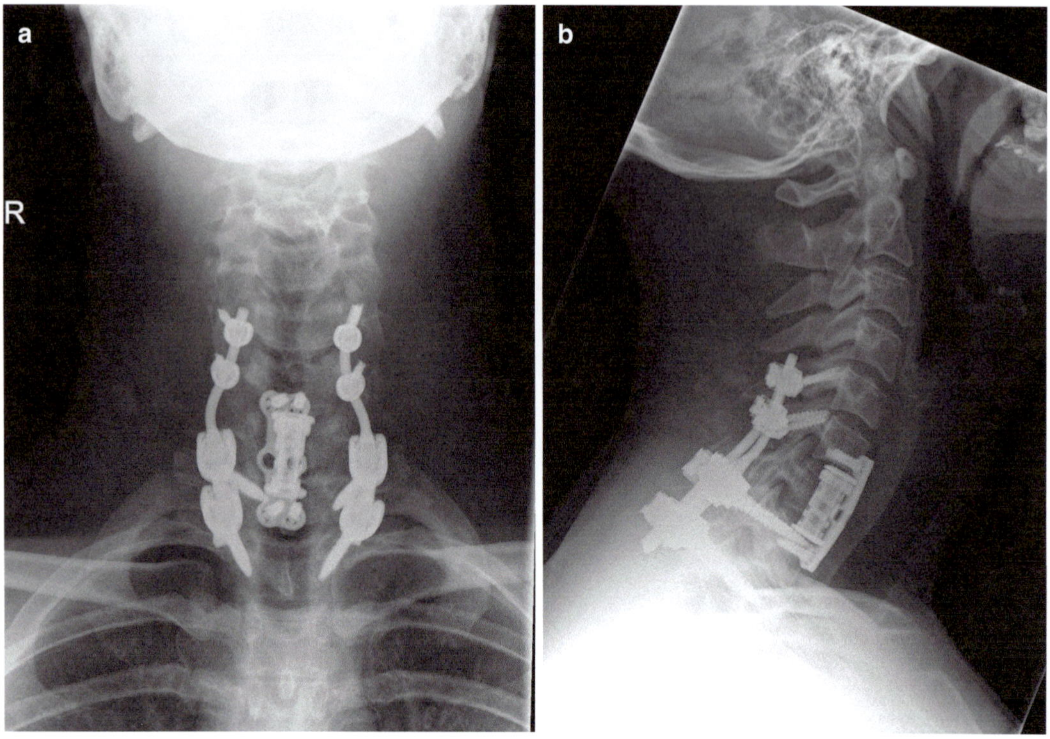

Fig. 6.9 Anterior cervical corpectomy cage and plate with posterior stabilisation. AP (**a**) and lateral (**b**) view

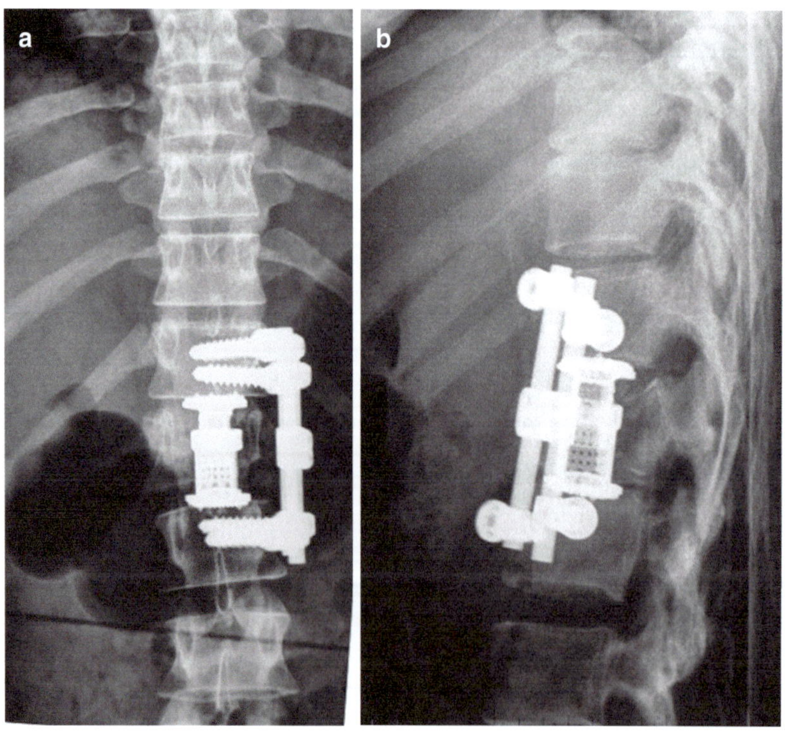

Fig. 6.10 Anterior vertebrectomy cage and stabilisation. AP (**a**) and lateral (**b**) view

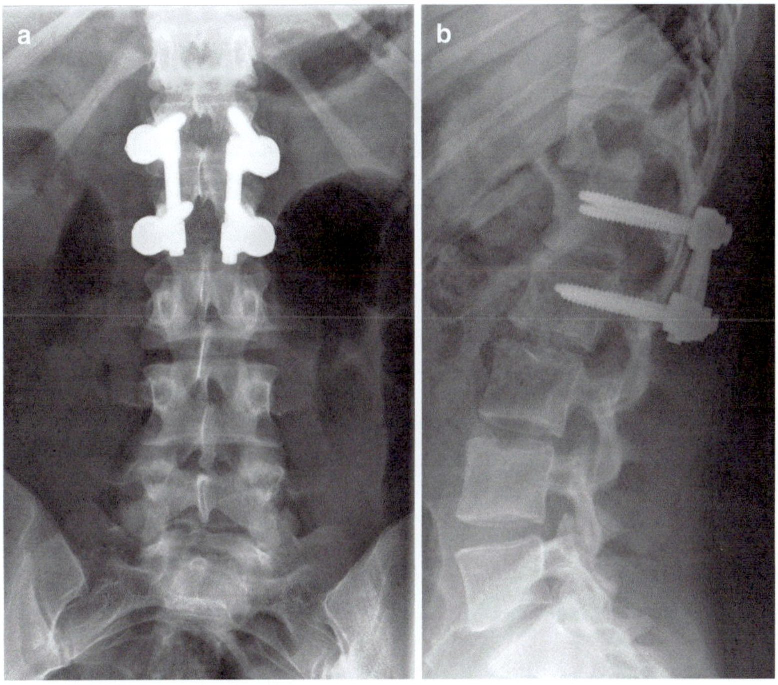

Fig. 6.11 Chance fracture fixation with pedicle screws. AP (**a**) and lateral (**b**) view

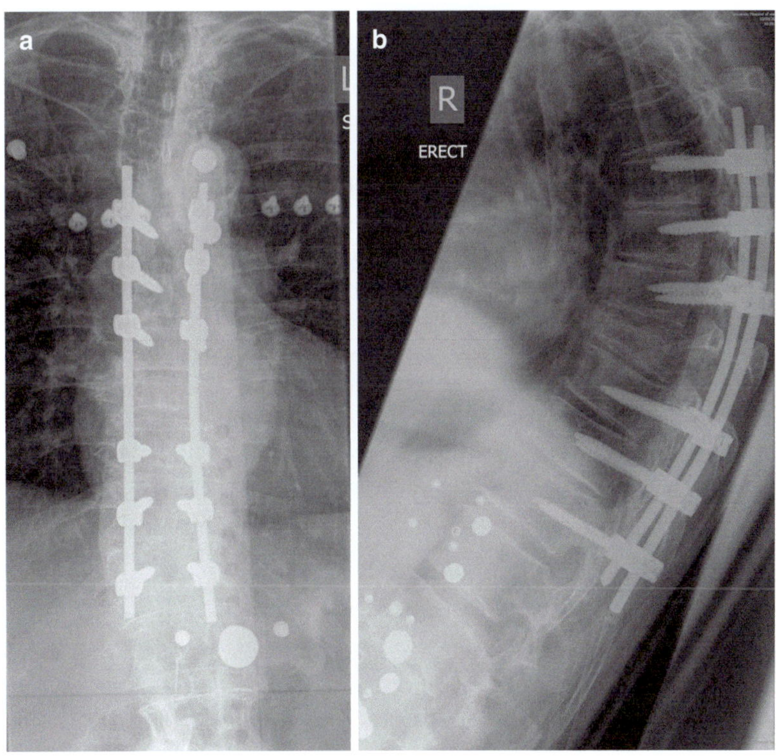

Fig. 6.12 Pedicle screw fixation post decompression for metastatic cord compression. AP (**a**) and lateral (**b**) view

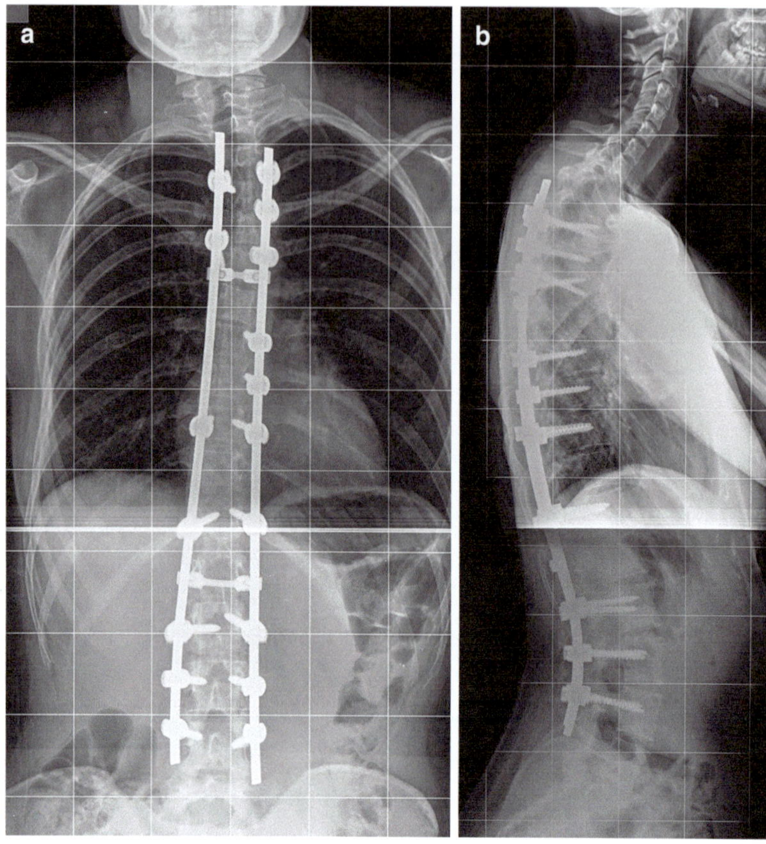

Fig. 6.13 Pedicle screw fixation post posterior only correction of scoliosis deformity. AP (**a**) and lateral (**b**) view

On both views, the level of the operation is confirmed. On AP view, the trajectory of the pedicle screw in the coronal plane is checked. The screws should not be medial to the medial wall of the pedicle or lateral to the lateral wall of the pedicle, i.e. missing the pedicle medially or laterally. The pedicle screws are usually directed medially but do not cross the midline of the vertebral column. The coronal alignment of the spine is assessed. The rods should be of adequate length and not impinge on the facet joint above or below.

On the lateral view, the pedicle screw should be in the position of the tract i.e. in the centre of the pedicle. The pedicle provides 80% fixation strength of the screw and the screws are expected to have adequate length. The screw should not breach the anterior wall of the vertebral body or reach the superior vertebral endplate. Restoration of the normal curvature of the spine is checked—thoracic kyphosis and lumbar lordosis. The primary purpose of the procedure, i.e. reduction of fracture and correction of deformity, is checked on both views.

Crosslink's are utilised to connect the two rods in a long construct to increase the torsional stability of the construct. Hybrid constructs formed by using hooks (sublaminar, transverse process hooks, hooks around ribs) wires or cables supplemented to pedicle screw fixation are employed to improve the stability of the construct.

Stabilisation for Lumbar Disc Degeneration

Spinal fusion is commonly performed in the management of lumbar disc degeneration. This is achieved by methods employing either anterior (interbody cage) fusion or posterior (pedicle screw fixation) fusion techniques. Often, to improve fusion rates, both these techniques are used in combination to provide global (360°) stabilisation.

Lumbar interbody cages, as the name implies, are placed in the disc space between the vertebral bodies. This can be achieved by different approaches and is named depending on the approach used, i.e. ALIF, anterior lumbar interbody fusion (Fig. 6.14); PLIF, posterior lumbar interbody fusion (Fig. 6.15); TLIF, transforaminal lumbar interbody fusion; or LLIF, lateral lumbar interbody fusion (Fig. 6.16).

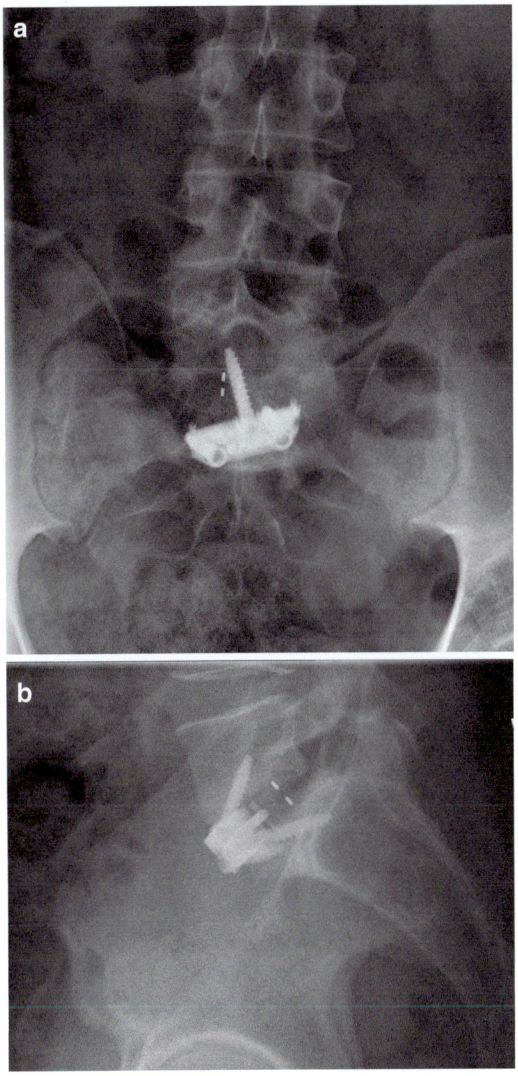

Fig. 6.14 ALIF—anterior lumbar interbody fusion. AP (**a**) and lateral (**b**) view

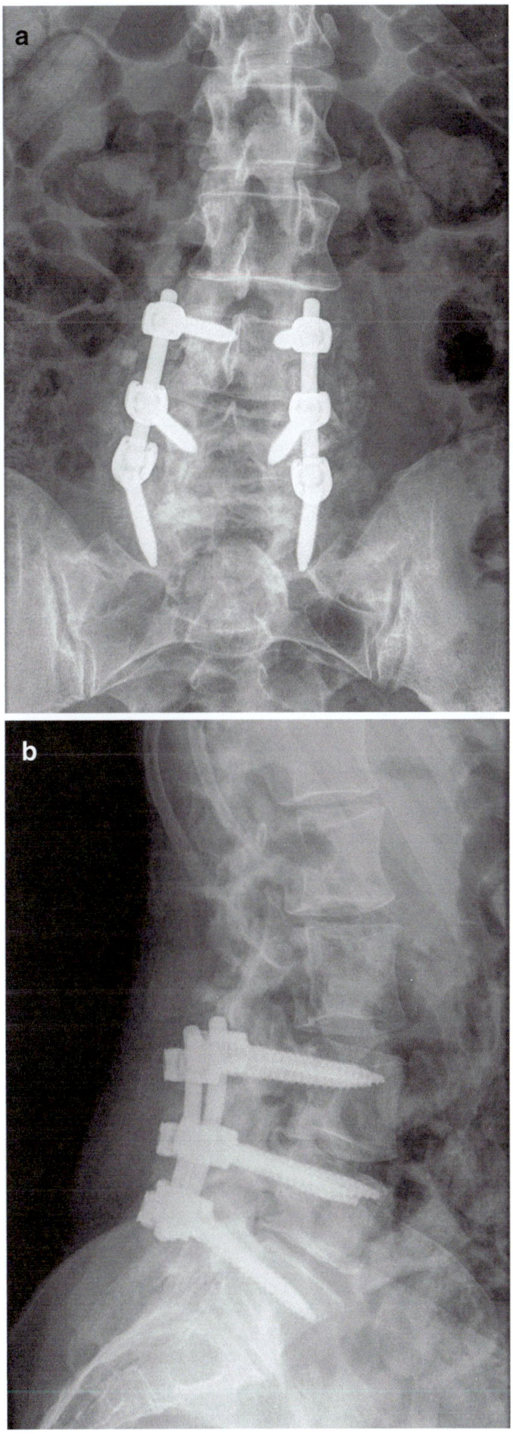

Fig. 6.15 Posterolateral lumbar fusion with pedicle screw fixation. AP (**a**) and lateral (**b**) view

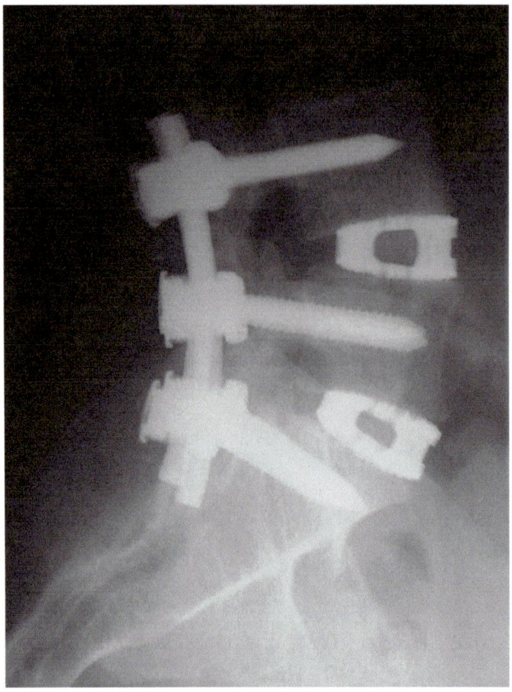

Fig. 6.16 Lumbar interbody cage with pedicle screw fixation—lateral view

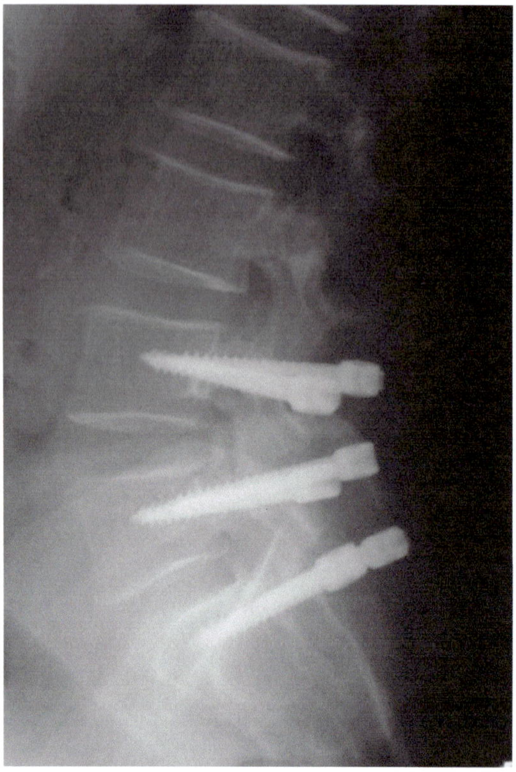

Fig. 6.17 Dynamic stabilisation of lumbar spine with pedicle screws and flexible rods—lateral view

In both views, the level of the operation is confirmed. On the AP view, checking the metal markers in a PEEK cage or the full cage profile in the case of titanium implants helps assess the position of the cage in the interbody space. Further features to note are adequacy of the fixation method, restoration of the disc height and bone graft/fusion mass especially in the posterolateral gutter in posterolateral fusion.

On the lateral view, the metal markers of the cage, or the cage itself with respect to the anterior and posterior vertebral lines, assess sagittal positioning of the cage. Restoration of the disc height, restoration of the foraminal height, adequacy of the segmental alignment, i.e. lordosis, and any surrounding soft tissue swelling are noted.

Dynamic Stabilisation

There are various modalities for dynamic stabilisation, which are also known as soft stabilisation or motion preservation. These can be pedicle screw-based devices. The assessment of the pedicle screws on the X-rays is similar to the description above.

These could be connected either with polyurethane radiolucent spacers (which would not be visible on plain X-rays—Fig. 6.17) or with spring-type devices, which connect the pedicle screws instead of rigid rods.

Interspinous Device

These devices are implanted in between the spinous processes and are usually made of PEEK with metal markers (Fig. 6.18), which helps to localise them on X-ray.

The level of operation is confirmed on both views. On the AP view, the implant should be positioned on either side of the spinous process.

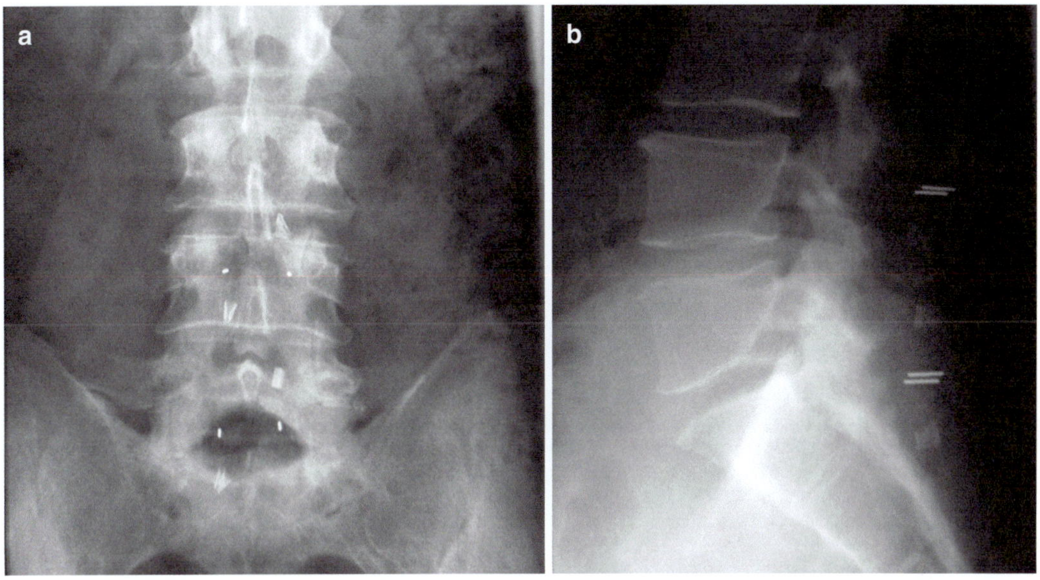

Fig. 6.18 Lumbar interspinous device. AP (**a**) and lateral (**b**) view

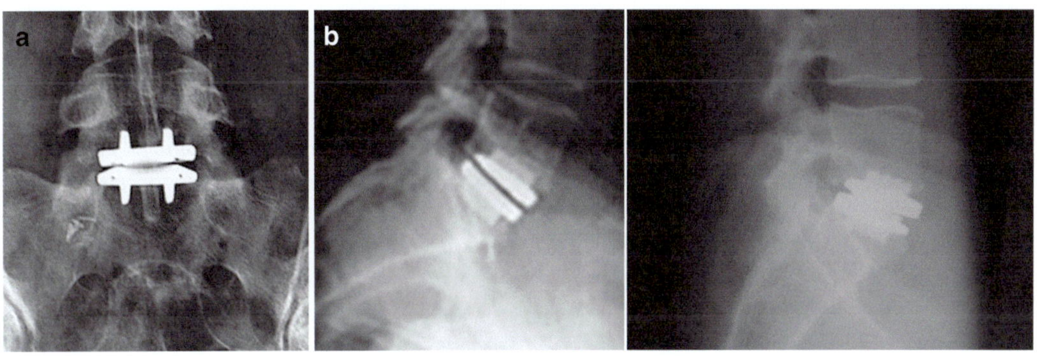

Fig. 6.19 Lumbar disc replacement. AP (**a**) and lateral (**b**) view

On the lateral view, the implant should be in between the spinous processes and not displaced posteriorly beyond the limits of the spinous process. The metal marker is helpful in determining the position of the implant.

Lumbar Disc Replacement

Imaging of lumbar disc replacement (Fig. 6.19) is similar to cervical spine disc replacement with regard to the AP and lateral view as described earlier.

Sacroiliac (SI) Joint Fusion

Fixations devices used for SI joint fusion (Fig. 6.20) may be hollow modular screws, cannulated compression screws, triangular wedges, etc. A minimum of two or three screws are used to stabilise the joint. The position of the implants is assessed on inlet and outlet views of the pelvis. The level and side of fusion is confirmed. In both views, the implant should be intraosseous, crossing the sacroiliac joint and not breaching the sacral foramen.

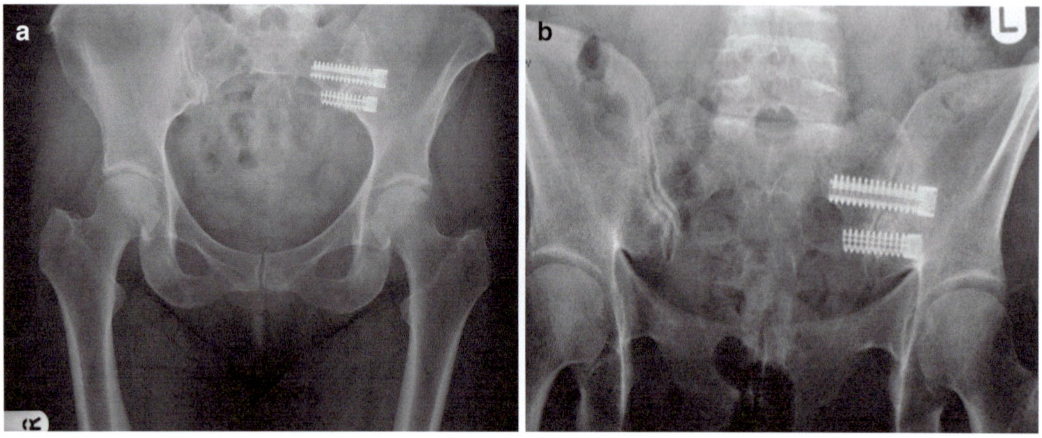

Fig. 6.20 Inlet view (**a**) and outlet view (**b**) of pelvis with sacroiliac joint fusion device in first and second sacral vertebra

Growth-Sparing Instrumentation for Paediatric Spine Deformities

Operative management of children with early-onset scoliosis, i.e. scoliosis identified below the age of 10, can be in the form of growth-sparing spinal instrumentation without fusion (Luque trolley, growing rod systems). These procedures involve multiple interventions consisting of correction of spinal deformity and holding the deformity in corrected position with instrumentation but without fusion, lengthening of instrumentation with growth to maintain correction until the need for definitive correction and fusion.

Other methods of operative management for early-onset scoliosis include selective fusion (hemiepiphysiodesis) and growth modulation with growth tethers or staples.

Luque trolley instrumentation (Fig. 6.21) consists of two U-shaped rods held by sublaminar wires. The distance between the ends of rods expands as the spine grows. Growing rod systems can be pedicle screw-based device (Fig. 6.22) with dual rods on each side connected with a tandem connector, e.g. paediatric isola. Tandem connectors holding the rods are operatively extended approximately every 6 months to facilitate growth.

The MAGEC® (Magnetic Expansion Control) system (Fig. 6.23) utilises a magnetic rod on either side, which are anchored proximally and distally with appropriate fixation device (pedicle screw, hooks with or without connectors). An external remote controller is used in an outpatient setting to allow growth of the spine by expanding the magnetic rods.

Chest wall deformity, e.g. congenital rib fusion, and scoliosis are co-dependent. Management of this form of scoliosis by VEPTR® (Vertical Expandable Prosthetic Titanium Rib) implant allows stabilisation of ribs post thoracoplasty, thereby promoting growth of the lung and spine.

VEPTR® device (Fig. 6.24) is attached to the proximal and distal fixation location (ribs, spine or pelvis). This device also needs lengthening at regular intervals like growing rods to accommodate growth.

X-ray assessment of early-onset scoliosis instrumentation is done to confirm the level and extent of operation, assess the fixation method and follow-up to confirm elongation of rods and potential for further extension. Definitive scoliosis correction X-rays are assessed similar to the earlier description in pedicle screw system for the thoracolumbar spine.

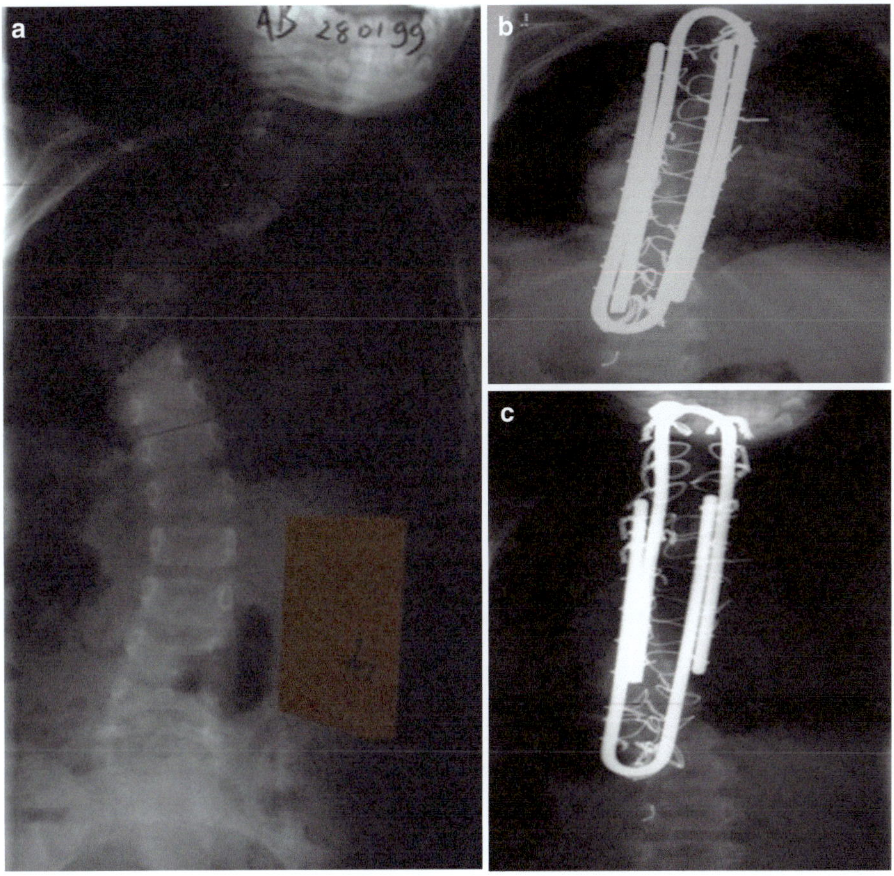

Fig. 6.21 Luque trolley method for correction of early-onset scoliosis. Pre-op (**a**), immediate post-op (**b**) and follow-up (**c**) radiographs

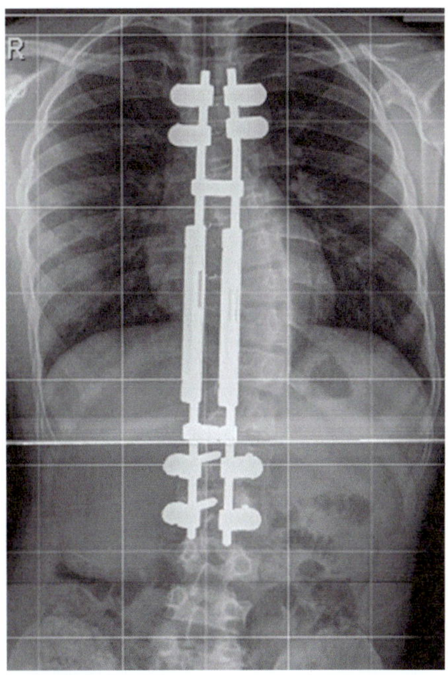

Fig. 6.22 Pedicle screw-based paediatric growing rod system. AP view of dorsolumbar spine

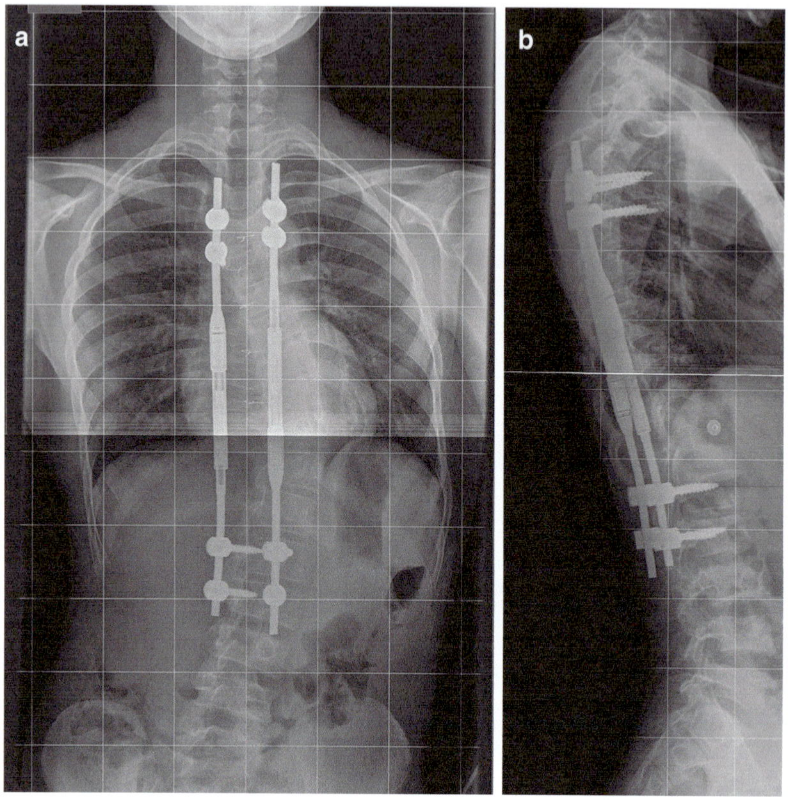

Fig. 6.23 MAGEC® (Magnetic Expansion Control) rods for early-onset scoliosis. AP (**a**) and lateral (**b**) view

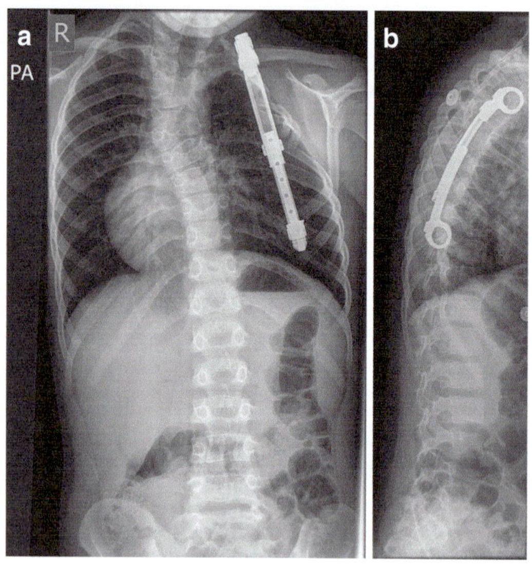

Fig. 6.24 VEPTR® (Vertical Expandable Prosthetic Titanium Rib) implant for thoracic deformities. AP (**a**) and lateral (**b**) view

7 Trauma

Juliet Clutton and James Lewis

Trauma is the leading cause of acute hospital admission in people under the age of 44 years (data from the Trauma Audit and Research Network, UK). Some traumatic fractures can be managed non-operatively with casts, splints, slings or braces. However, a significant proportion of patients require surgical implants to achieve a satisfactory outcome.

A huge variety of fixation methods exist, and the type of implant used depends on fracture location, type of fracture and patient factors such as age, mobility and bone quality.

Standard postoperative radiographs include AP and lateral views showing the entire implant, including the adjacent joint if relevant. The relevant features to note on trauma radiographs are as follows:

1. Fracture reduction
2. Position of implant relative to the bone
3. Number and type of screws used (locking or non-locking)
4. Position of screws in the bone
5. Length of screws relative to the bone
6. Evidence of implant loosening
7. Evidence of callus formation
8. Evidence of fracture migration, nonunion or malunion

J. Clutton · J. Lewis (✉)
University Hospital of Wales, Cardiff, UK

In many injuries, the method of treatment is determined by the classification of the fracture.

Fixation of the fracture can be achieved through internal fixation, external fixation or, rarely, a combination of the two. Various implants exist for achieving fixation.

Plates

There are many different types of plate available, each with specific functions and applications. Broadly, the plates can have either locking screws or non-locking screws and are consequently known as locking or non-locking plates. Many modern plates have options for either of these screws using elliptical 'combination holes', whereby one end of the hole accepts locking screws and the other part of the hole accepts non-locking screws.

The method in which the plates are used can vary with different situations. A standard dynamic compression plate (DCP) can be used in compression mode, neutralisation mode, bridging mode, antiglide mode or tension band mode.

Plates used in compression mode—known as compression plates—have specially shaped screw slots with an incline. Screws engage with this incline and shift the bone relative to the plate as they are tightened. These are designed to produce compression at the fracture site (Fig. 7.1). Plates used to fix simple transverse or simple

S. Agarwal, G. J. Bansal (eds.), *Radiology of Orthopedic Implants*,
https://doi.org/10.1007/978-3-319-76009-4_7

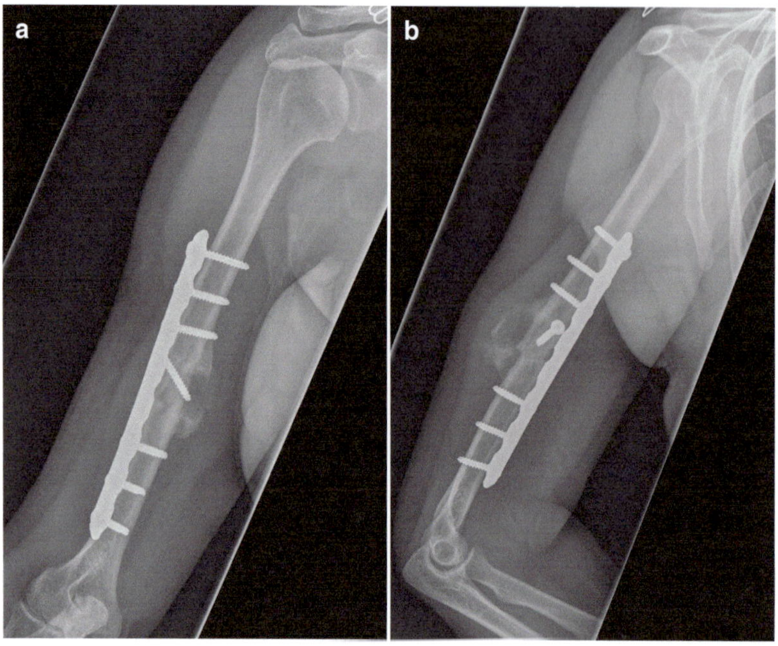

Fig. 7.1 Fixation of fracture of midshaft humerus treated with compression plating principle. AP (**a**) and lateral (**b**) views are demonstrated. The patient had a hypertrophic nonunion, as evidenced by extensive callus around the fracture site. The fracture has been stabilised with one compression screw, which is separate from the plate. The plate is a locking compression plate, and all screws are cortical screws. The plate has been used in neutralisation mode, as the lag screw provides the compressive force

short oblique fractures of the shaft of long bones are likely to be used in compression mode.

Plates used in neutralisation mode—also known as neutralisation plates—are used in conjunction with lag screws and resist bending and torsional forces. These reduce the force at the fracture site and are used to supplement the fixation provided by the lag screw. Long oblique or spiral diaphyseal fractures can be managed by compression (lag) screws and a neutralisation plate.

Plates in bridging mode are used in multifragmentary fractures. The plate is fixed to intact proximal and distal bone as an internal splint. The plate bypasses the fracture zone, leaving fracture fragments untouched and hence avoiding damage to the blood supply. No attempt is made to achieve compression. Buttress plates support and reinforce underlying bone without being fixed to the part of bone which needs support. Common sites for use of buttress plates are distal radius and proximal tibia.

Antiglide plates are secured at the apex of an oblique fracture to physically block shortening or displacement. A common site for their use is in lateral malleolus fractures.

Tension band plates convert tension forces to compressive forces when secured to the tensile surface of a bone.

Screws

A screw is an object that converts rotational force to longitudinal motion. Screws have been designed in a variety of types and diameters.

Cortical screws have threads that are designed to engage the cortex of the bone into which they are inserted. They are fully threaded and usually require the use of a tap to cut threads before they are inserted. Some cortical screws can be self-tapping. Self-tapping screws cut their own threads as they are inserted and do not require the use of a tap before insertion. Cancellous screws have a narrow core and a wide, deep thread. They are designed to achieve fixation in the relatively soft cancellous bone.

Locking screws have threads in the head, as well as in the shaft of the screw. The threads in the screw head are designed to lock into the plate. The holes of the plate are designed with corresponding threads, and the screw head locks into these holes. Hence, these screws engage with both the bone and the plate through which they are inserted (Fig. 7.2).

Fully threaded screws have threads from the tip to the head of the screw. These can be cortical or cancellous or locking screws. Partially threaded screws have threads at the tip of the screw, extending a set amount towards the screw head, with a smooth area of screw shaft between the head and the threads. Commonly, cancellous screws have the option of partial threads. These are helpful in gaining compression as the screw is tightened.

Cannulated screws are hollow, and are designed to be inserted over guide wires.

The term 'lag screw' refers to a technique whereby the screw is used to apply compression across a fracture site. For instance, a fully threaded cortical screw can be used as a lag screw (Fig. 7.3). The screw is inserted perpendicular to the plane of the fracture, and the near cortex (entry point of the screw into the bone) is 'over-drilled' to the outer width of the screw threads. As a result, the screw threads only engage in the far side of the bone and are free to slide in the proximal cortex. This applies compression across

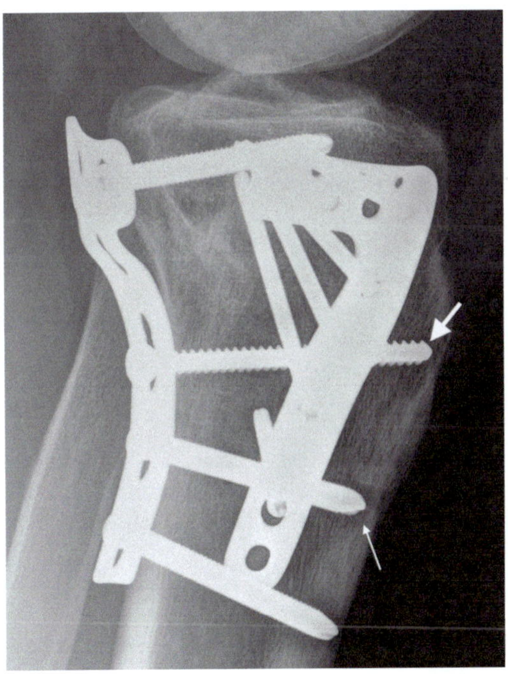

Fig. 7.2 Dual plating of proximal tibia. The posterior plate has a combination of cortical and locking screws. Note the tip of cortical screw is rounded (thick white arrow), and this screw requires the use of a tap before insertion. The tips of locking screws (thin white arrow) are designed to cut threads through the bone (self-tapping) as they are inserted

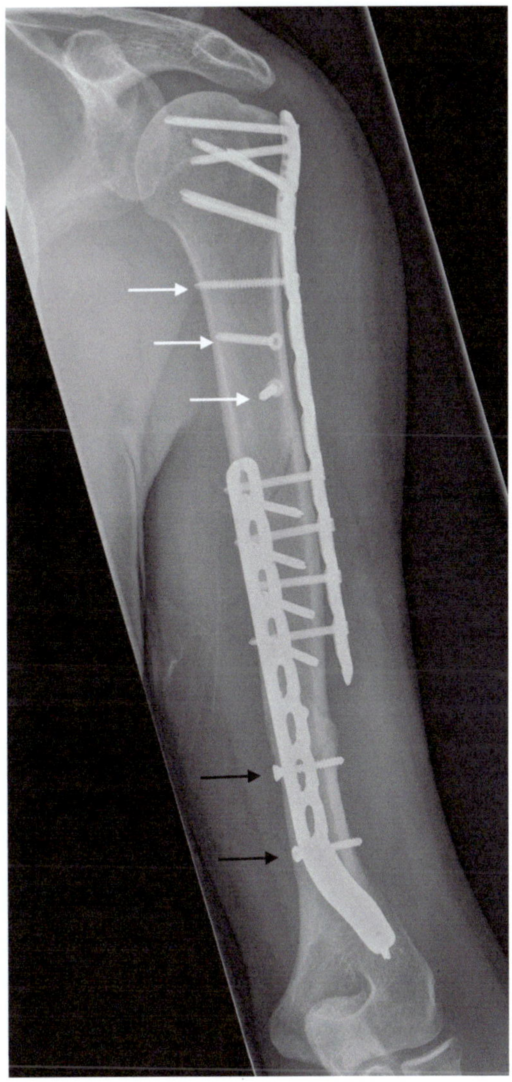

Fig. 7.3 Plating of the humerus using lag screws. This patient had a spiral distal humerus fracture that was treated with two lag screws (black arrows) and a distal humeral locking plate. He had a second injury 3 months after the initial injury, resulting in a spiral fracture above the plate, which was treated with a second plate, again with the use of three lag screws (white arrows) and a locking plate. Here, both the plates have been used in neutralisation mode

the fracture when the screw head engages with the cortex on the near side.

Intramedullary Nails

These devices have become the standard of treatment for many diaphyseal fractures, particularly in the lower limb. They are locked into place using screws to improve stability of the fracture. Static locking involves inserting screws into round holes in the nail, and these allow minimal movement. Dynamic locking involves inserting screws into oval-shaped elongated holes in the nail. This allows some movement at the fracture site and, in selected situations, can encourage callus formation.

Fracture Stability

Absolute stability means that there is no movement at the fracture site (or very little movement). This allows fractures to heal by direct bone healing, with no callus. Compression at the fracture site with a lag screw or dynamic compression plate helps achieve absolute stability.

Relative stability allows movement at the fracture site, whilst still stabilising the zone of injury. It allows fractures to heal by indirect healing, with the formation of callus. Intramedullary nail fixation is an example of relative stability.

Clavicle Fractures

Clavicle fractures are common injuries, often occurring in young individuals as a result of direct trauma or a fall onto an outstretched hand. Fractures are grouped into those involving the lateral, middle or medial third of the bone.

Plate fixation is the most common surgical treatment of clavicular fractures. The plate used can be either straight (see Fig. 7.4) or anatomically contoured (see Fig. 7.5), but in each case the idea of the plate is to bridge and stabilise the fracture. Either locking or cortical screws can be used, and the standard is to have fixation in six cortices (usually three screws) on either side of the fracture. The screws engage the cortex on the inferior surface of the bone to achieve bicortical fixation.

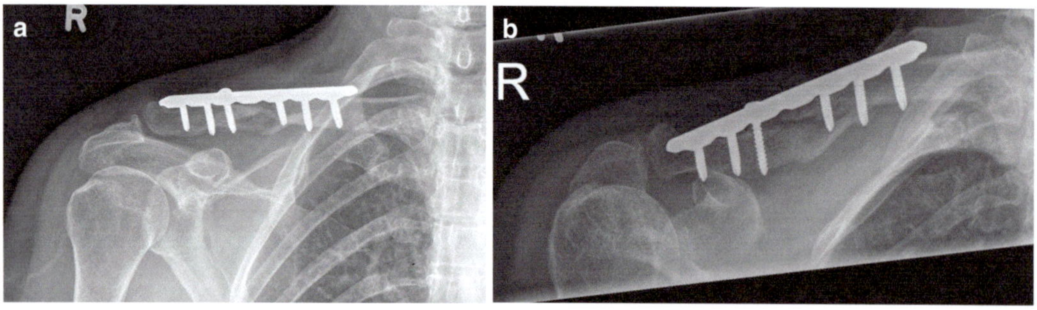

Fig. 7.4 Middle third clavicle fracture after internal fixation with a straight plate. The compression plate has six cortices fixation on either side of the fracture. AP (**a**) and oblique (**b**) view

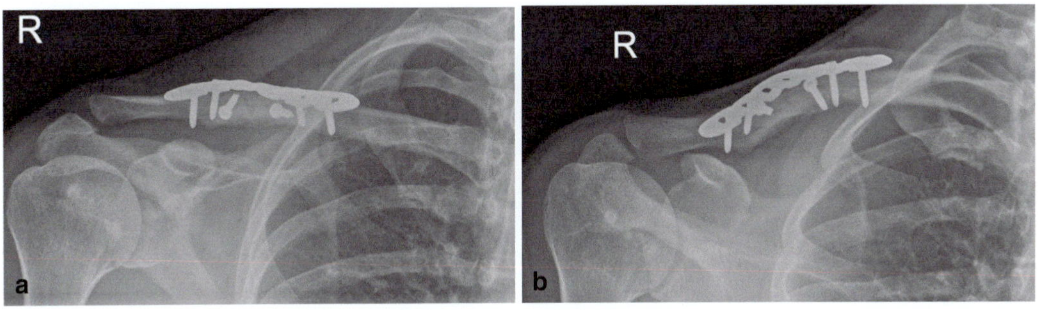

Fig. 7.5 Middle third clavicle fracture after internal fixation with an anatomically contoured plate with lag screws. In this fixation, only four of the six screws inserted go through the plate. The other two are lag screws, which have been inserted to apply pressure across the fracture sites. AP (**a**) and oblique (**b**) view

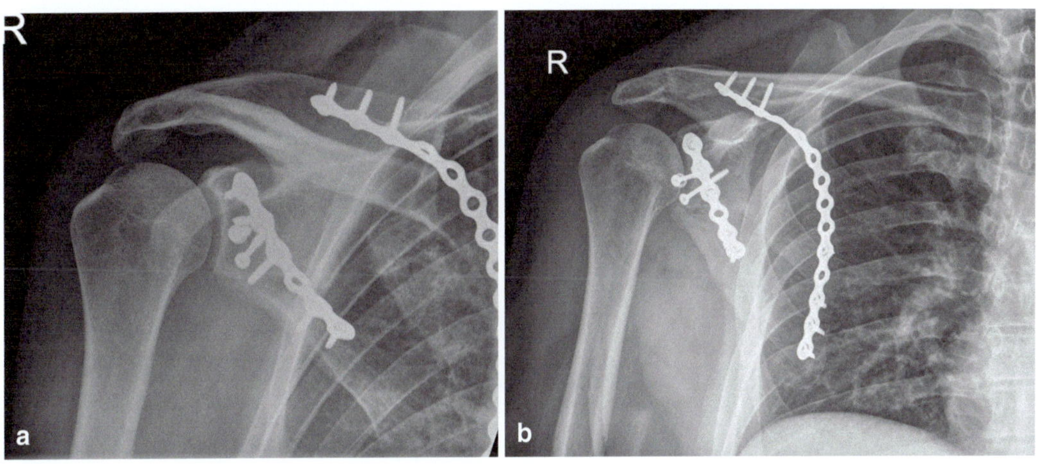

Fig. 7.6 Scapular fixation using anatomically contoured plates. There is a lateral and a medial plate, with the medial plate extending onto the inferior surface of the spine of scapula. AP (**a**) view of the shoulder and AP (**b**) view of the right hemithorax

Scapula Fractures

Most fractures of the body of the scapula are managed conservatively. The scapula is supported by its surrounding soft tissues, and therefore fractures are rarely displaced enough to warrant fixation. Anatomical plates can be used for scapular fixation (Fig. 7.6).

Proximal Humerus Fractures

Fractures of the proximal humerus are grouped according to Neer's classification, which is based on the relationship between the greater tuberosity, lesser tuberosity, articular surface and the shaft fragment. There are six fracture types, and each can be further split into two-, three- and four-part fractures.

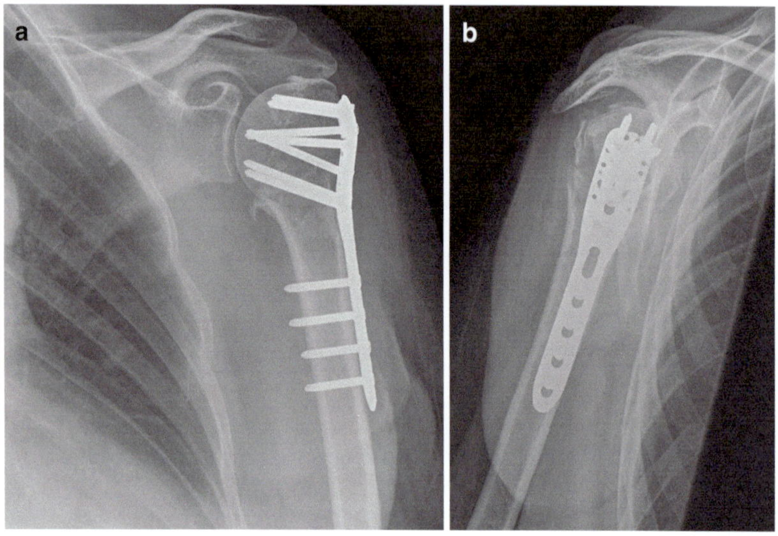

Fig. 7.7 In the locking proximal humerus plate, multiple screws are inserted at different angles into the humeral head. This multiple-angle construct increases stability and improves grip in osteoporotic bone and multipart fractures. AP (**a**) and scapular Y (**b**) view

Displaced fractures, head-splitting fractures, surgical neck fractures in young patients and fracture dislocations can be treated with open reduction and internal fixation using a locking plate (Fig. 7.7). In the example, the fracture has been anatomically reduced and fixed with the principle of absolute stability.

Mid-shaft Humerus

Mid-shaft humeral fractures should be treated operatively if they are open, have an associated vascular injury or are associated with fractures of the forearm (so-called floating elbow). These fractures can be managed with either plate fixation giving absolute stability (Fig. 7.8) or intramedullary nailing giving relative stability (Fig. 7.9). It is also recommended to fix pathological fractures or impending pathological fractures, usually with an intramedullary device.

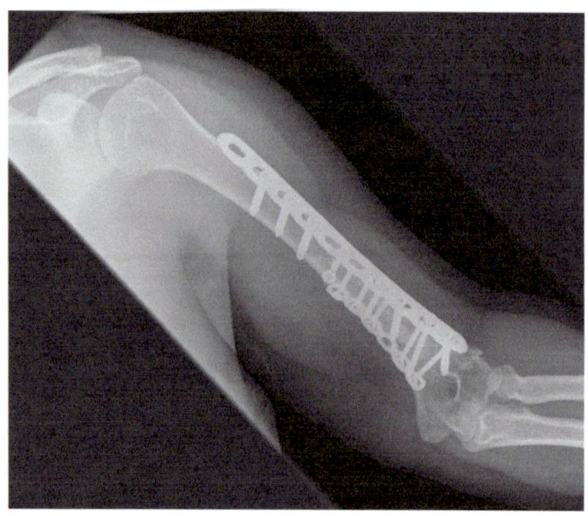

Fig. 7.8 Mid-shaft humerus fracture fixed using plates. Dual plating has been done to stabilise comminuted fragments

Distal Humerus Fractures

Capitellar fractures are rare and generally result from a coronal shear force. The posterior half of the capitellum is nonarticular and can be used for insertion of fixation devices. These should not extend beyond the anterior articular surface (Fig. 7.10).

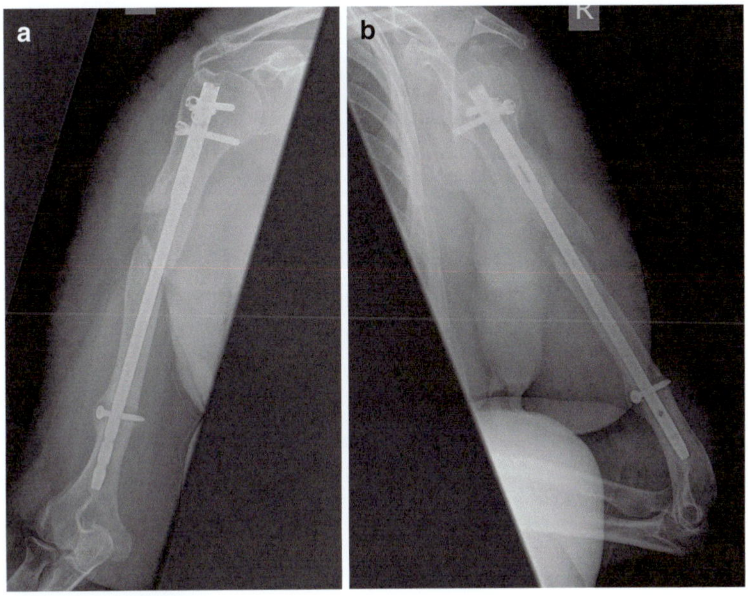

Fig. 7.9 IM nail for mid-shaft humerus fracture in AP (**a**) and lateral (**b**) view. Note that, despite having been fixed, the fracture is malaligned, and the distal fragment has some varus angulation. Note also the lucency around the distal locking screw, indicating relative movement between the implant and bone. The rounded appearance of the fracture site, and lack of bridging callus indicates nonunion

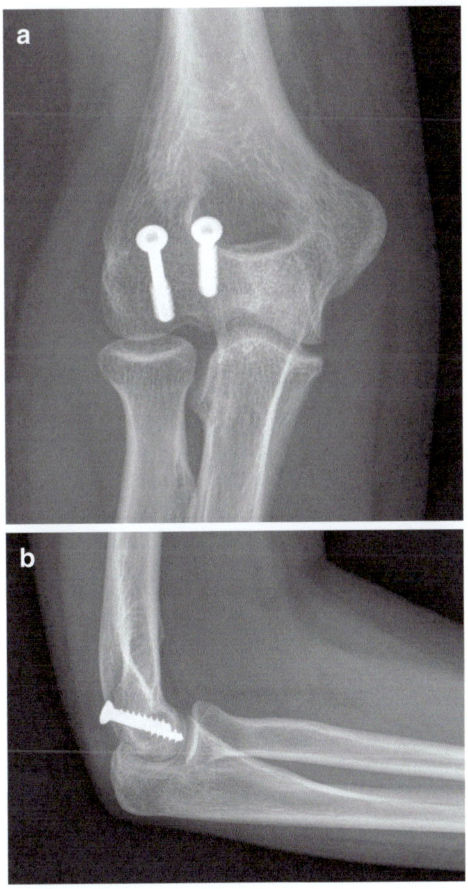

Fig. 7.10 Fixation of an isolated capitellar fracture AP (**a**) and lateral (**b**) view using two screws inserted from the nonarticular posterior aspect of the capitellum

Olecranon Fractures

Olecranon fractures almost always require fixation (except in elderly low-demand patients) because the fracture fragments are pulled apart by the action of the triceps. The two methods of fixation available use the tension band principle, which converts tensile forces crossing the joint into compressive forces and applies pressure to the fracture site.

The parallel wires are often engaged in the volar cortex of proximal ulna (Fig. 7.11). If the wires are prominent beyond the volar cortex of ulna, these can lead to injury to the anterior interosseous nerve. The wires should be less than 10 mm beyond the cortex [1].

In comminuted fractures, a locking plate is preferred to maintain length and restore stability (Fig. 7.12). The proximal screws should not penetrate into the humeroulnar joint.

Mid-shaft Fractures of Radius and Ulna

In adults, mid-shaft forearm fractures are almost always fixed to preserve length and rotational alignment (Fig. 7.13). The plate is positioned and contoured to the bone so as not to protrude and

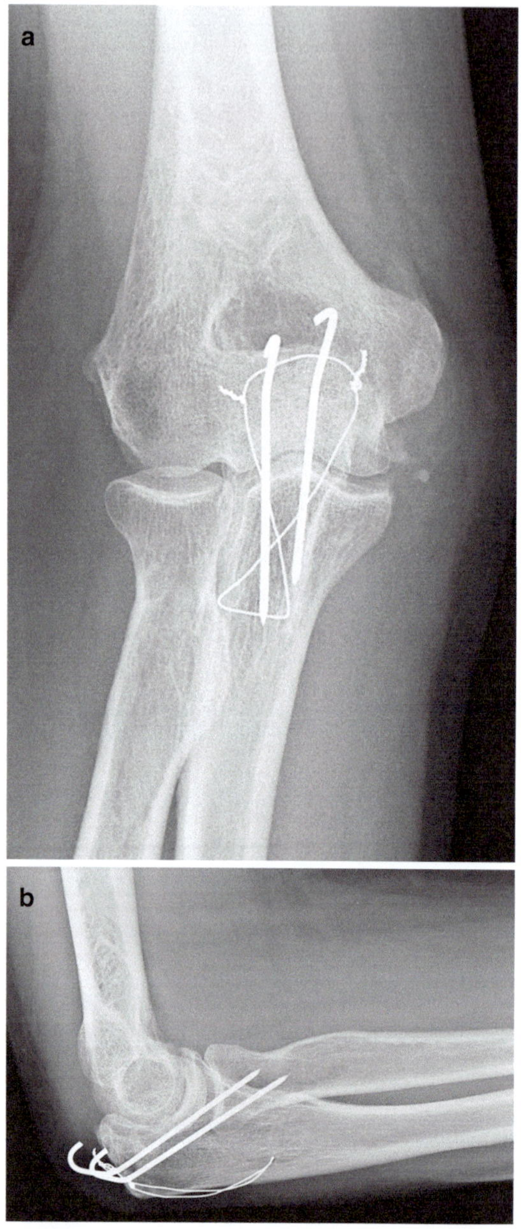

Fig. 7.11 Tension band wire fixation of the olecranon. The fracture has been fixed with a figure-of-eight tension band wire loop and two longitudinal K-wires. The twists in the wire loop (**a**) are used to tighten the loop in order to compress the fracture site intraoperatively. Note the prominent sharp ends of the two K-wires anterior to the anterior cortex of ulna in the lateral view (**b**). This can lead to anterior interosseous nerve problems if they protrude more than 10 mm from the cortex

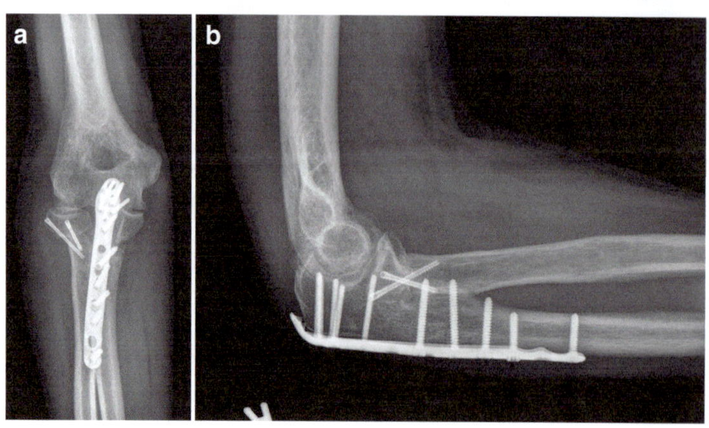

Fig. 7.12 Fixation of a proximal ulnar fracture and a radial head fracture using a locking plate AP (**a**) and lateral (**b**) view. A coexistent radial neck fracture has been stabilised using two headless screws

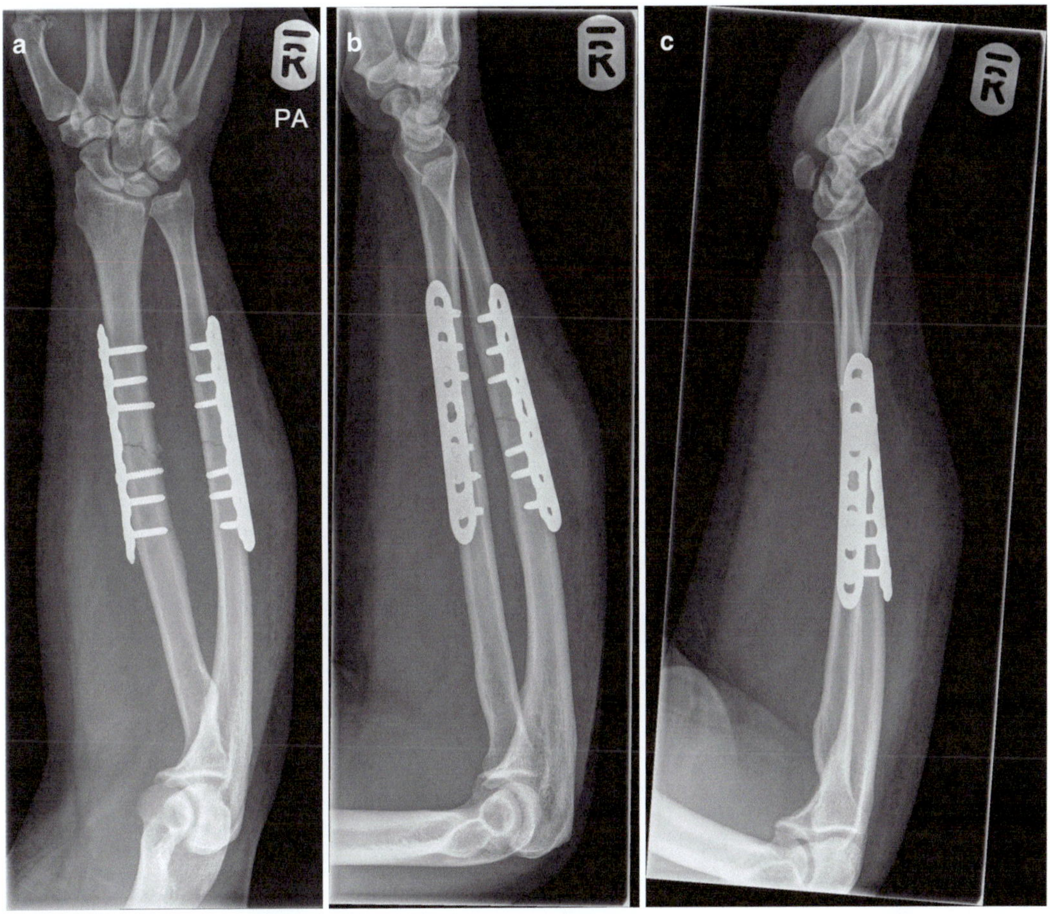

Fig. 7.13 Plate fixation of the radius and ulna in the AP (**a**), oblique (**b**) and lateral (**c**) view. In each plate, there are three screws on either side of the fracture site for optimum stability. Satisfactory length and rotational alignment have been achieved. It is important to note the proximal and distal radio ulnar joint on the radiographs and check for any subluxation/dislocations in forearm injuries

cause irritation. Screw length is also very important here, as screws that are too long can impinge on the ulna or soft tissues and cause problems with pronation and supination.

Distal Radius Fractures

Simple extra-articular distal radius fractures can be fixed with closed reduction and percutaneous pinning (Fig. 7.14). Two or three K-wires are inserted to hold and stabilise the fracture, along with a plaster cast for added support. However, K-wires may not provide enough stability to adequately stabilise comminuted intraarticular fractures, and these are therefore managed by plate fixation (Fig. 7.15).

There are many different plate constructs available. Some provide absolute stability (such as T-plates and variable angle locking plates) whilst some are inserted to support comminuted fractures and prevent 'drifting' of the distal fragment without the use of screws in the distal fragment—known as the buttress principle.

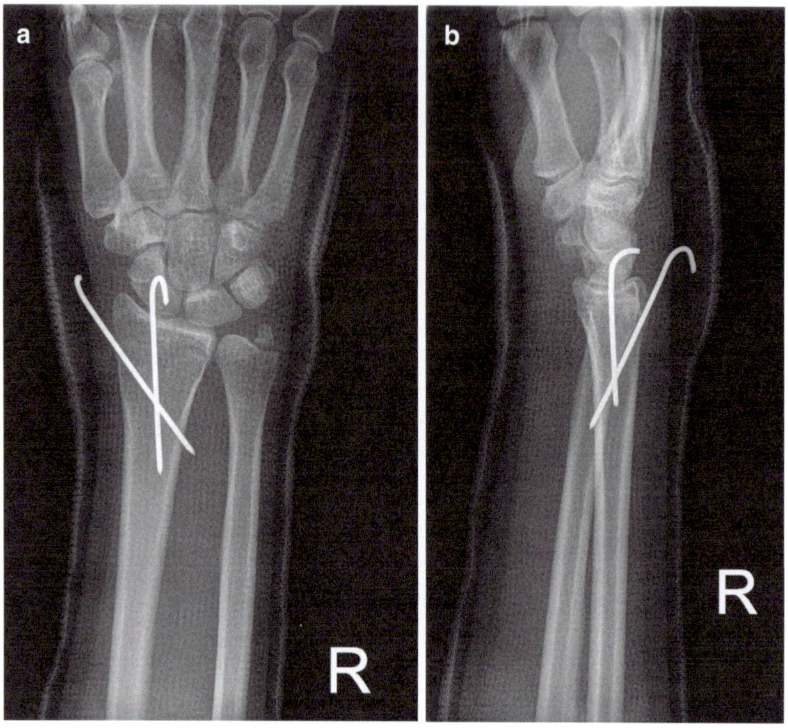

Fig. 7.14 K-wire fixation of the distal radius. Two wires have been used, one from the dorsal aspect and one from the radial styloid AP (**a**) and lateral (**b**) view. Both wires engage the opposite cortex. A plaster cast is required for support, despite the use of wires. Note the ulnar styloid fracture, which has not been surgically stabilised

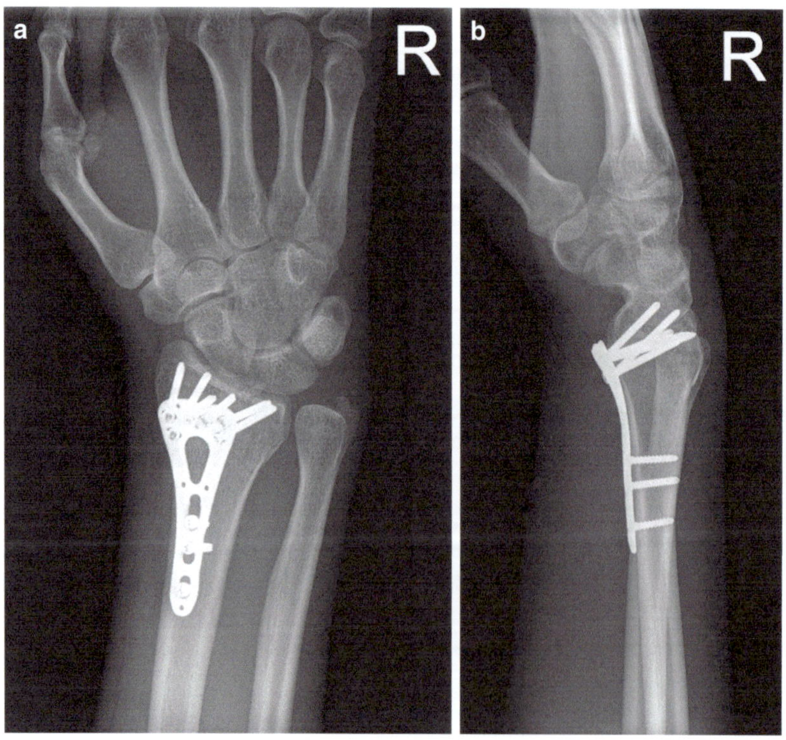

Fig. 7.15 Plate fixation of the distal radius using a volar locking plate. Care should be taken that no screws protrude into the joint (**a**). This should also be carefully assessed on the post-op X-rays. The screws should engage the dorsal cortex of radius, but excessive prominence of screws will cause irritation/injury to the extensor tendons (**b**)

Acetabular Fractures

Acetabular fractures are frequently high-energy injuries, and displaced fractures require reduction and internal fixation to achieve a congruent articular surface and allow early mobilisation.

Acetabular fractures are classified according to whether they involve the anterior column (from symphysis pubis and obturator foramen, through the acetabulum to the ASIS and iliac crest), the posterior column (from inferior pubic ramus, through obturator foramen, through the posterior aspect of the weight-bearing dome to the greater sciatic notch) or both.

Plates used in pelvic fractures are usually precontoured but can be altered by the operating surgeon to provide a close contact between the plate and bone. They are low-profile and should be long enough to provide stability across the entire fracture site (Fig. 7.16a–c). Posterior column plates (Fig. 7.17) applied through a posterior approach usually act as bridging plates, gaining fixation above and below the acetabulum.

In very comminuted fractures, multiple plates may be required (Fig. 7.18).

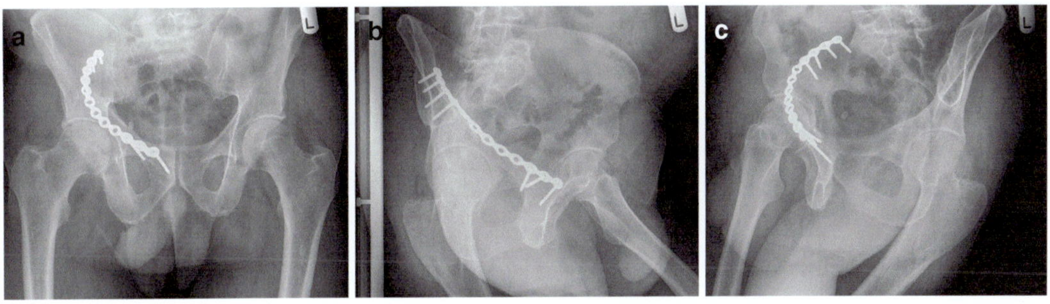

Fig. 7.16 Anterior column acetabular fracture fixed with a precontoured plate. AP (**a**) and Judet (**b**, **c**) views

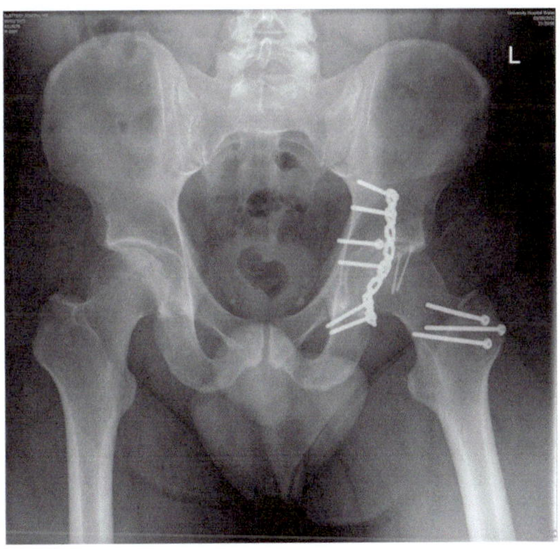

Fig. 7.17 Plate fixation of the posterior column. Two lag screws have been used to stabilise a posterior wall fracture. The plate is fixed proximally and distally to buttress the fragment. This patient had a fracture of the femoral head as well. A trochanteric osteotomy was used for access and has been fixed with three cortical screws. There are two headless screws in the femoral head

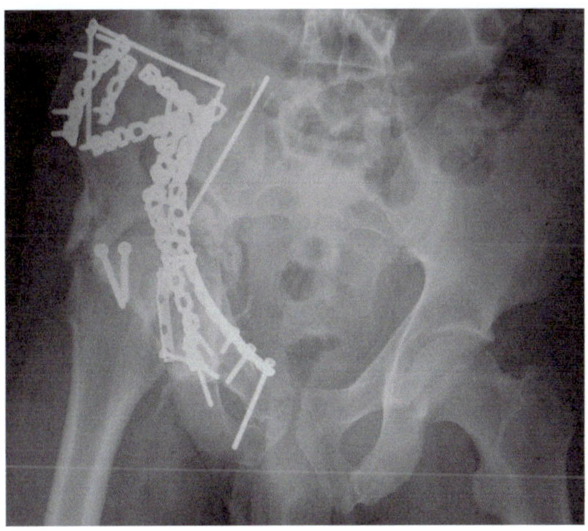

Fig. 7.18 Highly comminuted fracture of the right acetabulum stabilised with multiple plates covering the anterior column, posterior column and the iliac wing. Despite extensive fixation, the acetabulum was not reconstructible and required a hip replacement

Pelvic Ring Injuries

In all three types of pelvic fractures (lateral compression, AP compression and vertical shear), the SI joint and pubic symphysis are often involved. The affected SI joint (or joints) are stabilised with screws, whilst the anterior disruption can be managed with either a plate (Fig. 7.19) or an internal fixator (Fig. 7.20).

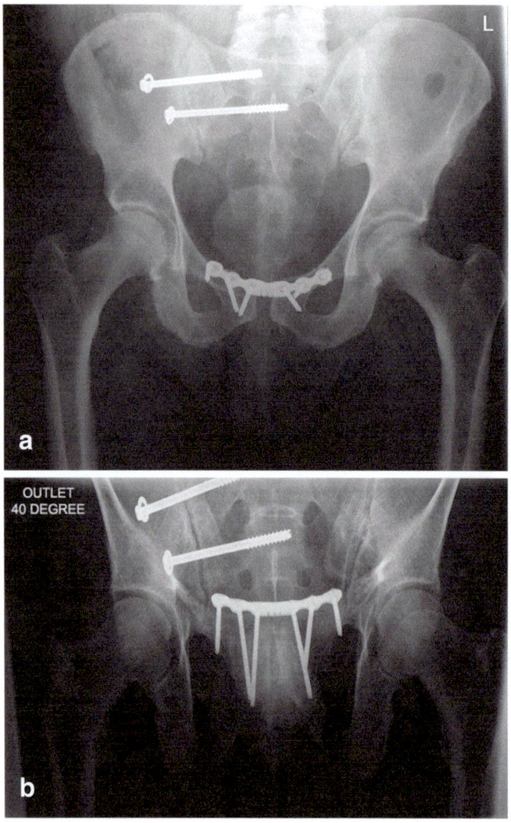

Fig. 7.19 The anterior pelvis has been fixed with a plate and screws, and the posterior fracture fixed with ilio-sacral screws as seen in the AP (**a**) and outlet (**b**) view. The ilio-sacral screws should not penetrate through the sacral foramen. CT scans may be helpful to determine the screw position

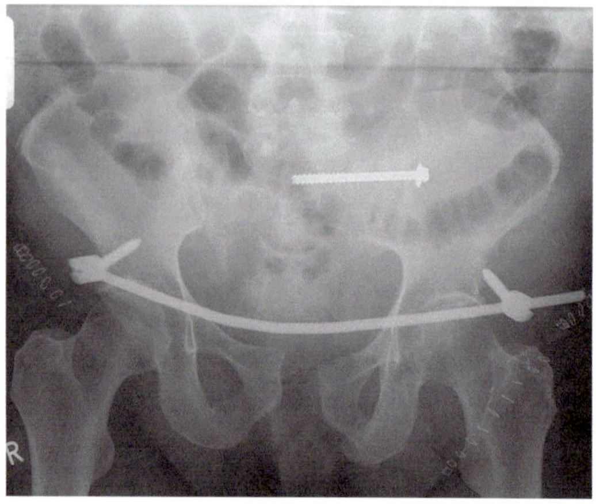

Fig. 7.20 Open book pelvic injury stabilised with in-fix (internal fixator) anteriorly and SI joint screw posteriorly. There is inadequate fixation of the left iliac screw

Intracapsular Fracture of the Neck of Femur

Intracapsular fractures of the neck of femur are treated according to the degree of displacement. Undisplaced fractures are usually managed by internal fixation. Displaced fractures in young patients are treated by reduction and internal fixation. Relatively older patients may require a replacement procedure with either a hemiarthroplasty or a total hip replacement.

Fixation for undisplaced fractures, or after reduction of displaced fractures, is accomplished usually with the use of three screws (Fig. 7.21). These are inserted parallel to each other and in a triangular configuration with two superior and one inferior screw. The entry point of the screws should be above the level of lesser trochanter on the lateral cortex. An inferior entry point may increase the risk of subtrochanteric fracture. The screws should engage the subchondral bone in the head avoiding superior and anterior placement in the head. The threads should cross the fracture site in order to achieve compression. Despite a satisfactory AP and lateral view showing the screws to be contained within the head, it is still possible for screws to protrude beyond the femoral head (Fig. 7.22) and any doubtful appearance should be evaluated with a CT scan.

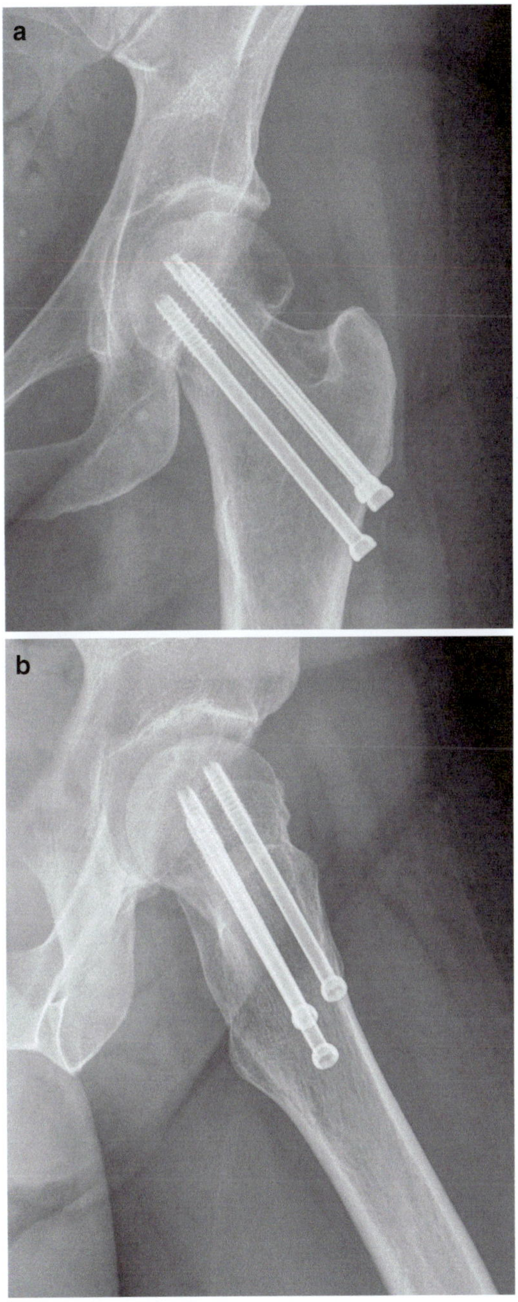

Fig. 7.21 AP (**a**) and lateral (**b**) view of an minimally displaced (valgus impacted) intracapsular hip fracture, which has been fixed with cannulated screws. These pictures show the 'two screws, two views' principle. Three screws have been inserted, but their orientation is such that it appears only two screws are visible on both the AP and lateral views

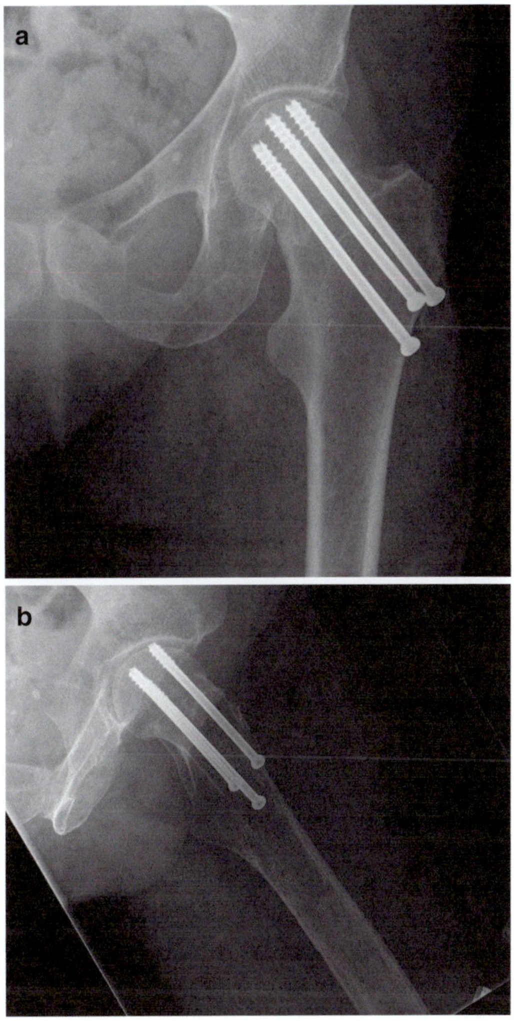

Fig. 7.22 Prominent screw which can damage the articular surface of the femoral head or acetabulum. The screws appear satisfactory on the AP (**a**) view, but the anterior screw is protruding into the joint in the lateral (**b**) view. This requires removal and insertion of a shorter screw to prevent ongoing damage to the joint

Reduction parameters for cannulated screw fixation are:

- No varus (results in increased rates of nonunion)
- Maximum 15° of valgus acceptable (increases bony stability; however, excessive valgus increases the rate of avascular necrosis)
- Anteversion of 0–15°

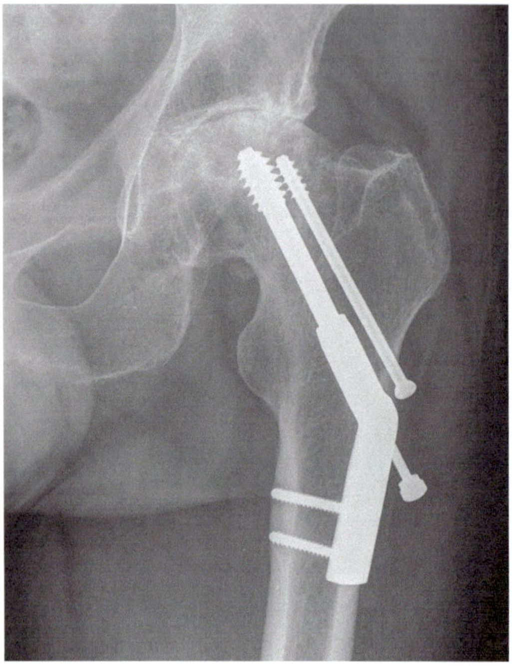

Fig. 7.23 AP view of the hip showing fixation of intracapsular femoral neck fracture using a dynamic hip screw with two-hole side plate. There is a de-rotation screw proximal to the dynamic compression screw for rotational stability. There has been loosening and backing out of the screw from the barrel. The fracture is healed, but there are arthritic changes in the hip

The screws should have a wide spread in the lateral view [2]. A reduced spread on the lateral view is associated with a higher risk of failure of fixation and nonunion.

Dynamic hip screw, with a two-hole side plate (Fig. 7.23), can be used for fixation of intracapsular femoral neck fractures. This implant is frequently supplemented with an additional screw superior to the compression screw. The superior screw provides another point of fixation and also reduces the risk of loss of reduction as the compression screw is tightened in the femoral head. There is little evidence to suggest the superiority of screws over dynamic compression screw, but screws are generally a more popular choice.

Hemiarthroplasties (Figs. 7.24 and 7.25) can be either unipolar (stem, neck and head of the implant are a single block) or bipolar (mobile head on a fixed neck and stem). Most hemiarthroplasty implants are designed for cementation as this provides firm fixation in the bone. Uncemented implants such as Austin Moore

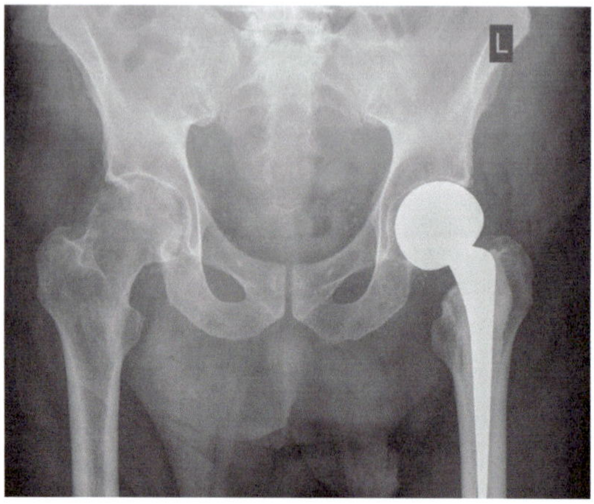

Fig. 7.24 Cemented unipolar hemiarthroplasty of left hip

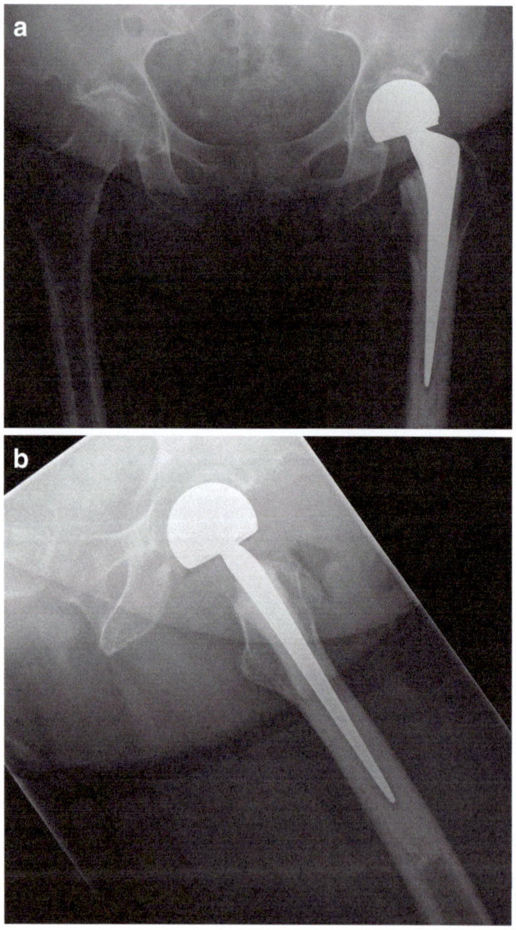

Fig. 7.25 Cemented bipolar hemiarthroplasty of the left hip in AP (**a**) and lateral (**b**) view

prosthesis (Fig. 7.26) were designed before the development of porous coating technology.

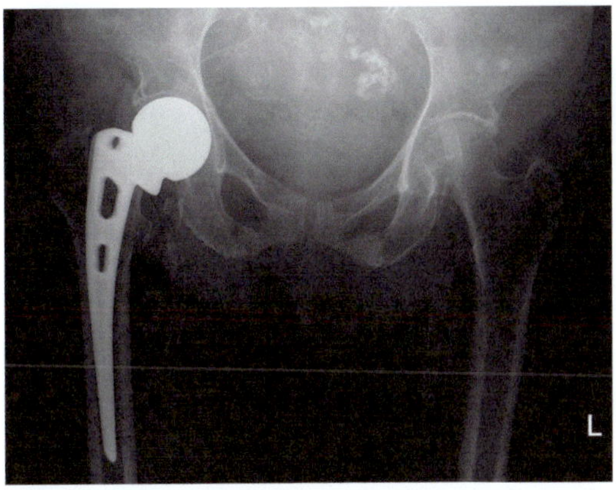

Fig. 7.26 Austin Moore uncemented hemiarthroplasty of the right hip. This operation is rarely performed now as the stability of the stem is generally poor

These provide inadequate fixation and are no longer in general use. Modern uncemented hemiarthroplasty prostheses have a porous coating on the surface, which allows bone ingrowth, and this provides secondary stability of the stem.

Features to note on radiographs of hemiarthroplasty are the type of prosthesis, cemented or cementless fixation, the quality of the cement mantle, presence of cement restrictor and the size of prosthetic head in relation to the acetabular socket. The restoration of leg length is determined by drawing a horizontal line through the inferior end of the tear drop on both sides. The relative perpendicular distance of a fixed point, commonly the lesser trochanter, is compared on both sides in relation to the horizontal line. A careful check should be made for any periprosthetic fracture and any retained cement.

Total hip replacement for displaced femoral neck fractures is indicated for patients who are independently mobile, cognitively intact and medically well enough to withstand the procedure.

Extracapsular Fracture of the Neck of Femur (Intertrochanteric Fracture)

The vast majority of extracapsular fractures of the proximal femur are managed by internal fixation. These fractures do not disrupt the blood supply to the femoral head, and therefore the risk of avascular necrosis is low.

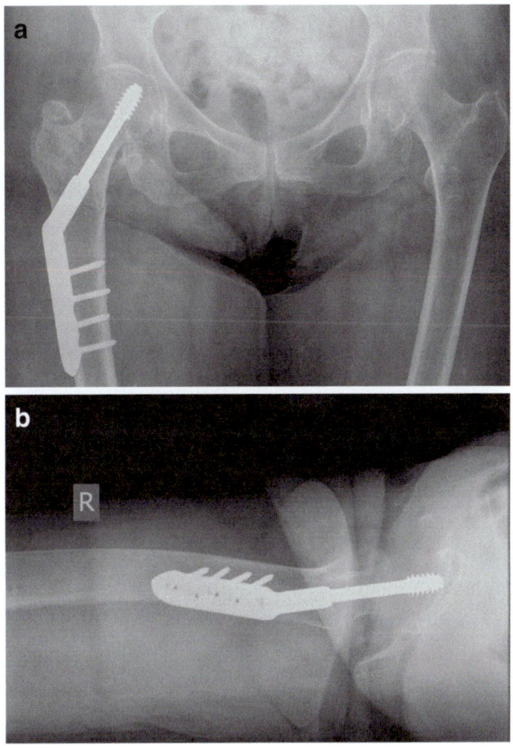

Fig. 7.27 An extracapsular fracture of the right hip, which has been fixed with a dynamic compression screw. Note that the screw is low in the neck on the AP (**a**) view, which helps achieve the position of the screw tip in the centre of the femoral head. The tip-apex distance is less than 20 mm, which is calculated by adding the distance between the AP and lateral (**b**) view

Most extracapsular fractures can be managed with a dynamic hip screw (Fig. 7.27), which encourages compression at the fracture site as the patient mobilises. The implant is in two parts: a screw inserted along the femoral neck and into the femoral head, and a plate attached to the lateral surface of the femoral shaft through which the screw can glide. This construct stabilises most extracapsular fractures, as these fractures are usually orientated obliquely between the greater and lesser trochanters.

Many factors determine the rate of success of the implant construct; however, one of the key factors is the tip-apex distance. This is a measurement proposed by Baumgaertner in 1997 [3, 4] and is the sum of the distance, measured on the AP and lateral views of the hip, between the tip of the screw and the apex of the femoral head. Tip-apex distance of less than 20 mm is associated with a much lower rate of cutout of the screw compared to those where the distance is greater than 20 mm (Figs. 7.28 and 7.29). Adequate reduction of the fracture is associated with a reduced failure of fixation.

For accurate determination of tip-apex distance, the magnification of the radiograph has to be accounted for. The dynamic hip screw is 12.5 mm at the widest point of the threads, and this measurement can be used to correct for magnification. In some situations, where there is a fracture of the greater trochanter, it can be stabilised with an additional plate fixed to the side plate of the dynamic hip screw (Fig. 7.30). The additional plate allows multiple screw placements for fixation of the greater trochanter fragment.

Extracapsular fractures that are orientated in the opposite direction (so-called 'reverse oblique' fractures) will not be sufficiently stabilised by a

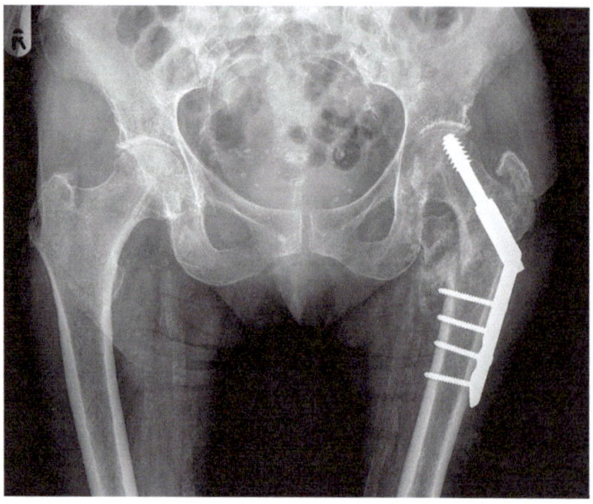

Fig. 7.28 An improperly positioned dynamic hip screw. In this case, note that the screw is high in the neck, and the tip is far superior to the apex of the femoral head. This screw is at high risk of cutting out

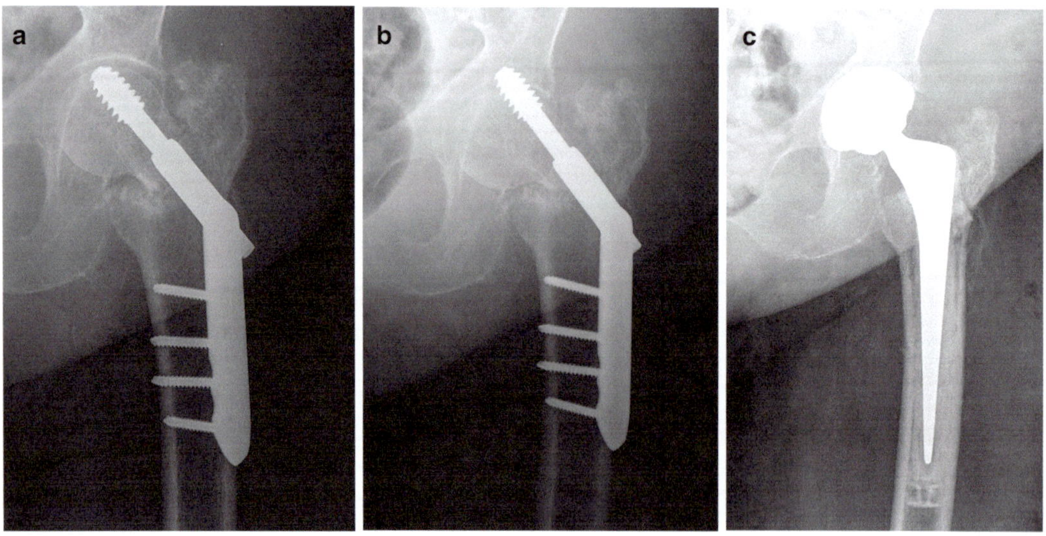

Fig. 7.29 Dynamic hip screw positioned in the superior part of the femoral head (**a**) with a large tip-apex distance. The fracture is not well reduced and femoral neck is shortened. On follow-up, the screw cut through the femoral head and penetrated into the acetabulum (**b**). This was managed by removal of the screw, bone grafting of the contained defect in the acetabulum and total hip replacement (**c**)

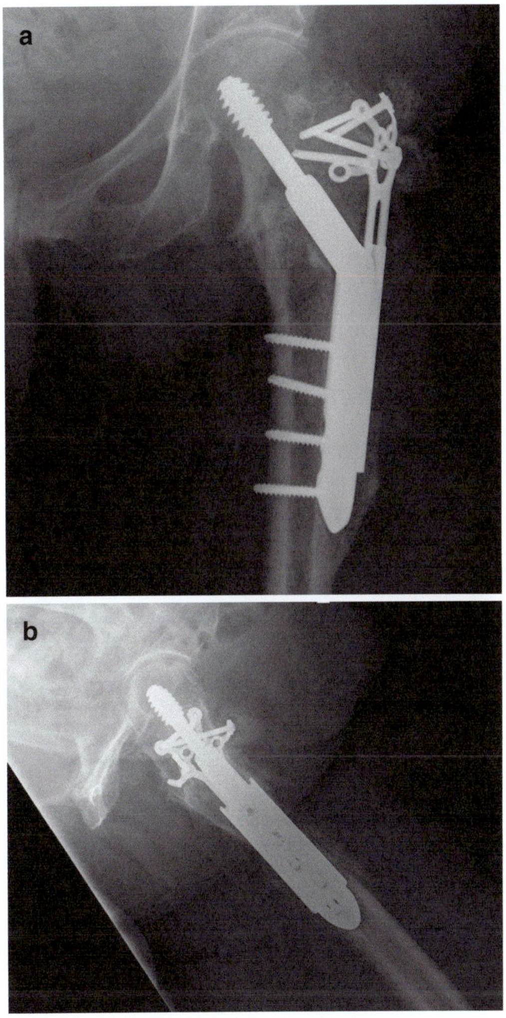

Fig. 7.30 Side plate used with the dynamic hip screw to fix greater trochanter fragment in the AP (**a**) and lateral (**b**) view

dynamic hip screw. This is because shear forces acting on the fracture are parallel to the compression screw. These fractures are better managed with an intramedullary device (Fig. 7.31) with a screw placed along the femoral neck and into the head. Similar to the DHS, the screw into the femoral head is dynamic to allow compression at the fracture site. The presence of intramedullary nail avoids excess shortening at the fracture site. The nail is fixed distally with one or two distal interlocking screws. If more movement at the fracture site is required, only the oval-shaped dynamic hole is used. However, more often than not, a screw is inserted into both the dynamic and static (round) holes in order to achieve static stability.

Mechanical failure of the cephalomedullary nail can be predicted by the absence of three-point contact [5]. The three points are the tip of the screw in the femoral head, the contact between the lateral end of screw and the lateral cortex of femur, and the contact point between the proximal end of the nail and its entry point in the femur (Fig. 7.32).

Mid-shaft Femur Fractures

Mid-shaft femoral fractures in adults are often high-energy injuries that require early stabilisation to prevent severe complications. In the elderly, it is possible to sustain low-energy fractures due to poor bone quality

These fractures are most often fixed with either antegrade (proximal to distal) or retrograde

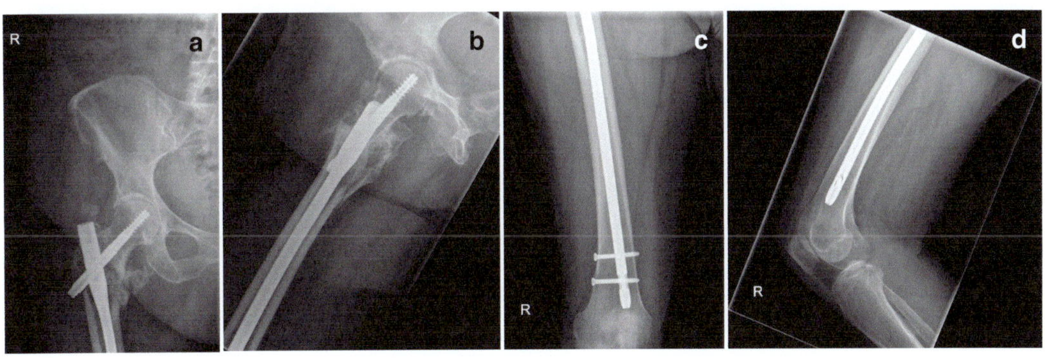

Fig. 7.31 Extracapsular fracture of the hip, which has been fixed with an intramedullary nail in AP (**a**) and lateral (**b**) view. AP (**c**) and lateral (**d**) views of the knee should be obtained to check implant position postoperatively

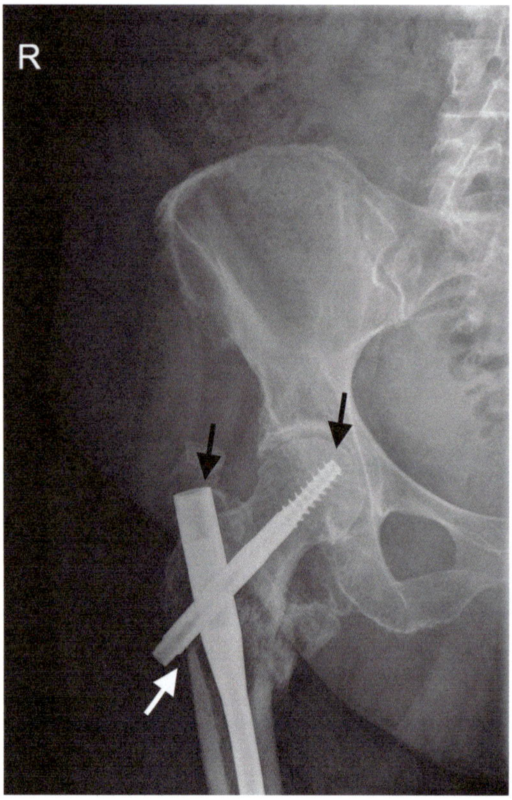

Fig. 7.32 Three-point fixation of the intramedullary nail. The two black arrows represent fixation in the femoral head and the entry point of the nail. The white arrow signifies contact on the lateral cortex

(distal to proximal) intramedullary nailing of the femur (Figs. 7.33 and 7.34). There are a variety of implants used for this purpose, but the basic construct is the same with an intramedullary nail fixed into position in the bone with proximal and distal locking screws. These nails provide relative stability to fractures, and on postoperative X-rays, evidence of callus formation indicates fracture healing.

Distal Femur Fractures

In distal femoral fractures, the aim of surgery is to restore the anatomy of the knee joint and provide rigid fixation if the fracture is intraarticular. This is usually achieved by open reduction and internal plate fixation (Fig. 7.35). Commonly, the plates are applied to the lateral aspect of distal femur, although fractures involving only the medial condyle may be best managed by medial fixation (Fig. 7.36).

Tibial Plateau Fractures

Tibial plateau fractures are intraarticular and are graded in terms of severity by the Schatzker

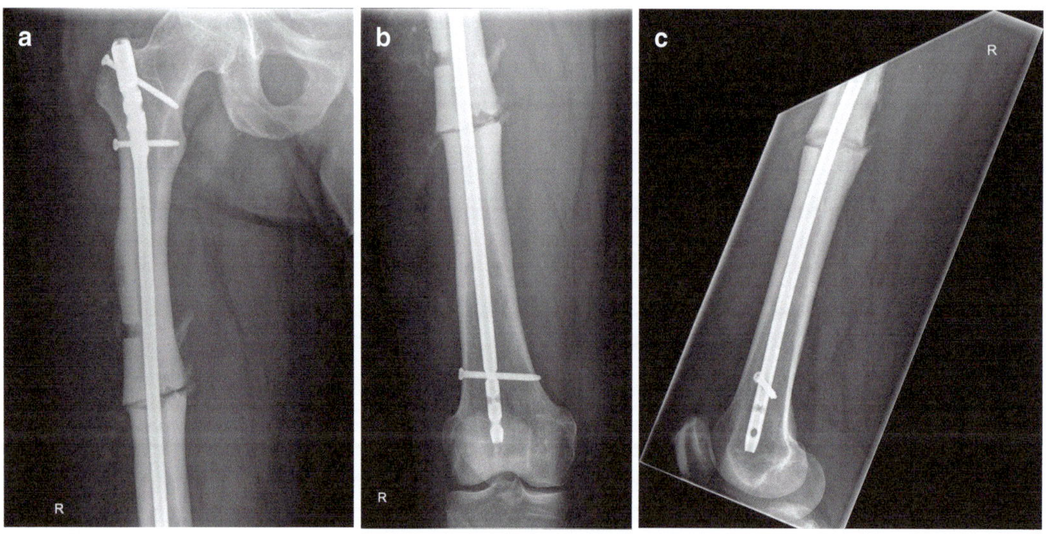

Fig. 7.33 Antegrade femoral nail for correction of a previous fracture malunion. Note that there are multiple options for screw fixation of the nail at both the proximal (**a**) and distal (**b**, **c**) ends

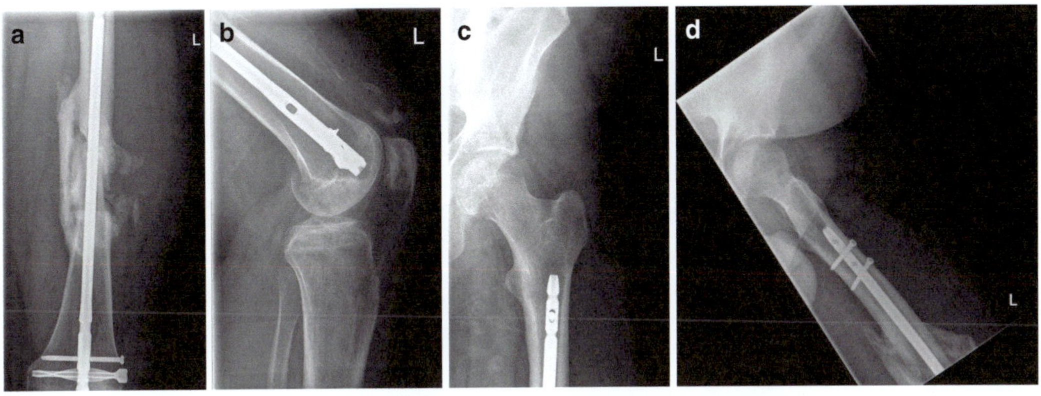

Fig. 7.34 Retrograde femoral nail AP (**a**) and lateral (**b**) view. Note that this nail has been fixed distally with both a cortical screw and a spiral blade. The spiral blade gives added stability in comminuted fractures, or in patients with osteoporotic bone. Proximally, the nail is locked (**c**, **d**) using two anteroposterior locking screws

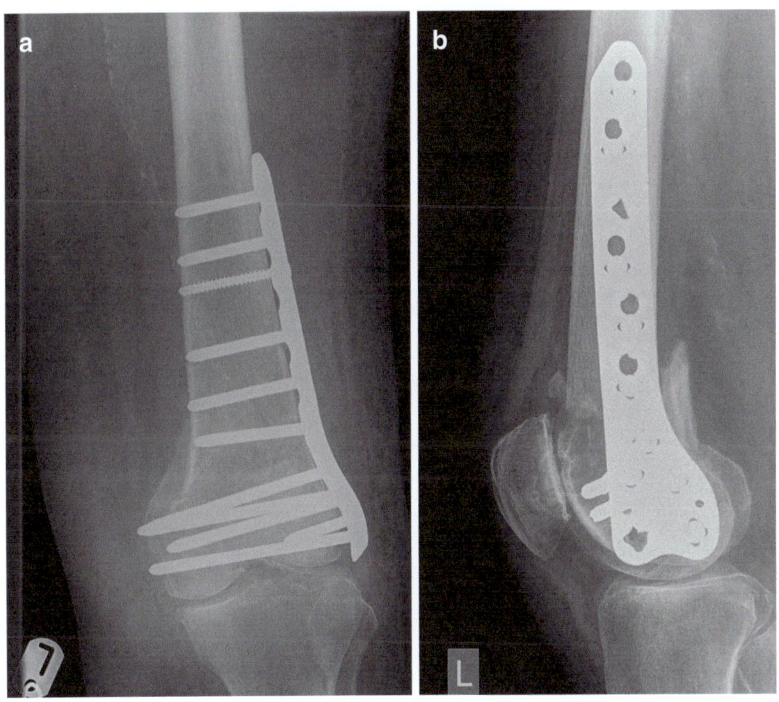

Fig. 7.35 A very distal fracture of the left femur, fixed with a locking plate on the lateral surface of the bone. The plate allows multiple screws in the distal fragment, all of which are locking and act as fixed angle devices providing far superior fixation compared to non-locking screws. AP (**a**) and lateral (**b**) views are demonstrated

classification [6]. They are usually managed with open reduction and internal fixation in order to provide absolute stability. There are multiple methods of fixing a tibial plateau fracture, as illustrated in the examples (Figs. 7.37, 7.38, 7.39 and 7.40). The approach and the use of plates depend on the pattern and severity of injury. In some situations, a combination of limited internal fixation along with external fixation helps to restore articular surface and bridge the metaphyseal comminution (Fig. 7.41).

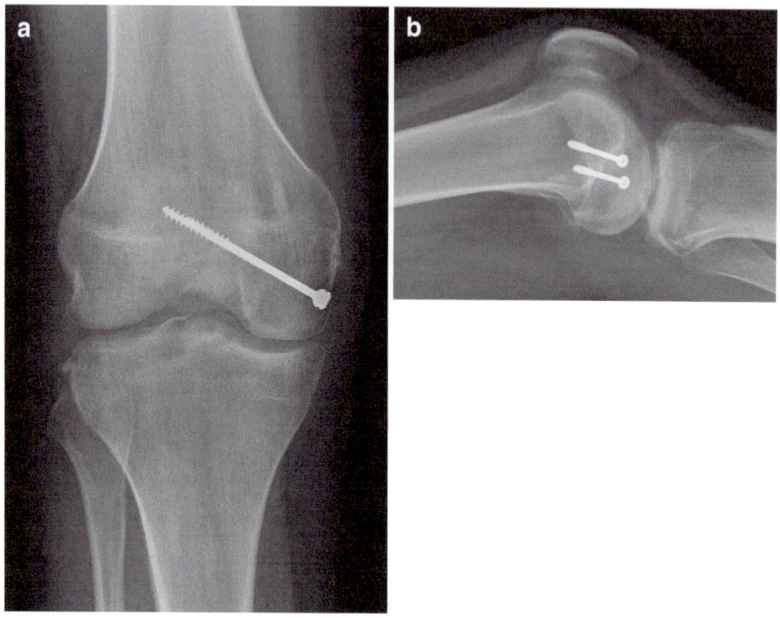

Fig. 7.36 Fracture of the medial femoral condyle stabilised with screws inserted from a medial approach—AP (**a**) and lateral (**b**) view

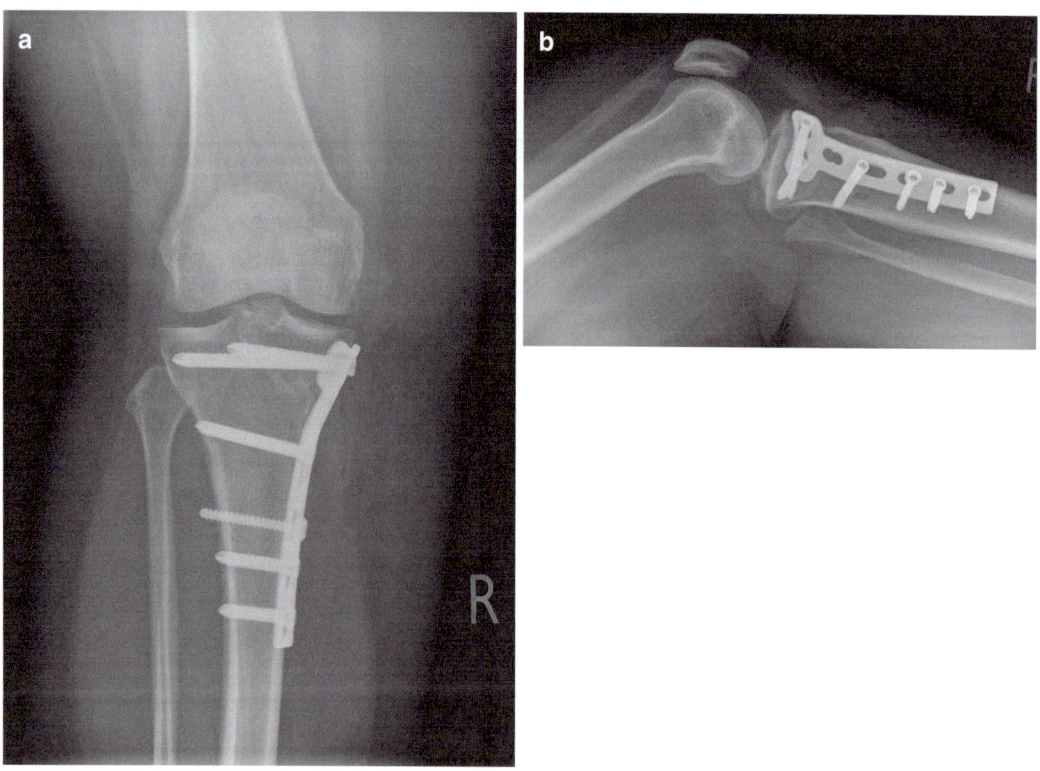

Fig. 7.37 Tibial plateau fracture fixed with a medial plate. The third screw from distal end is a non-locking screw (**a**). This helps to pull the plate close to the bone. All other screws are locking screws for better fixation (**b**)

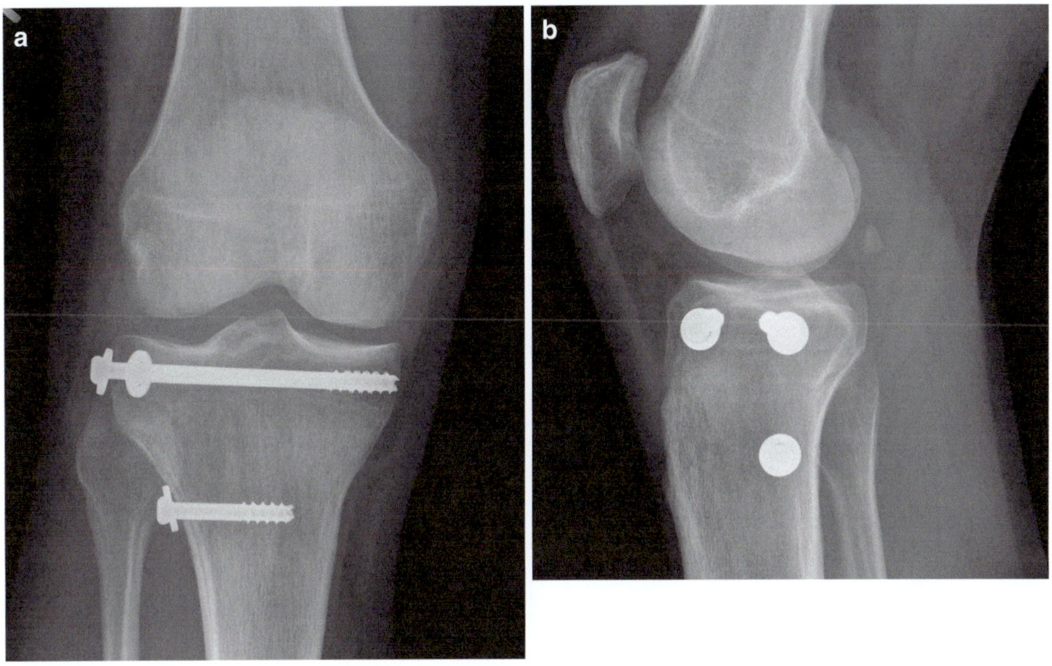

Fig. 7.38 Tibial plateau fracture fixed with three screws from lateral to medial side AP (**a**) and lateral (**b**) view. This method is suitable for fractures with a longitudinal split, without significant depression. The distal screw functions as an antiglide screw

Fig. 7.39 Tibial plateau fracture fixed with a posterior plate. The restoration of articular surface on the AP (**a**) view and tibial slope on the lateral (**b**) view is satisfactory

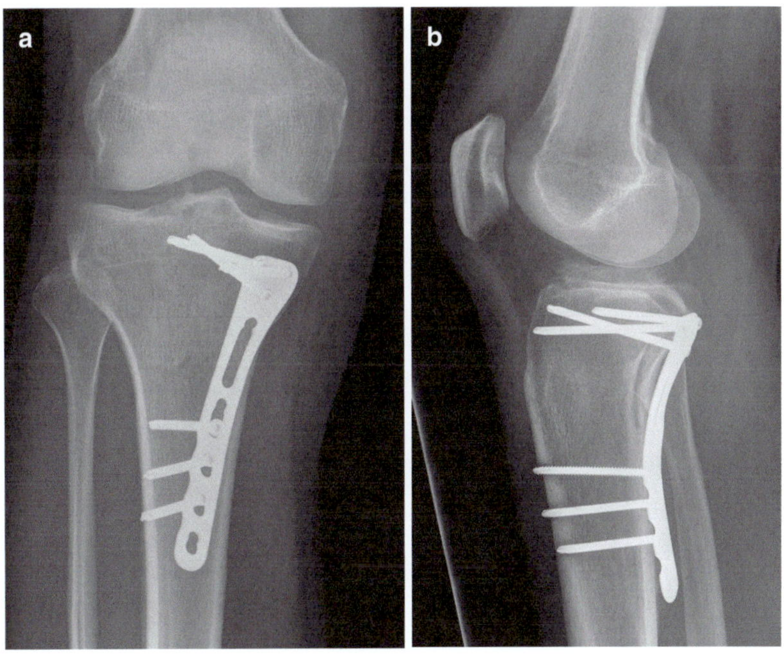

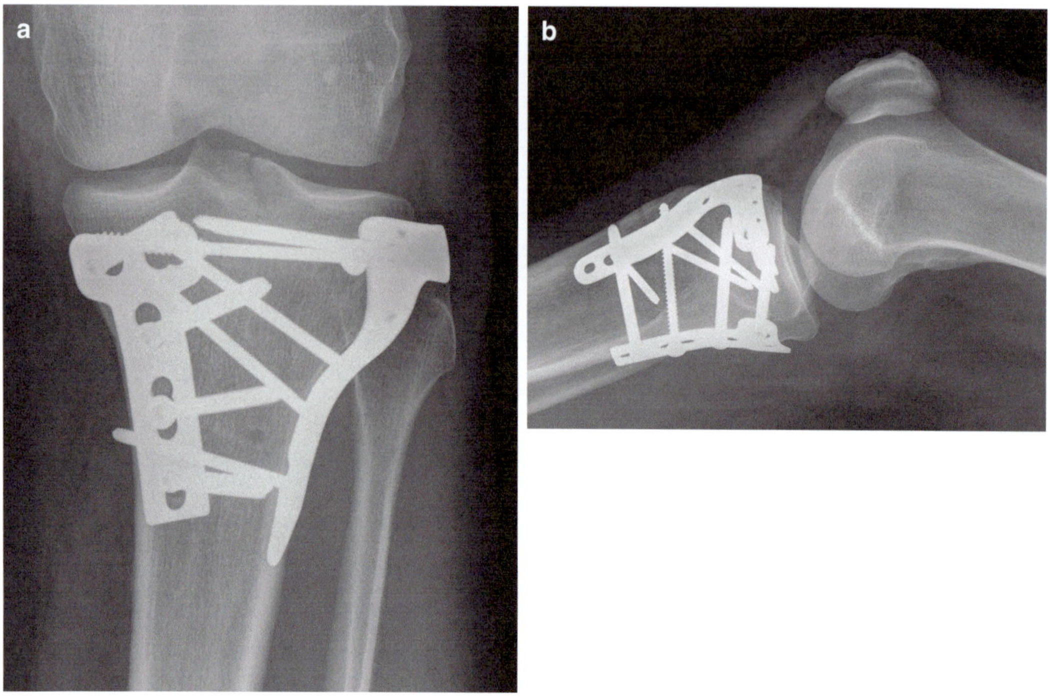

Fig. 7.40 Double plating of the proximal tibia using an anterolateral locking plate and a posteromedial buttress plate. AP (**a**) and lateral (**b**) views. The posterolateral plate does not provide locking option and is used purely in buttress mode

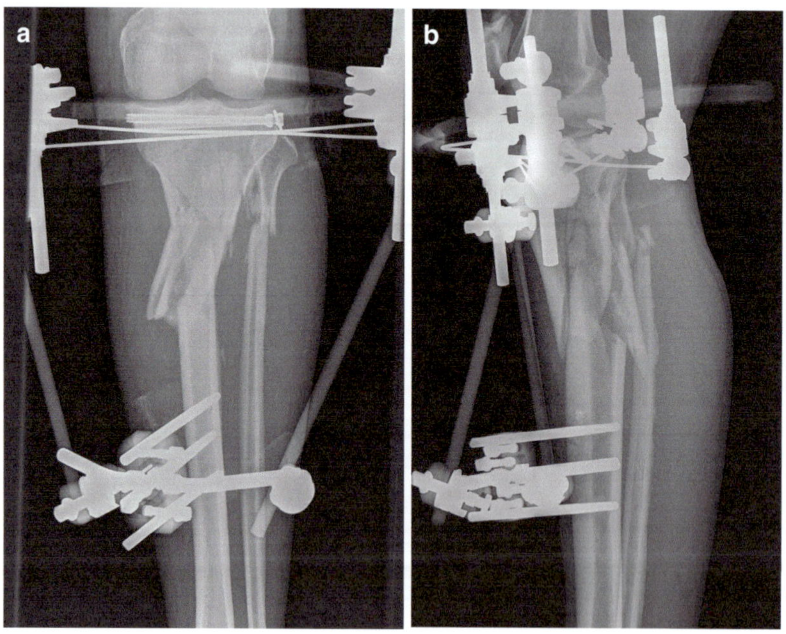

Fig. 7.41 Combined internal and external fixation of the proximal tibia. The two cannulated screws inserted lateral to medial in the proximal tibia help to restore the articular surface continuity as seen in AP (**a**) and lateral (**b**) view. Extensive metaphyseal comminution has been bridged using an external fixator. The fixator uses fine wires in the proximal tibia and half pins in the tibial shaft

Patella Fractures

Patella fractures are fixed if they are open, if there is displacement of fracture fragments or if there is failure of the extensor mechanism. The method of fixation commonly uses a tension band construct, which converts the tensile forces across the knee joint into compressive forces, and draws the two fragments together. The wire loop on the anterior aspect of the patella is the actual tension band, with the parallel wires acting to provide stability to the fixation. As an alternative, two parallel cannulated screws can be used in place of wires (Fig. 7.42).

Mid-shaft Tibia Fractures

Tibial shaft fractures in adults are commonly fixed with an intramedullary nail in order to achieve and maintain good alignment and prevent malunion.

Tibial intramedullary nails (Fig. 7.43) are inserted antegrade and are statically locked (with screws through the round holes) at both the proximal and distal ends. There are usually one or two proximal screws (inserted from lateral to medial) and two distal screws (inserted from medial to lateral).

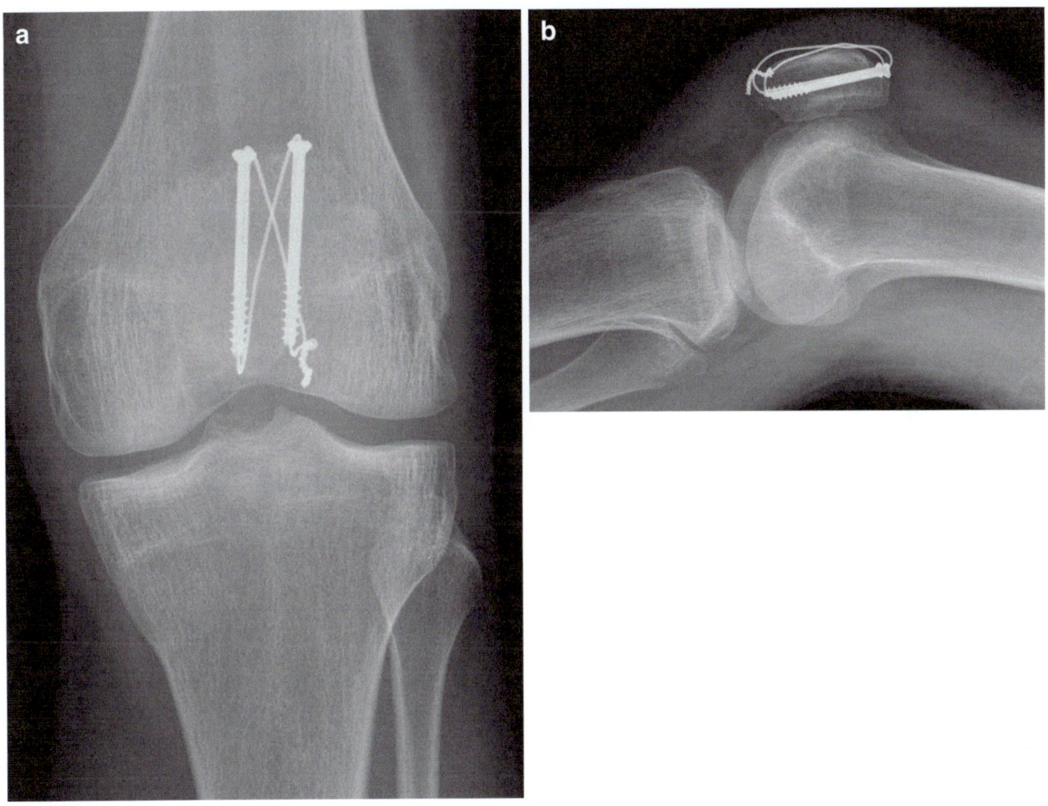

Fig. 7.42 Patella fracture treated with two cannulated screws and a wire loop used in 'tension band principle'. Unlike in the elbow (Fig. 7.11), the construct here uses two cannulated screws through the patella, through which the wire loop is threaded. AP (**a**) and lateral (**b**) view. Either method is acceptable although screws provide some degree of interfragmentary compression

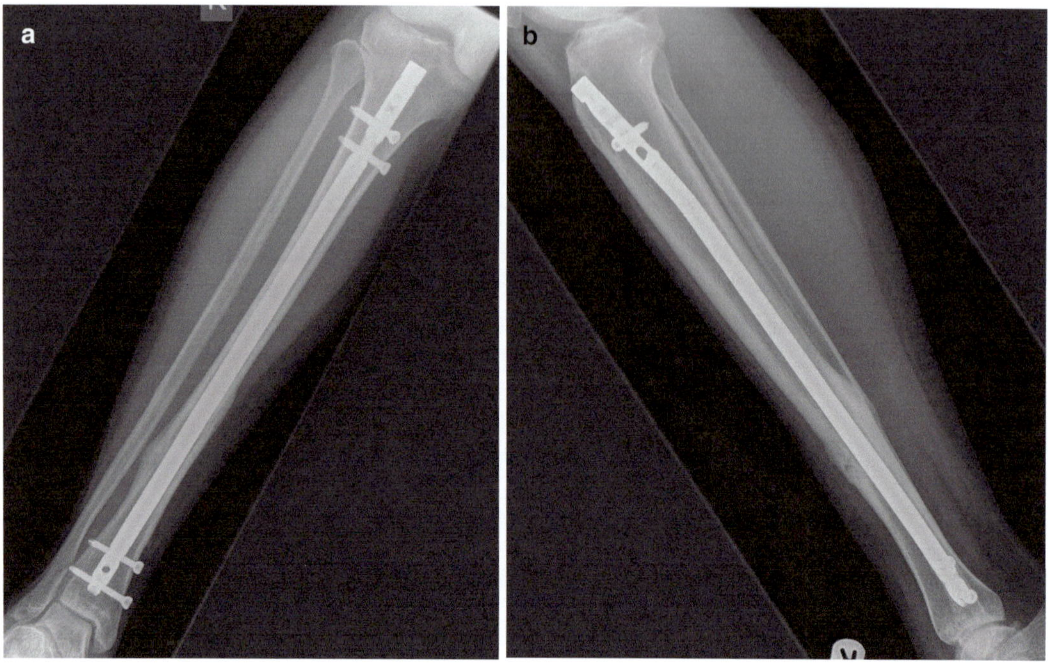

Fig. 7.43 Tibial intramedullary nail. Note the presence of two locking screws proximally and two distally in the AP (**a**) and lateral (**b**) view. There is evidence of callus formation at the fracture site due to indirect bone healing

Distal Tibia Fractures

Extra-articular fractures of the distal tibia can be managed by intramedullary nail or plate fixation (Fig. 7.44). Ring fixators are also an option.

Pilon Fractures

Pilon fractures are usually the result of axial loading injuries and involve the articular weight-bearing surface of the distal tibia. The pattern of fracture configuration determines the approach and choice of fixation (Figs. 7.45 and 7.46).

Ankle–Bimalleolar Fractures

Fractures involving the ankle can be classified according to the number of malleoli involved. Bi- and tri-malleolar fractures are almost always fixed in order to stabilise the ankle joint.

The other important classification in ankle fractures is Weber's classification of distal fibular fractures. This is based on the level of the fracture relative to the syndesmosis between the tibia and fibula. Weber A (below the syndesmosis) fractures are inherently stable and can be managed conservatively. Weber B fractures (at the level of the syndesmosis) may be stable or unstable, depending on the presence or absence of an injury on the medial side, and should be fixed on the basis of this (Fig. 7.47). Weber C fractures (above the syndesmosis) are inherently unstable and require fixation (Fig. 7.48).

External Fixators

An external fixator is a device that stabilises a fracture at a point distant from the focus of injury. There are many different constructs, all of which involve an external frame of bars and connectors,

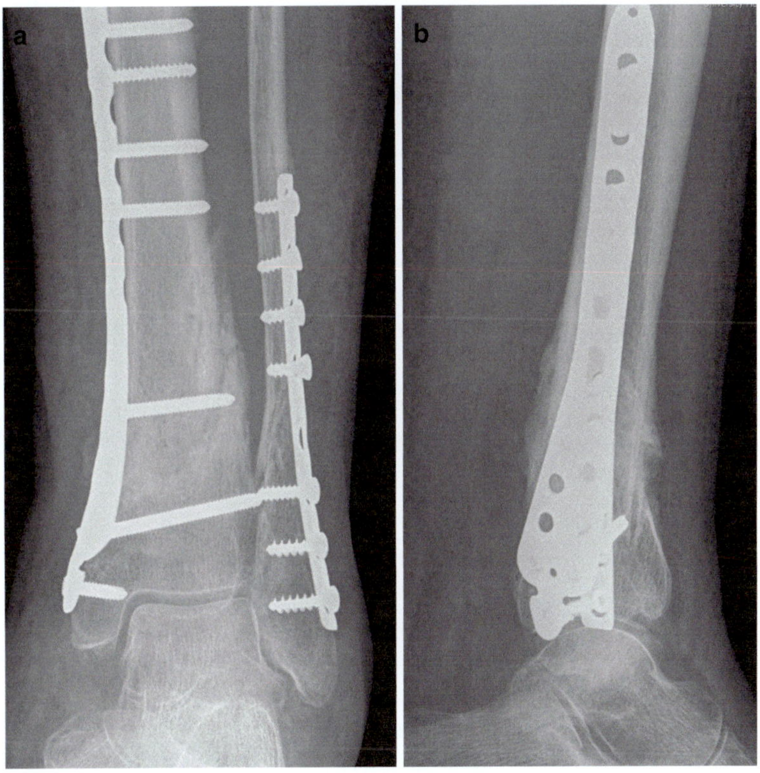

Fig. 7.44 Medial locking plate for a distal tibial extra-articular fracture. AP (**a**) and lateral (**b**) view show locking plate on the tibia, and a non-locking one third tubular plate on the tibia. The syndesmosis was stable and hence has not been surgically stabilised

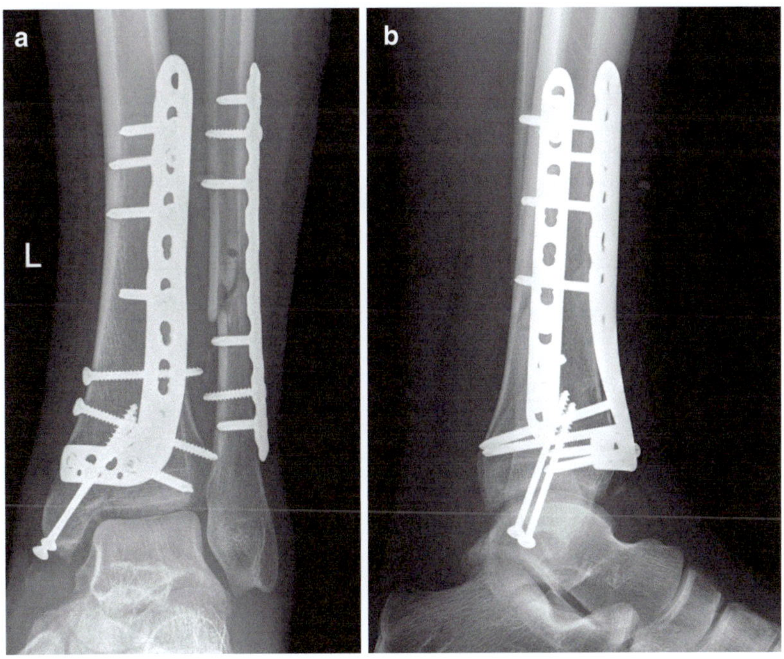

Fig. 7.45 Anteromedial locking plate of distal tibia. There are two lag screws inserted from medial to lateral direction for compression seen in the AP (**a**) and lateral (**b**) view. Two further screws have been used to stabilise the medial malleolus. The locking plate acts like a neutralisation plate. The fibula has been fixed with a locking plate, which is used in neutralisation mode as the fibular fracture is comminuted

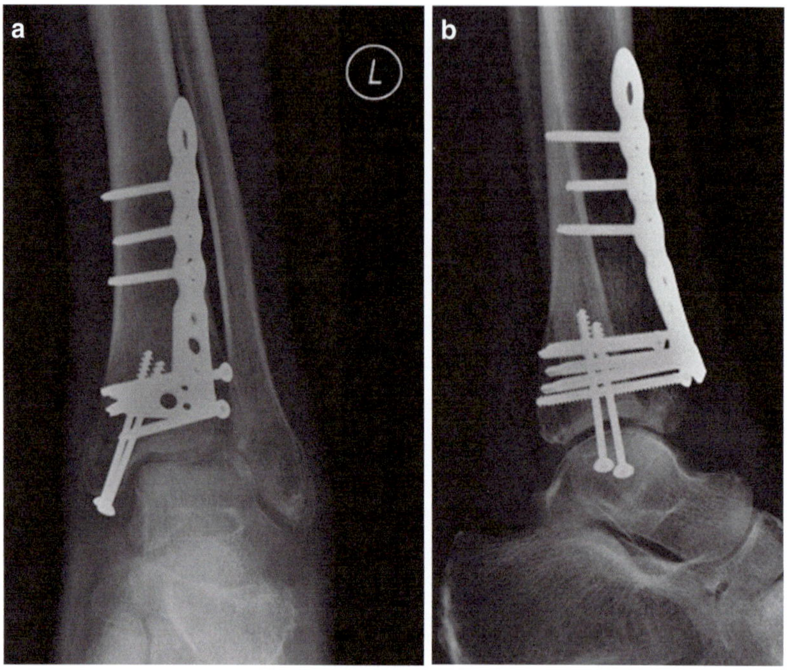

Fig. 7.46 Pilon fracture of the left ankle. This has been fixed with a plate on the anterolateral surface of the tibia, and two screws to fix the medial malleolus. There are multiple screws holding the anterior fragments in place, along with a T-plate which is acting as a buttress to prevent the fracture fragment migrating proximally. AP (**a**) and lateral (**b**) view

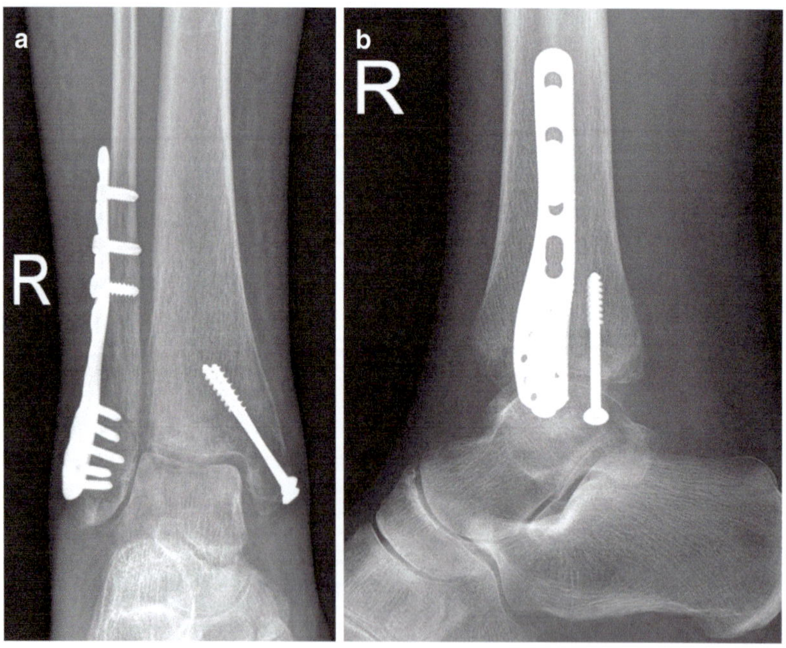

Fig. 7.47 Bimalleolar fracture of the ankle fixed with a contoured fibular plate and two screws in the medial malleolus. This plate is a specially designed contoured locking plate, allowing multiple screw options in the distal fragment. AP (**a**) and lateral (**b**) view. There are no washers on the medial screws. Washers are needed in osteopenic bone. There was no syndesmotic injury, hence no fixation across the distal tibio-fibular joint

with pins or wires fixed into or traversing the bone. External fixators can be used either as a temporary stabilisation measure to rest the soft tissues prior to definitive fixation or as definitive fracture management.

'Quad Frame'

A quadrilateral frame is a simple external fixation construct consisting of pins through and through the proximal tibia and calcaneum in the coronal plane,

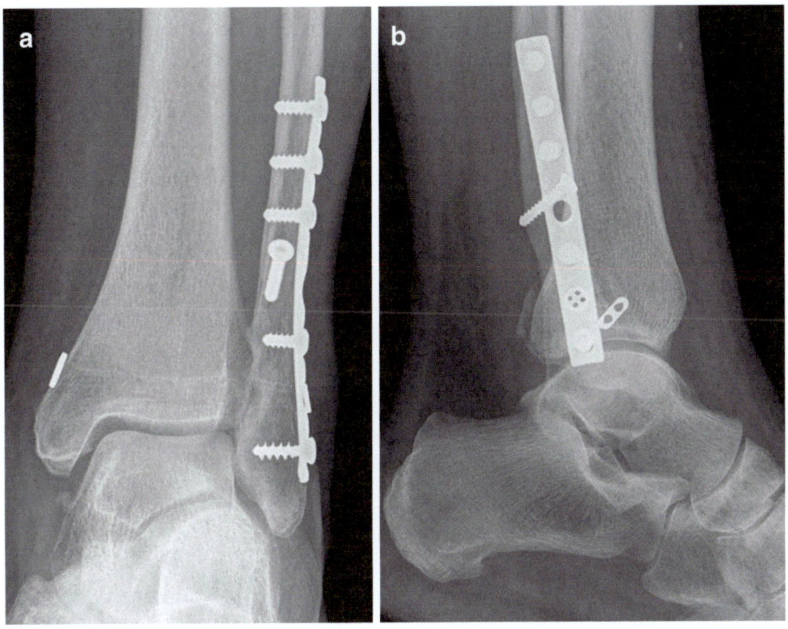

Fig. 7.48 Weber C of the lateral malleolus fracture fixed with a fibular plate and a TightRope implant system to stabilise the syndesmosis. The fibula has been fixed with a lag screw across the fracture site, and a neutralisation plate with three screws proximal to the fracture, and two screws distally. Where the middle distal screw would have been placed, there are buttons on the medial side on the tibia, and another adjacent to the plate seen in the AP (**a**) and lateral (**b**) view from the TightRope implant used to stabilise the syndesmotic injury. There is also a small posterior malleolus fragment, which has not been fixed

parallel to the sole of the heel (Fig. 7.49). Clamps to a bar on either side of the leg connect these pins. The frame can be strengthened by the addition of two further pins, one from the medial bar into the medial side of the proximal tibia and a further pin into the first metatarsal. There are helpful temporary measures whilst the swelling reduces.

Delta Frame

A delta frame is an A-shaped (or delta-shaped) external fixation construct used for stabilisation of distal tibial fractures (Fig. 7.50).

An important concept in the use of delta frames is the 'tibial safe zone'. In the tibial shaft, this is the area between the sagittal plane anteriorly and the coronal plane medially. In the distal tibia, this zone starts just medial to the sagittal plane (to avoid the anterior tibial artery and vein) and runs medially for 120°.

For a delta frame, two pins are inserted anteriorly in the tibial shaft (one in the mid-shaft region, and one more distally). These two pins are connected by a multi-pin clamp, which is then connected by bars to a Steinmann pin through the calcaneum (inserted in the same way as for a quadrilateral frame).

Circular Frame

Circular frame external fixators can be used for complex injuries including where there is deformity or limb length discrepancy requiring correction. The device consists of at least two circular frame ring elements connected to the bone by pins or wires (Fig. 7.51). The frame components are attached by adjustable rods, which allows for gradual lengthening and/or correction of angular deformity. This construct allows correction to be achieved in multiple planes.

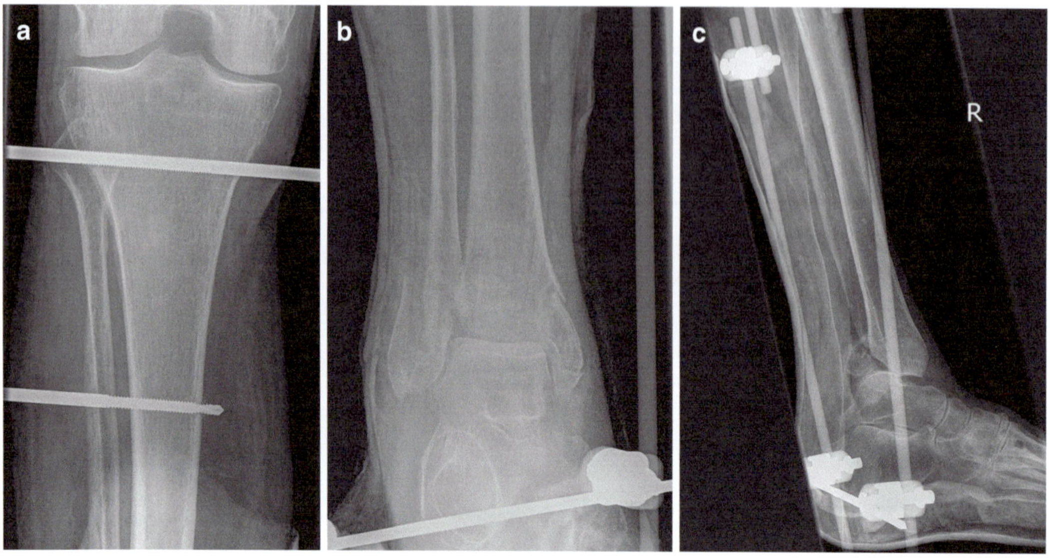

Fig. 7.49 'Quad frame' across the right ankle. There is a Steinmann pin through the proximal tibia (**a**) just distal to the flare of the metaphysis and a half pin in the tibial diaphysis providing extra fracture stability in the sagittal plane (**b**). A third pin has been inserted through the calcaneum. Connecting the three pins to rods running parallel to the lower leg forms a stable rectangular construct. There is a plaster support to prevent equinus deformity. There is residual subluxation of the talus seen in the lateral view (**c**) posteriorly, which is not acceptable and had to be corrected urgently

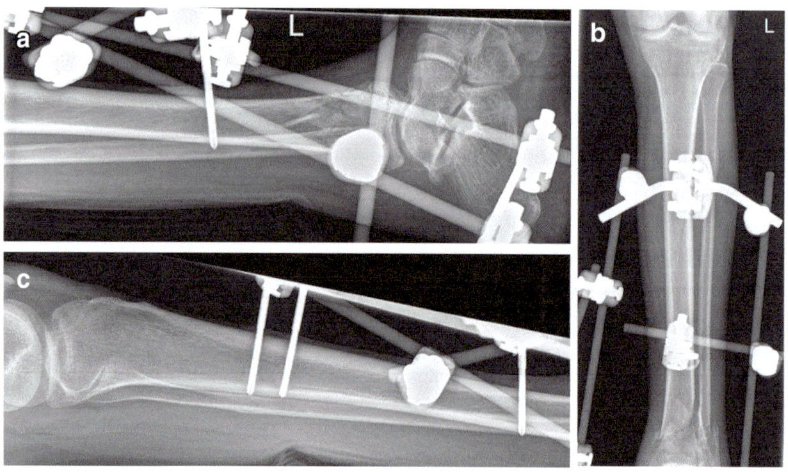

Fig. 7.50 Delta frame—there is a multi-pin clamp attached to the pin in the tibial shaft seen in the lateral (**a**) and AP view (**b**). This allows both lateral rods to be attached to a single tibial pin. In this case, a half pin has been inserted more distally in the tibial shaft, to improve stability (**c**)

The Masquelet Technique

The Masquelet technique is a procedure that can be used to manage traumatic bone defects and infected non-union. The technique involves the debridement and stabilisation of the bone and insertion of a temporary cement spacer impregnated with antibiotics (Fig. 7.52). This construct is left in place for several weeks to allow the formation of an induced pseudo-membrane around the cement spacer.

Once the membrane has formed, the second stage of the procedure involves the gentle removal of the cement spacer and insertion of bone graft into the induced membrane space (Fig. 7.53). The bone graft encourages the formation of new bone, whilst the induction membrane prevents resorption and acts as a 'bone-forming chamber' (Fig. 7.54).

The Masquelet technique can also be used in more distal fractures, such as Tibial Pilon frac-

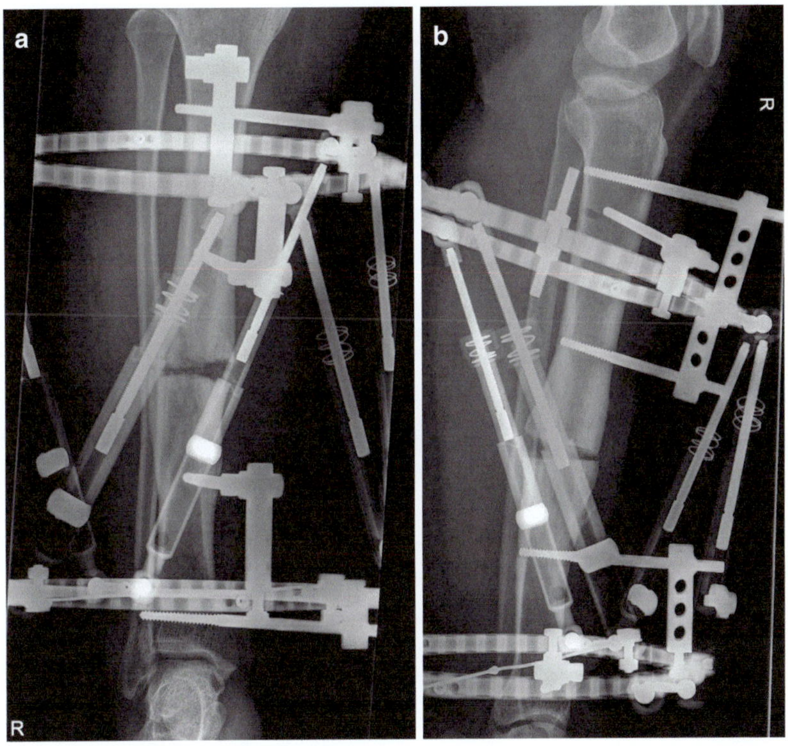

Fig. 7.51 Circular frame used to stabilise the tibia AP (**a**) and lateral (**b**) view. There is an osteotomy in the mid third of the tibial shaft at the site of a previous fracture malunion. Correction is achieved with the frame and maintained until sufficient bony union

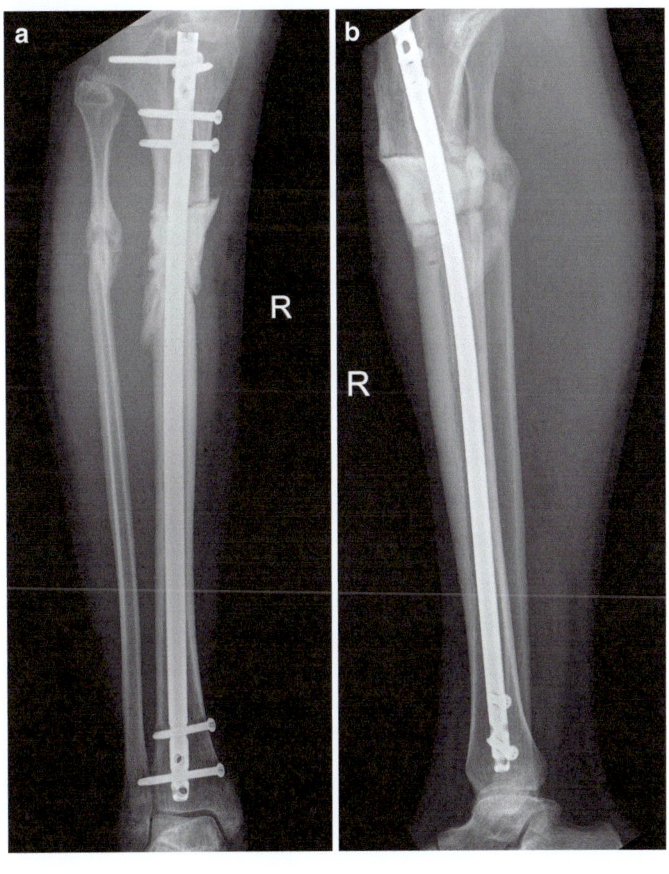

Fig. 7.52 Masquelet technique stage 1. There is cement at the fracture site in the proximal tibial metaphysis. This was the site of an infected nonunion. The infected bone has been removed, local debridement done and the gap filled with a cement spacer. AP (**a**) and lateral (**b**) view shown. There is also a fibular fracture at the same level, which is healing by secondary (indirect) bone healing

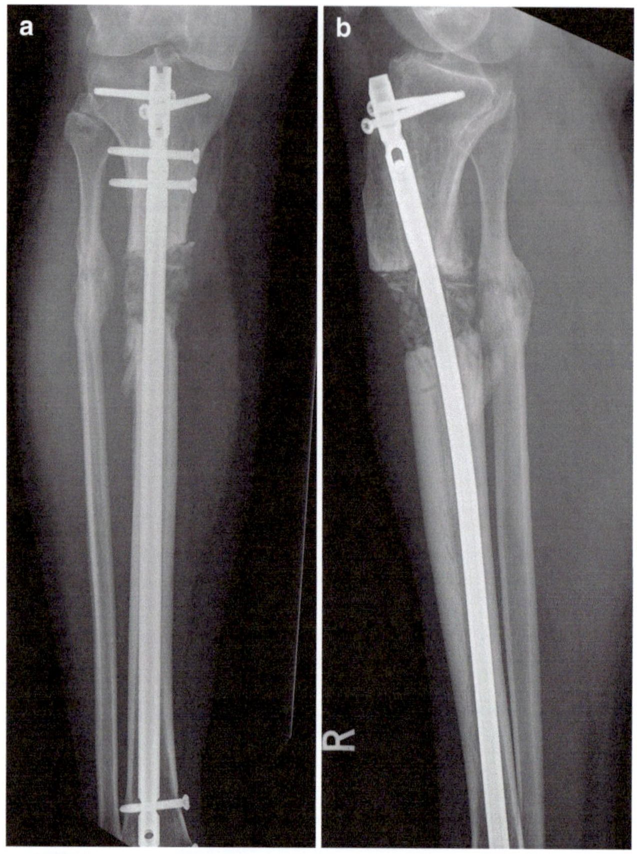

Fig. 7.53 Masquelet technique stage 2. The cement has been removed, and length has been maintained with the nail AP (**a**) and lateral (**b**) view. The gap at the fracture site is packed with bone graft

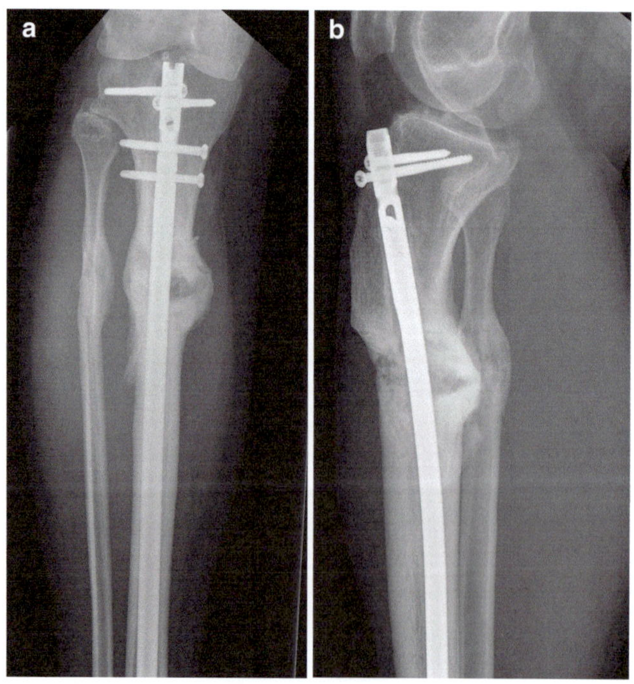

Fig. 7.54 Masquelet technique—end result. Note that tibial length has been maintained, and there is evidence of fresh bone filling the gap in the fracture site AP (**a**) and lateral (**b**) view

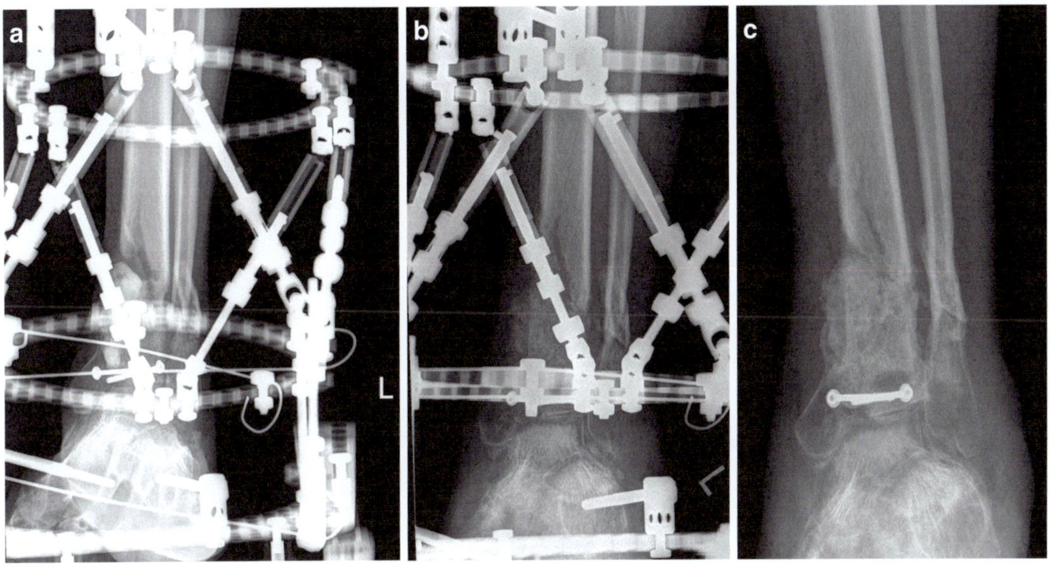

Fig. 7.55 Masquelet technique used in a Pilon fracture. (**a**, **b**) demonstrate the Taylor-Spatial frame with cement at the fracture site, and subsequently the presence of the induction membrane. (**c**) shows evidence of new bone formation at the fracture site. Two screws used to stabilise the articular block have been left in situ

tures with loss of significant bone stock (Fig. 7.55). In these cases, an external fixator is often used to immobilise the fracture during stages one and two of the procedure.

References

1. Prayson MJ, Iossi MF, Buchalter D, Vogt M, Towers J. Safe zone for anterior cortical perforation of the ulna during tension band fixation: a magnetic resonance imaging analysis. J Shoulder Elbow Surg. 2008;17(1):121–5.
2. Gurusamy K, Parker MJ, Rowlands TK. The complications of displaced intracapsular fractures of the hip: the effect of screw positioning and angulation on fracture healing. J Bone Joint Surg Br. 2005;87(5):632–4.
3. Baumgaertner MR, Curtin SL, Lindskog DM, Keggi JM. The value of tip-apex distance in predicting failure of fixation of peritrochanteric fracture of the hip. J Bone Joint Surg Am. 1995;77A:1058–64.
4. Baumgaertner MR, Solberg BD. Awareness of tip-apex distance reduced failure of fixation of trochanteric fractures of the hip. J Bone Joint Surg Br. 1997;79(6):969–71.
5. Abram SGF, Pollard TCB, Andrade AJMD. Inadequate three point proximal fixation predicts failure of Gamma nail. Bone Joint J. 2013;95(B):825–30.
6. Schatzker J, McBroom R, Bruce D. The tibial plateau fracture. The Toronto experience 1968-1975. Clin Orthop Relat Res. 1979;138:94–104.

Hand and Wrist Implants

8

Tamsin Wilkinson, Ryan Trickett, and Carlos Heras-Palou

The development of arthroplasty in the hand and wrist lags behind that of the larger joints, and as yet, there is no clear consensus on the best overall material or configuration for most joint replacements. As a result, there is a proliferation of replacements on the market, most of which have only short-term results available. This chapter is, therefore, not a comprehensive atlas of all replacements but endeavors to provide an idea of radiological appearances. Some specialized fusions have been included as well.

The Hand

Replacements in the small joints of the hand consist of either resurfacing arthroplasty, or spacers, which are usually made of silicone. The arthroplasties are very dependent on the availability of bone stock for implant fixation and soft tissue integrity for joint stability, which are commonly both destroyed in the inflammatory arthropathies. Arthroplasty is therefore generally reserved for posttraumatic or osteoarthritis. To date, the available evidence suggests that resurfacing arthroplasties provide pain relief but do not improve range of motion. Both metal and pyrocarbon resurfacing arthoplasties exist. The biomechanical properties of pyrocarbon mimic that of cortical bone more closely and thus theoretically should lead to less stress shielding and therefore less loosening of the implant. However, a non-progressive lucent line is frequently noted around these implants.

In the presence of an inflammatory or post-infective arthritis, where there is significant bone loss or loss of soft tissue integrity, resurfacing arthroplasty is contraindicated and a choice must be made between a silicone spacer or fusion of the joint. When making this decision, the functional requirements of the different parts of the hand should be considered. In general terms, the radial half of the hand is used for pinch, tripod, and key grip. This involves holding the digits in slight extension, with significant lateral loading, so fusion of the index and middle fingers provides strength and stability with limited effect on function. Similarly, the thumb can be considered a stable post that the fingers grip against, and fusion of the thumb is usually tolerated well. The ulnar half of the hand, however, is used predominantly for power grip, and this relies on the ability to curl the fingers into deep flexion. Fusion of the ring and little fingers is therefore much less tolerated, and silicone spacers should be considered.

In general, no replacement in the hand allows the patient to regain much in the way of movement, and in the presence of an already stiff, but painful joint, fusion is a more reliable long-term option than replacement. However, in very

T. Wilkinson (✉) · R. Trickett
University Hospital of Wales, Cardiff, UK
e-mail: admin@valehandsurgery.com

C. Heras-Palou
Pulvertaft Hand Centre, Derby, UK

S. Agarwal, G. J. Bansal (eds.), *Radiology of Orthopedic Implants*,
https://doi.org/10.1007/978-3-319-76009-4_8

mobile but painful proximal inter phalangeal joints (PIPJ) or metacarpophalangeal joints (MCPJ), the patient will find it hard to adapt to the loss of movement, and arthroplasty should be considered.

Metacarpophalangeal Joints

The history of MCPJ replacement dates back to the 1950s, when initially, metal hinges were used. These rapidly loosened, with bone erosion and metal debris abounding. Following the success of the early hip replacements, a similar design was used for the MCPJ, incorporating a metal head within a high-density polyethylene cup. Again, breakage and erosion were problematic. Interest then moved to the silicone spacer, and a variety of metal/silicone devices were developed. Of these, the Swanson [1] has proved the most durable and is still in use today. The principle of Swanson's joint replacement is a flexible silicone spacer which is inserted into the medullary canal of the bone on either side of the joint, following resection of the articular surfaces. This acts as a constrained prosthesis to maintain joint alignment, but the combination of the implant flexibility and the ability of the tapered stems to piston in and out of the medullary canal permits the joint to maintain range. The silicone promotes the formation of a fibrous capsule, thus increasing the joint stability (Fig. 8.1).

These spacers do not, however, replicate the normal rotating and gliding action of the MCPJ and thus do not restore normal function. They also have a tendency to fracture at the hinge over time (although fracture does not invariably

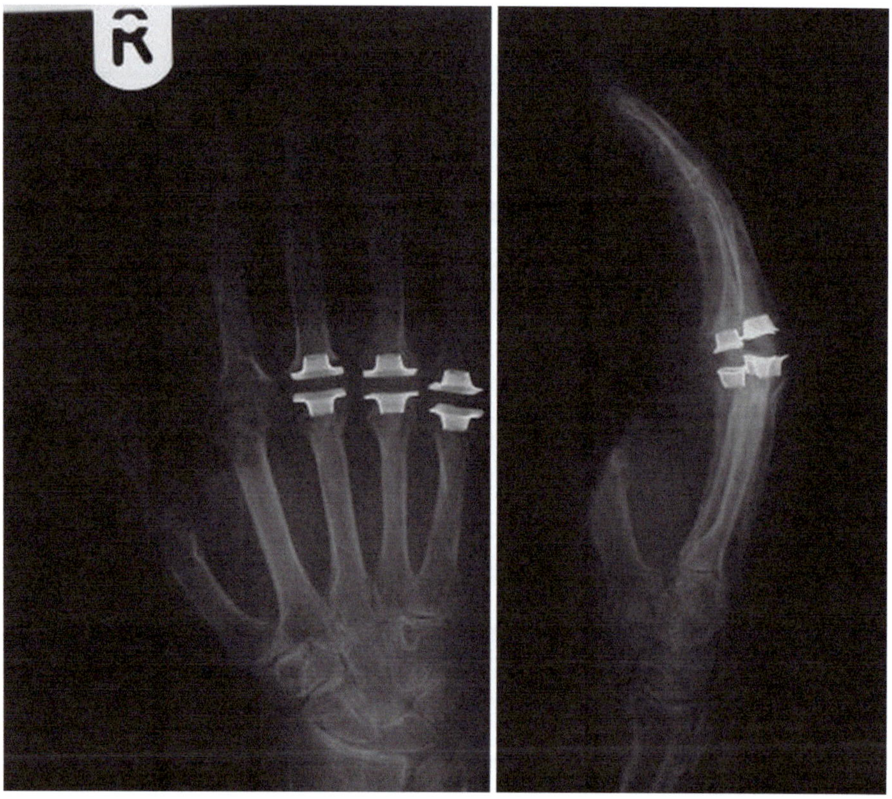

Fig. 8.1 Silicone metacarpophalangeal joint replacements in the middle, ring, and little fingers of the right hand. The flat cut of the resected joint surfaces is noted, compared to the irregular erosions on the index finger MCPJ. The silicone spacer is not visible on X-ray. The metal components are cuffs, called grommets, which sit just within the medullary canal, around the neck of the spacer, and were originally designed to strengthen the implant. Their use has been largely abandoned as they offer no protection against implant fracture of the silicone

necessitate revision) and, although still the most commonly used type of implant, are now generally reserved for lower-demand patients.

The motion of the MCPJ varies depending on its position. In flexion, it moves predominantly in the sagittal plane, but in extension, some adduction and abduction in the coronal plane are permitted. This complex action is best replicated by two separate articulating components. For these to function as a joint, there must be sufficient soft tissue stability to maintain the alignment of the components throughout their range of motion.

Cobalt-chrome and ultrahigh molecular weight polyethylene (UHMWPE) MCPJ replacements have been designed to replicate the three-dimension shape of the native anatomy [2]. They consist of a proximal cobalt-chrome head and a distal polyethylene cup. They are cemented in situ, and this makes revision difficult due to subsequent loss of bone stock. Results are equivalent to those for silicone arthroplasty. They are highly dependent on intact soft tissue for stability and coverage.

More commonly used, but still with relatively short-term follow-up, are pyrocarbon resurfacing arthroplasties. These consist of two, uncemented (press fit) pyrocarbon implants, which are designed to replicate the native anatomy. They rely on intact soft tissues for stability, but the absence of cement makes revision easier, as bone stock is preserved (Fig. 8.2). They seem to provide reasonable

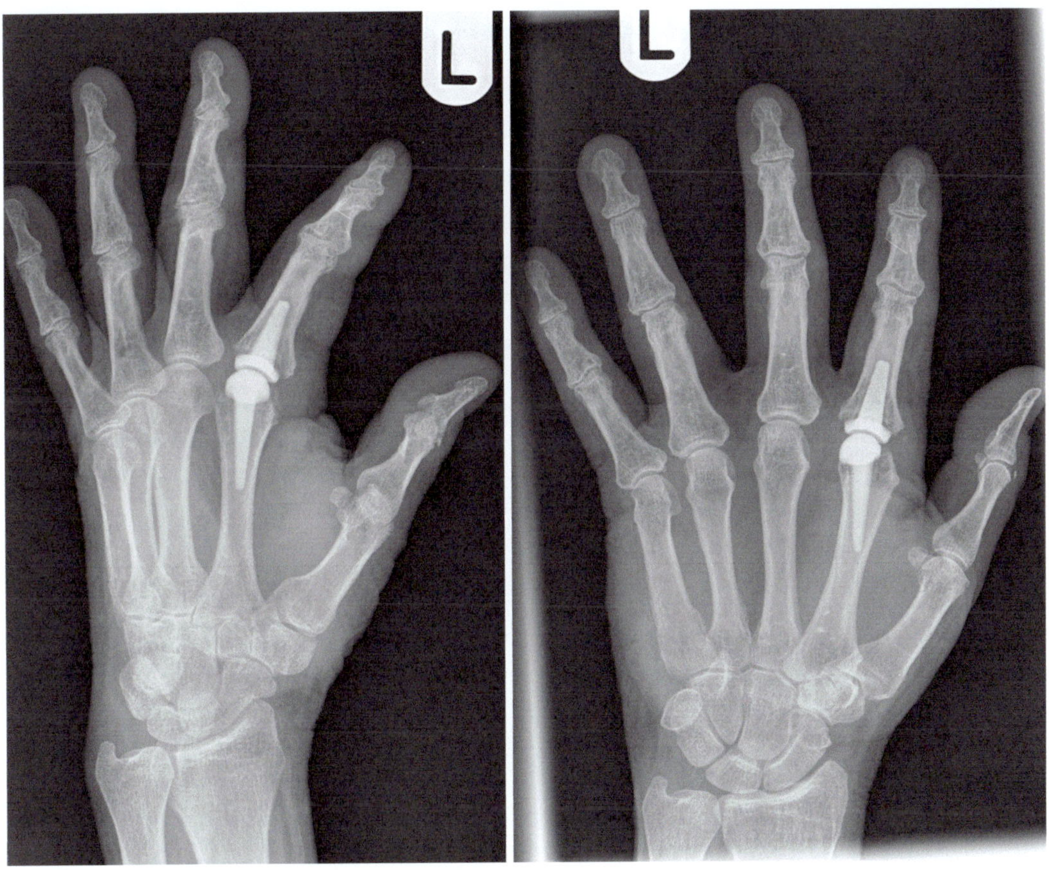

Fig. 8.2 Pyrocarbon metacarpophalangeal joint replacement of the left index finger. The pyrocarbon is a similar density to cortical bone on X-ray, as distinct from ceramic or metal, which look completely white. The area which has been reamed to allow the press fit of the components can be seen as a halo around the implants. It should be noted that the metacarpal head component has not been inserted centrally, but instead, replicates the load bearing articulation of the native joint

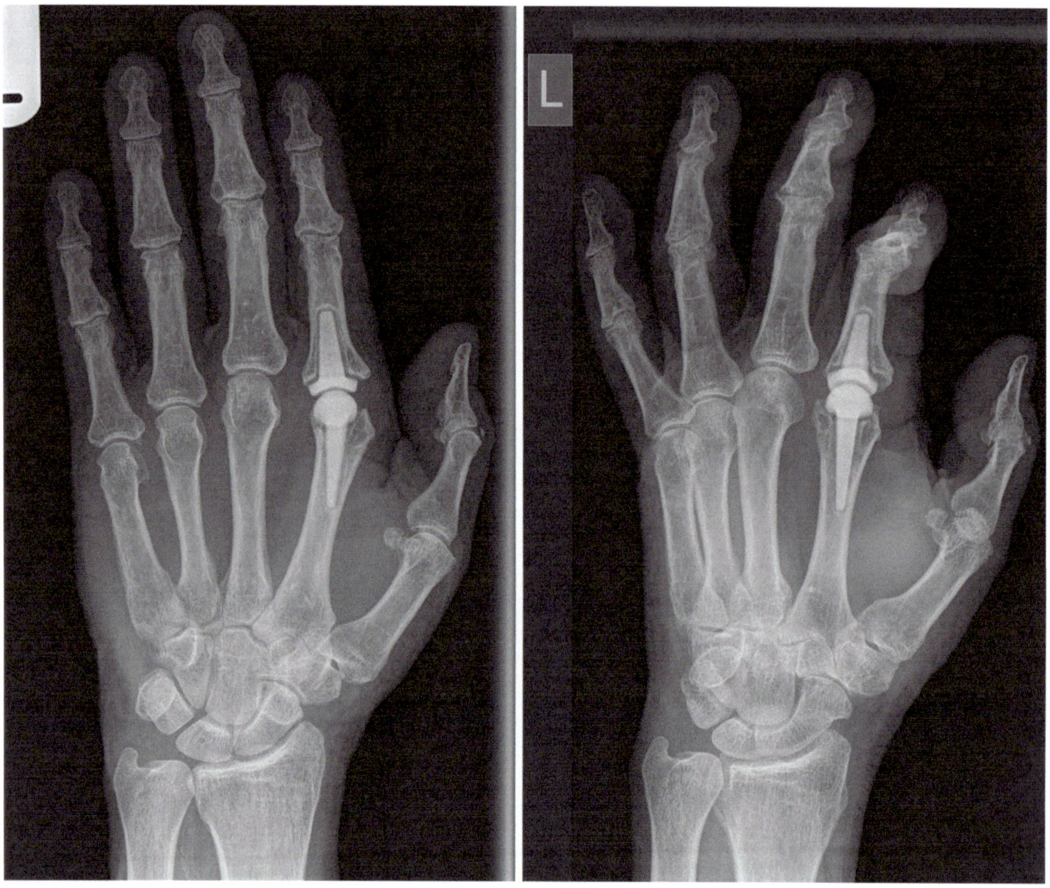

Fig. 8.3 Lysis around the pyrocarbon MCPJ replacement. Subsequent X-rays of the same patient show a clear area of lysis around the implants. The edges of this lysis are clearly defined and well demarcated, with no surrounding erosions or bone reaction. This is commonly seen in these joint replacements and should be followed up radiographically. A nonprogressive lytic region of up to 1 mm surrounding the prosthesis is not considered pathological

pain relief and, in the MCPJ, a slight increase in range of movement of about 10°. Evidence of nonprogressive lysis around the components is common, as is subsidence (Fig. 8.3). In asymptomatic patients, these radiographic changes do not necessitate revision. Stability of these implants relies on adequate soft tissues (Fig. 8.4). If these joints are revised, they are usually exchanged for a silicone arthroplasty. Most studies report average follow-up of 5 years, with reasonable patient satisfaction [3–5].

Proximal Interphalangeal Joint

The development of proximal interphalangeal joint replacements has followed a similar path to the MCPJ, with silicone spacers remaining the gold standard. However, the even smaller size of the joint, and the complex soft tissue balancing, often on a background of degenerate soft tissues preoperatively, means that results have been less satisfactory overall. The joints have to withstand large loads, particularly during pinch grip, and the surgical approach requires release and subse-

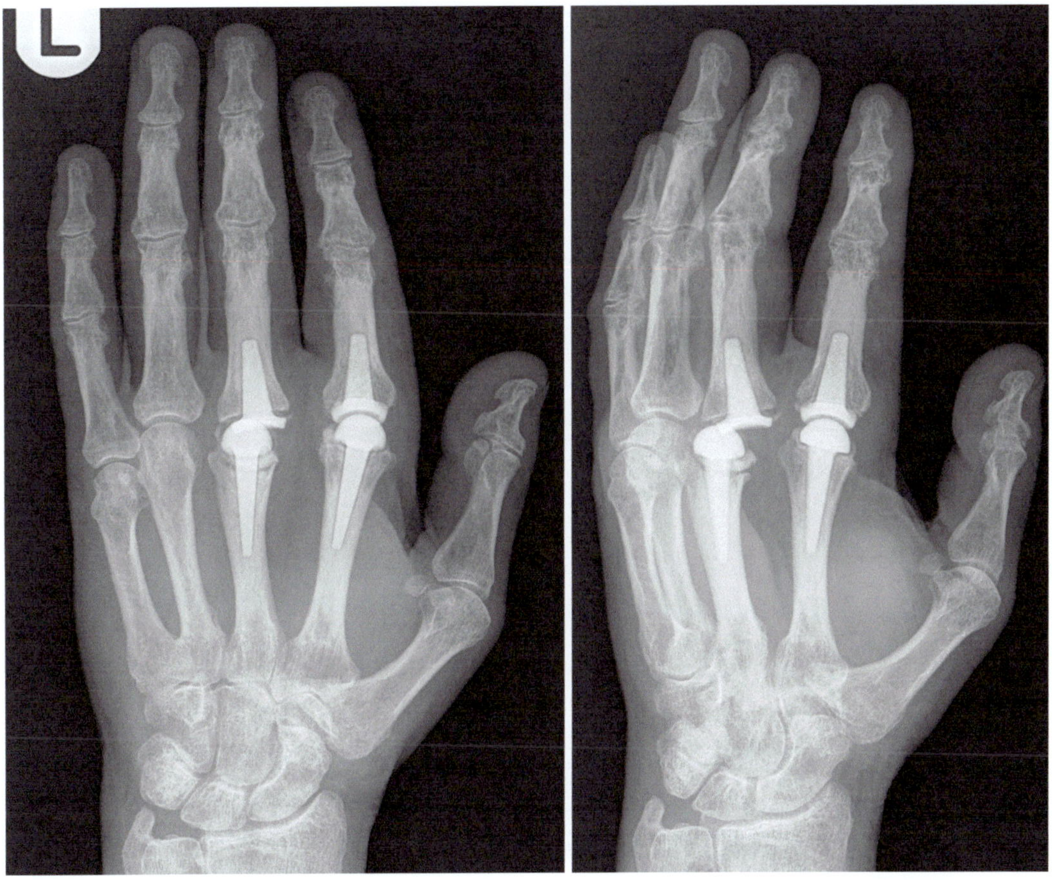

Fig. 8.4 Dislocated pyrocarbon MCPJ replacement. In this X-ray, the index and middle MCPJ have been replaced with pyrocarbon resurfacing components. Alignment of the index MCPJ is maintained, but the middle MCPJ has dislocated. There is no inherent stability to the resurfacing arthroplasty, and joint congruency is entirely dependent on the soft tissue constraints. These are often damaged by the underlying pathology preoperatively (such as soft tissue erosions from rheumatoid arthritis), and the extensive surgical approach weakens them still further. Dislocation is a common complication and is usually managed with revision to a silastic implant. In common with Fig. 8.3, a narrow lytic line can be seen surrounding the components. Note also the areas of heterotopic ossifications surrounding the prosthesis

quent repair of the collateral ligaments. Failure of these often leads to unsatisfactory results.

The silicone spacers, by necessity being smaller, are less stiff and less able to resist lateral loading. Particularly in the radial digits, fracture rate of the implant is high and they are very intolerant of preexisting deformity (such as swan neck deformity). They do not show any increase in range of motion from preoperative measurements, but in selected patients, satisfaction is generally good [6].

Pyrocarbon resurfacing of the PIPJ replicates the anatomy of the native joint, and because of the bicondylar design, it provides more lateral stability than the silicone spacers. The surgical approach, however, is similarly unforgiving, and good soft tissue structure preoperatively is a necessity. Numerous studies have shown that preoperative range of motion is preserved, but not increased, following pyrocarbon joint replacement [7], and significant bone erosion and implant subsidence have been demonstrated radiographically. This latter phenomenon is thought to cause a gradual loss of range in these joints but doesn't appear to be associated with

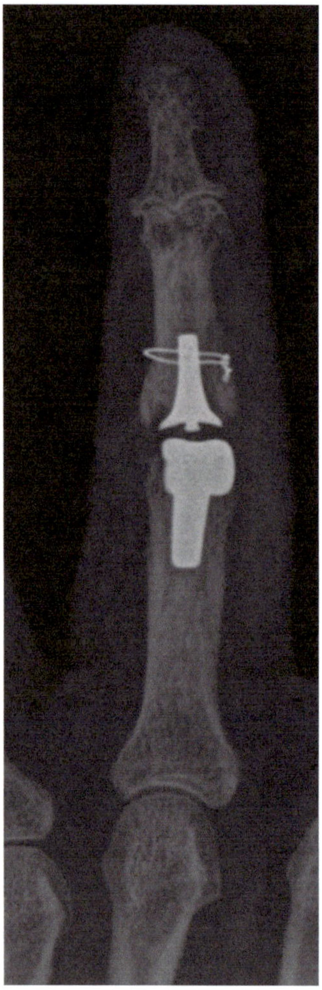

Fig. 8.5 Pyrocarbon proximal interphalangeal joint replacement. The size of the components in the PIPJ is determined by the size of the medullary canal. In this case, it can be seen that the joint surface has expanded in response to the osteoarthritis, and the surface replacements look undersized. However, the stems of the components are well fixed and centrally located in the medullary canal, and it would not have been possible to insert a larger component. The cerclage wire around the middle phalanx has been placed there intraoperatively to treat a split in the cortex which occurred during reaming. When managed in this way, these splits usually go on to unite, as in this case, without resulting in instability of the components

either pain or dissatisfaction (Fig. 8.5). A slightly unusual complaint is an audible squeak from the joint, which has not been fully explained. Revision is sometimes requested for this! Titanium semiconstrained implants have a high failure rate due to extensive osteolysis and consequent loosening (Fig. 8.6).

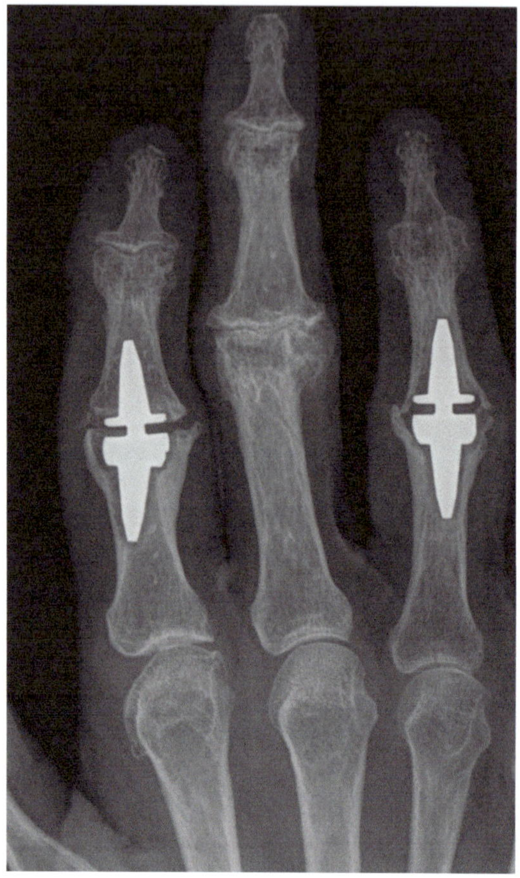

Fig. 8.6 Failure of the titanium semiconstrained PIPJ replacement. The LPM PIPJ replacement was introduced in 2000. The two titanium implants are constrained by a central hinge. Nearly 50% were showing signs of failure within 6 years. In this image, massive lysis around the components can be seen. Unlike the well-demarcated lysis seen in Fig. 8.3, the cortices here are being eroded and there is significant subsidence of the components

Distal Interphalangeal Joint

There are no resurfacing arthroplasties available for the distal interphalangeal joint (DIPJ), but there are Swanson's silicone spacers in use. Radiographic appearances are similar to other silicone spacers. However, fusion of the DIPJ remains the gold standard and by far the most commonly used surgical treatment for arthritis of this joint.

Carpometacarpal Joint of the Thumb

The carpometacarpal joint of the thumb (CMCJ) is the most commonly operated on joint for arthritis in the hand. It has an incredibly complex articular shape, often described as “saddle shaped,” with two arcs of curvature which enable circumduction of the thumb metacarpal. The combination of high load on gripping and flexibility of the surrounding soft tissues leads to a high rate of arthritis in this joint (30% of women and 12% of men).

The gold standard for surgical treatment of arthritis in the thumb CMCJ remains excision of the trapezium. Soft tissue stabilization procedures at the same time are popular, but have not been found to lead to superior results [8]. Satisfaction is generally high, but some patients complain of weakened grip strength, and in patients with ongoing pain following trapeziectomy (15%), there are few salvage options.

For these reasons, the search for an acceptable joint replacement has been ongoing. The unique articular shape of the CMCJ has proved challenging to replicate, and numerous articulations have been trialed, some with more success than others. Two implant types will be discussed, the total joint replacement and the interposition arthroplasty.

Interposition arthroplasty is appealing, as it has the potential to maintain thumb length and grip strength, with minimal surgical exposure and limited bone resection, thus facilitating subsequent revision. Implants are commonly made of pyrocarbon and are usually either spherical or disc shaped. They most frequently fail by dislocation. The disc-shaped implants have a hole through the center to allow a ligamentous constraint to be passed through, with the aim of preventing this. As yet, they have not been shown to have superior clinical results to simple trapeziectomy (Fig. 8.7).

There has been more success with joint replacements, but the design of these still has its

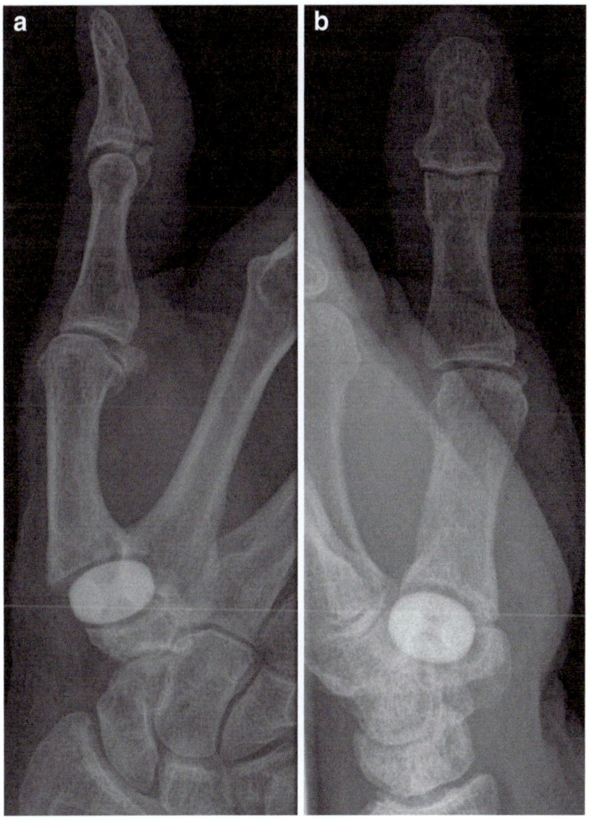

Fig. 8.7 Pyrodisc thumb carpometacarpal joint interposition prosthesis. This pyrocarbon prosthesis is shaped like a doughnut, with a central hole. This allows a section of tendon to be passed through to hold the prosthesis within the resected joint space. The curved resections of the base of the thumb metacarpal and trapezium match the surface contours of the pyrodisc. Height of the thumb metacarpal (and thus length of the thumb) has been maintained. There has been only limited bony resection required. Results of implant arthroplasty of the thumb CMCJ remain mixed. AP (**a**) and lateral (**b**) view

limitations. The older designs consist of monoblock "spacers," with stems inserted into the thumb metacarpal. These can either be silastic or titanium. More recent designs usually consist of a stemmed ball, fitted into the thumb metacarpal, and a screw-fit hydroxyapatite-coated socket in the trapezium. The articulation of these implants is usually a cobalt-chrome metal on metal design and is unconstrained (Fig. 8.8). Nineteen different types have been recorded, none of which have shown superior results to trapeziectomy [9]. A review of total arthroplasties from the Norwegian Joint Registry found a total of five different implants used, with an average survival rate of 91% at 5 years and 90% at 10 years. However, they stress that survival was defined as not having been revised and did not necessarily imply that the implants were functioning well [10]. Implants fail by dislocation, loosening, or periprosthetic fracture. In those implants that survive, however, patients report good pain relief, range of motion, grip strength and high satisfaction [11].

It is clear that CMCJ arthroplasty requires considerable development before it can match simple trapeziectomy in efficacy; however, the more recent designs have promising early results, and they may become more popular in the future.

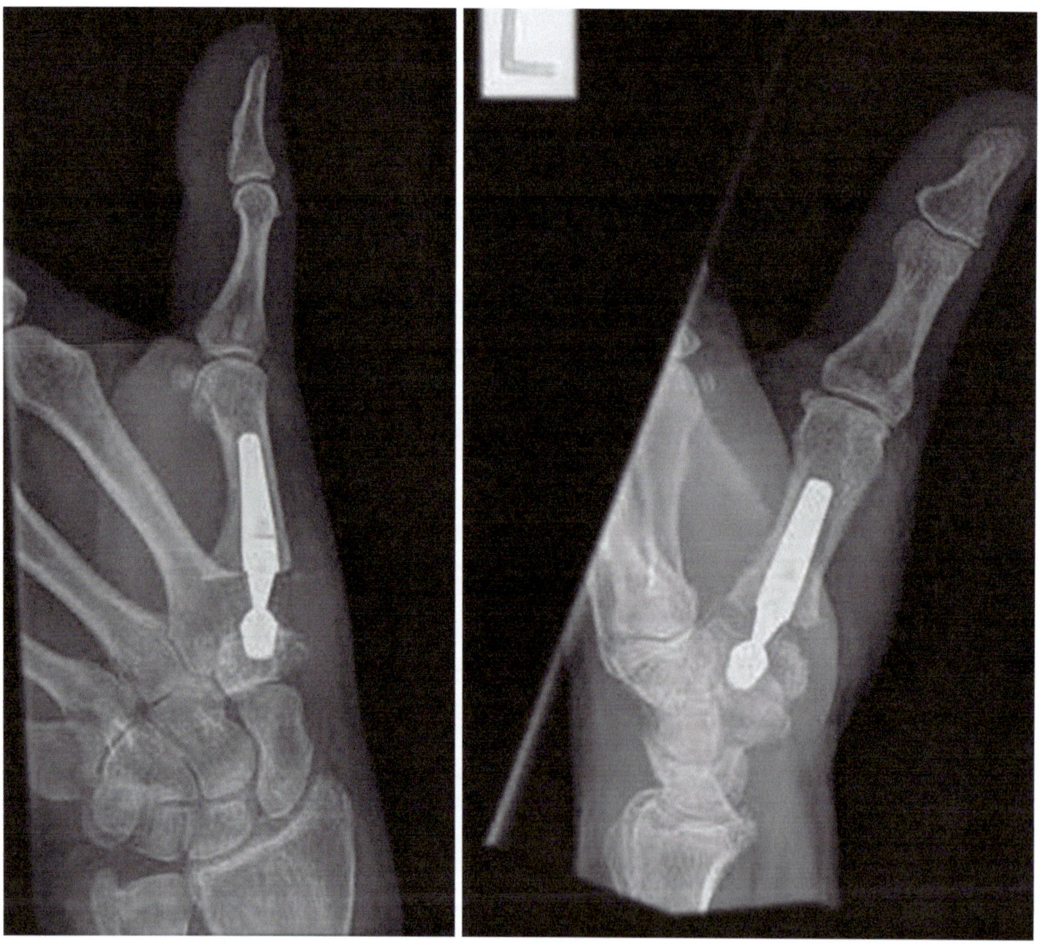

Fig. 8.8 The Elektra thumb CMCJ prosthesis. The proximal thumb metacarpal has been resected and a modular stemmed head has been inserted. In the trapezium, a hydroxyapatite-coated threaded cup has been impacted. There is little mechanical constraint to this prosthesis and the small bone size means that periprosthetic fracture is a risk. It can be seen that the height of the thumb metacarpal has been maintained, and the axis of the thumb articulation is well aligned, meaning that subsequent Z deformity should not occur

The Wrist

The wrist consists of three separate articulations, the midcarpal joint, the radio and ulnar carpal joint, and the distal radioulnar joint (DRUJ). A discussion regarding the biomechanics and the consequent effects of arthroplasty of these joints is beyond the scope of this chapter, but some examples will be illustrated.

The midcarpal and radioulnar carpal joints are primarily responsible for flexion and extension of the wrist, approximately 50% of the range coming from each articulation. The radioulnar carpal joint is largely responsible for radial and ulnar deviation of the wrist. The distal radioulnar joint (DRUJ), the proximal radioulnar joint, and the diaphysis of each bone, held by the interosseous membrane, in combination, permit pronosupination of the forearm. The DRUJ should therefore be considered separate from the wrist, although it is often involved in wrist joint pathology.

Radio Carpal and Midcarpal Joints

Arthritis of the midcarpal and radio carpal joints is most commonly treated with fusion of the affected joints. Numerous implants exist to fuse the small joints in isolation, but they can also be fused using headless compression screws or simple k-wires. Non-union is becoming less common as locking implant technology allows greater compression and stability but should be considered in a patient with ongoing pain.

Fusion across either the radio carpal joint or the midcarpal joint will sacrifice 50% of the flexion-extension range but is well tolerated (Fig. 8.9).

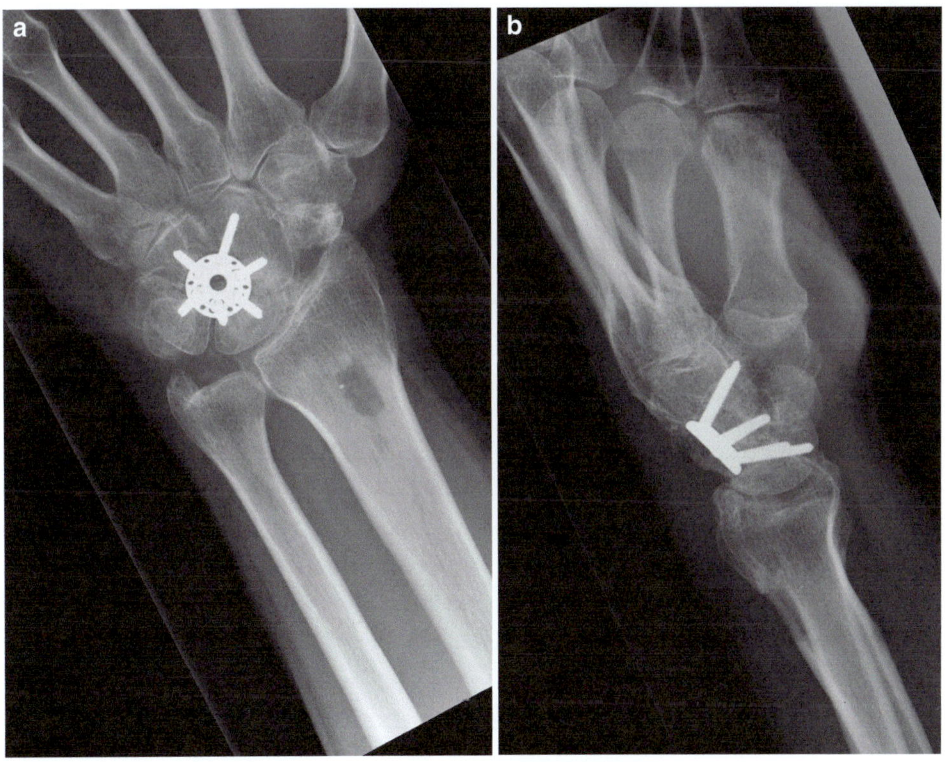

Fig. 8.9 The four-corner fusion. This plate has locking screw holes to allow rigid fixation of the midcarpal, lunotriquetral, and capitohamate joints. The scaphoid has been excised to treat either a non-union, AVN, or radioscaphoid osteoarthritis, and the remainder of the carpus have been fused to prevent collapse of the carpal height. The defect in the distal radial metaphysis is iatrogenic and is the site where bone graft has been taken to fill the intercarpal spaces. AP (**a**) and lateral (**b**) view

Total wrist arthrodesis spans the radio carpal, midcarpal, and usually the third carpometacarpal (CMCJ) joints. It abolishes all flexion and extension and radial and ulnar deviation at the wrist but provides excellent long-term pain relief and good strength. The wrist is usually fused in 15° of extension, to facilitate power grip (Figs. 8.10 and 8.11). Unilateral wrist arthrodesis is well tolerated, but lack of flexion is disabling when bilateral wrist arthrodesis is performed. Non-union of the third CMCJ is common, and more recent plate designs abolish the need to span this joint.

Total wrist replacement is predominantly used for low demand patients, often with a contralateral wrist fusion. The indication is pain relief where some preservation of movement is required [12]. It is typically used in patients with rheumatoid arthritis.

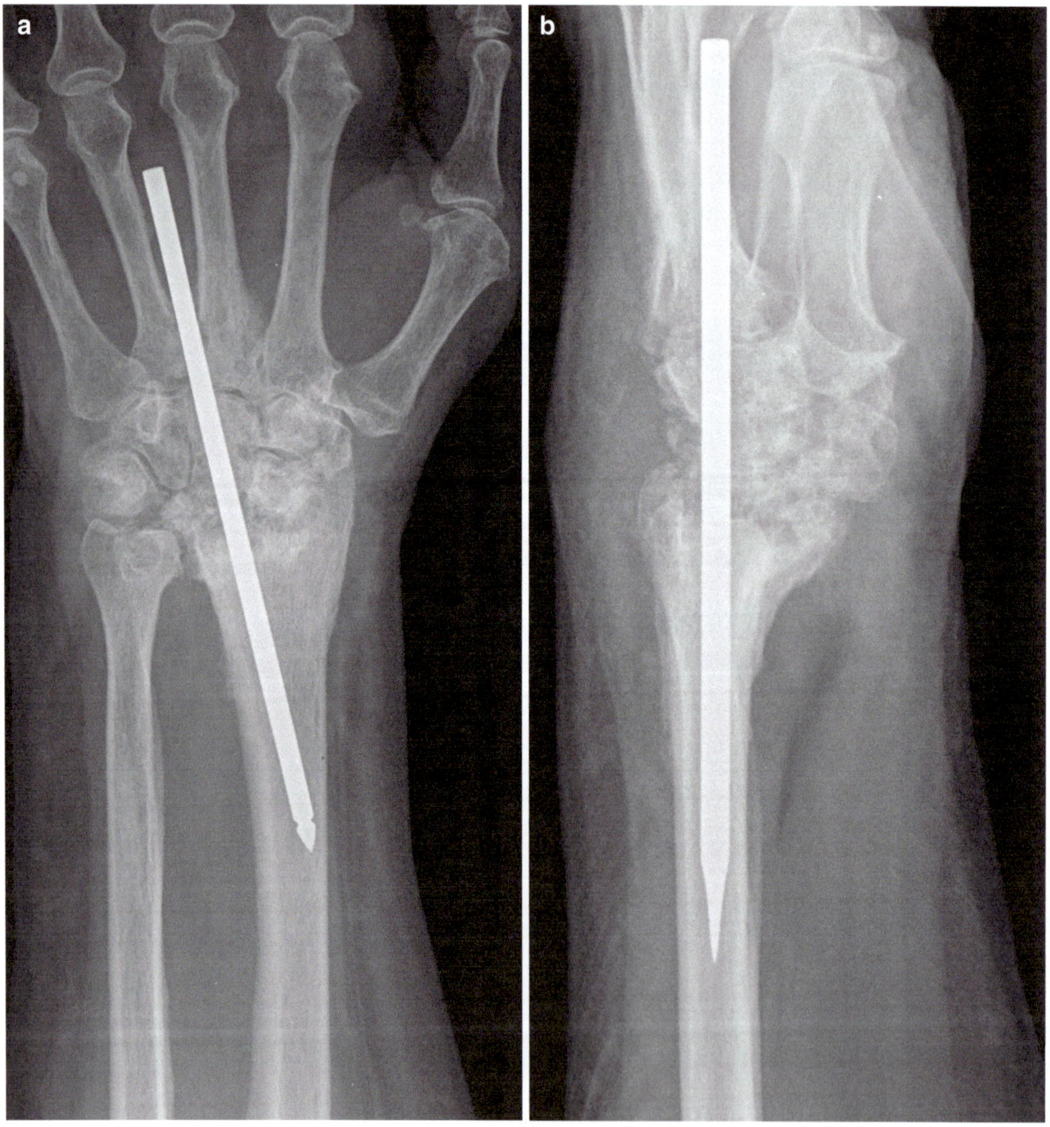

Fig. 8.10 Wrist fusion using a Steinman pin. This patient with severe erosive arthritis from rheumatoid disease has had a wrist fusion using a Steinman pin to stabilize the carpus onto the distal radius. The Steinman pin can also be inserted through the head of the third metacarpal. AP (**a**) and lateral (**b**) view

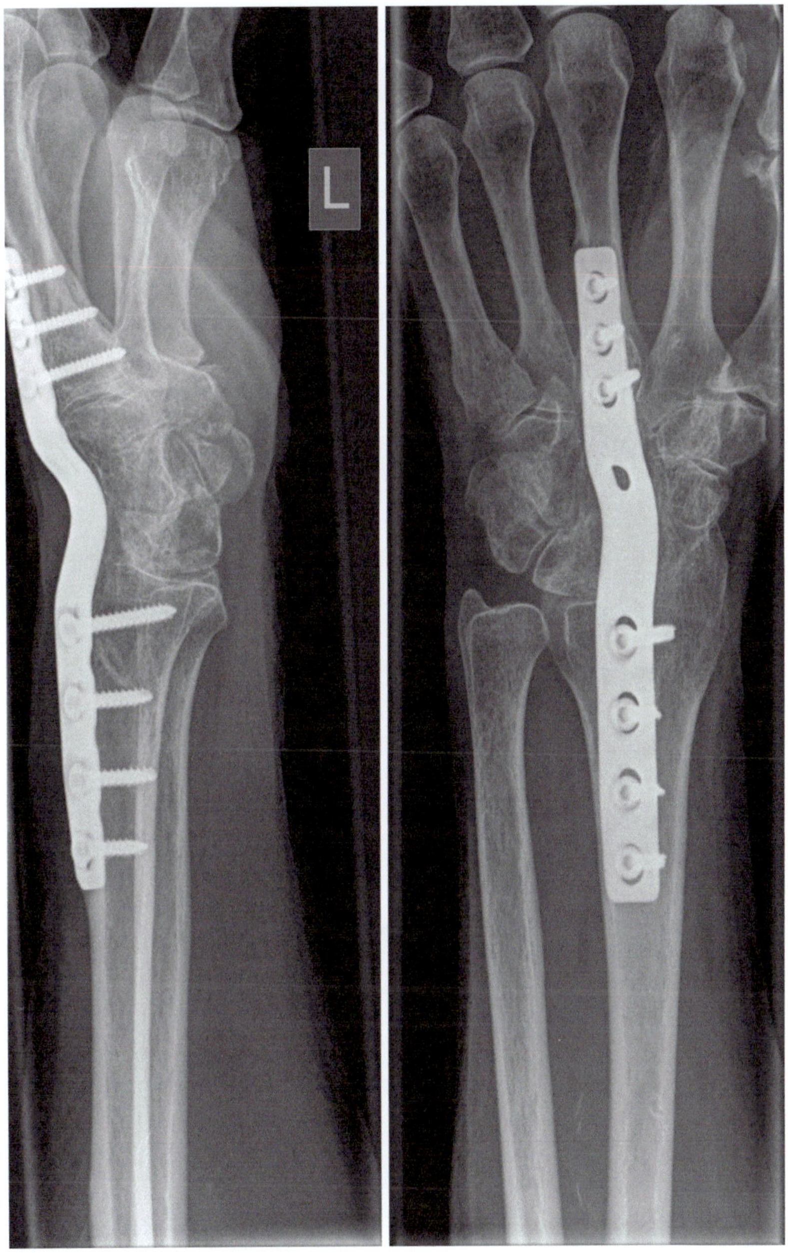

Fig. 8.11 The Synthes wrist fusion plate. This patient with osteoarthritis and well-preserved carpal height has had a dorsal wrist plate, spanning the radius, carpus, and third metacarpal. The third carpometacarpal and lunotriquetral joints have not been excised. The radioscaphoid and scapholunocapitate joints have fused. Note that the wrist is fixed in slight extension to enable power grip

Early wrist replacements have developed along similar lines to the hand arthroplasties. The earliest examples are Swanson's silastic spacers. These demonstrated considerable problems with instability of the hand, implant breakage, and synovitis and have now been abandoned. In the 1970s, cemented prostheses with a ball and socket design were introduced. These have also been abandoned due to poor soft tissue balancing, loosening, and periprosthetic fracture. More recent designs utilize an offset articulation to mimic the dual plane of motion of the wrist and to preserve the soft tissue balancing. Further developments have reduced the amount of bone resection required, thus making subsequent revision or fusion more feasible. The current generation of total wrist replacements is coated with hydroxyapatite and relies on osseous integration in the proximal component and screw and peg fixation with osseous integration distally. The majority employ a metal on polyethylene bearing and are designed to replicate the anatomical shape of the distal radius and proximal carpal row. A modular design allows different thicknesses of polyethylene to be selected to enable better soft tissue balancing. These designs allow flexion and extension and radial and ulnar deviation at the wrist but permit only very limited or no pronosupination at the carpus, which many rheumatoid patients rely on for function (Figs. 8.12 and 8.13).

A recent review of the evidence for total wrist replacement looked at the results for seven different manufacturers. Follow-up was reported up to 10.8 years (for the Universal). Survivorship ranged from 50% at 7.3 (5–10.8) years to 100% at 5.5 (3–9) years. All prostheses demonstrated improved pain scores postoperatively, although when compared to arthrodesis, pain scores do not improve as much. Only one,

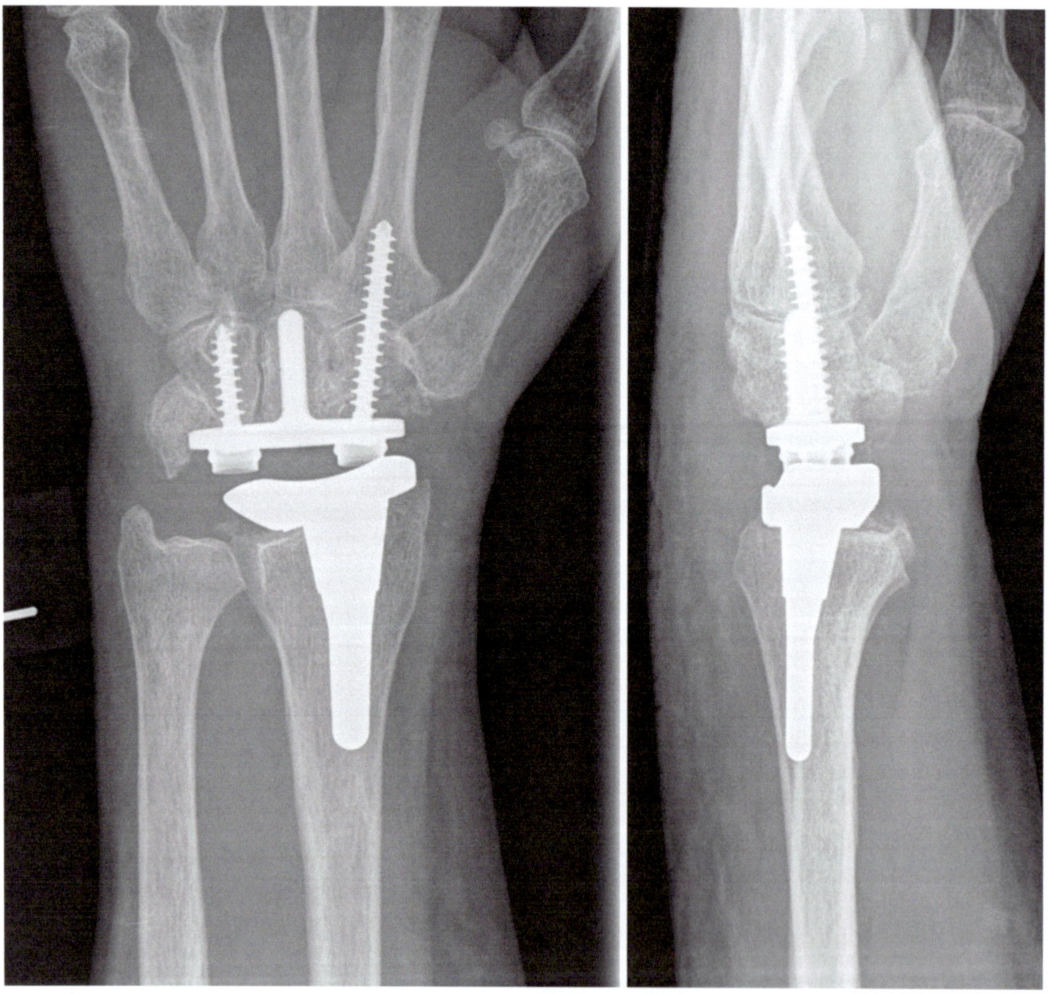

Fig. 8.12 Total wrist replacement. The proximal carpal row has been excised and an oblique cut has been made at the distal radius. The proximal part of the prosthesis is coated with hydroxyapatite and impacted into the shaft of the radius. The distal part is held in place with a hydroxyapatite-coated peg and two screws, one into the hamate and one crossing into the index metacarpal. Between the two cobalt-chrome prostheses, there is a polymer-bearing surface which fixes onto the distal component and articulates with the proximal component. The curvature of the articulating surfaces copies the normal articular dynamics of the radiocarpal joint. AP (left) and lateral (right) view

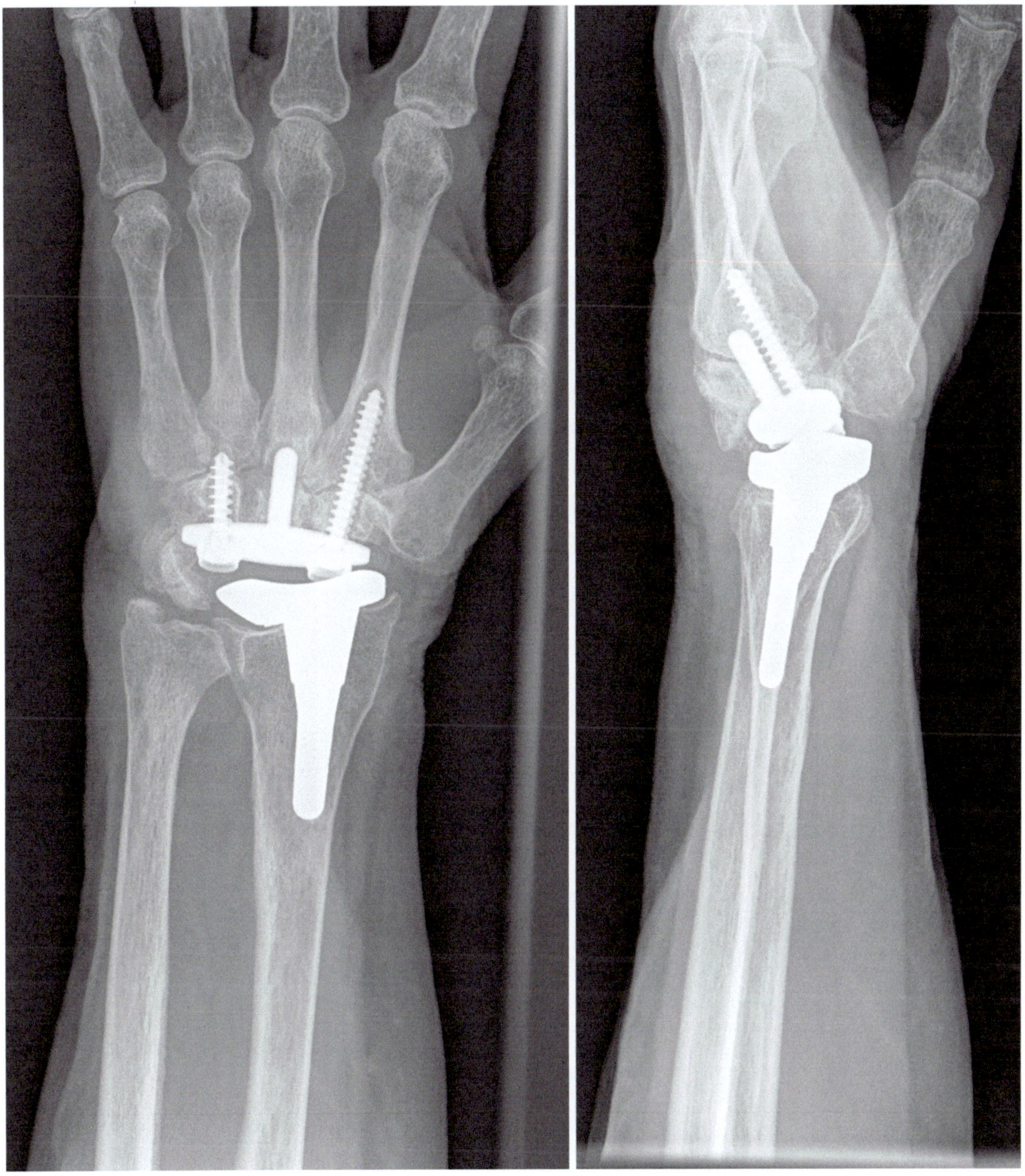

Fig. 8.13 Comparing these images with Fig. 8.12, lysis has developed around the distal component. The screws and pegs have areas of bone loss around them, and the component has subsided into the distal carpal row. The proximal component remains well fixed, with trabecular bone extending up to the metal-bone interface

the Maestro, demonstrated a functional range of motion. The remainder tended to show that the preoperative range of motion was preserved but not improved. Data for grip strength was insufficient [13]. It is clear that total wrist replacement currently lags significantly behind that of larger joints in its efficacy, and fusion remains the gold standard.

The Distal Radioulnar Joint

The distal radioulnar joint (DRUJ) has a complex gliding and rolling motion with stability largely provided by the soft tissue constraints of the triangular fibrocartilaginous complex (TFCC) and the tension in the interosseous membrane. Pathology of the DRUJ consists of either arthritis, leading to pain and loss of forearm rotation, or instability, which can cause pain and loss of grip strength and a feeling of "giving way."

Traditional approaches to management of DRUJ pathology were to either excise the distal ulna (Darrach's procedure) or to fuse the DRUJ and perform an osteotomy proximal to the DRUJ articulation to allow forearm rotation (Sauve-Kapandji procedure). Both of these procedures can lead to instability of the ulnar stump and painful abutment between the ulna and radius (Fig. 8.14). The salvage options for these patients are a soft tissue stabilization procedure, arthroplasty, or a one-bone forearm,

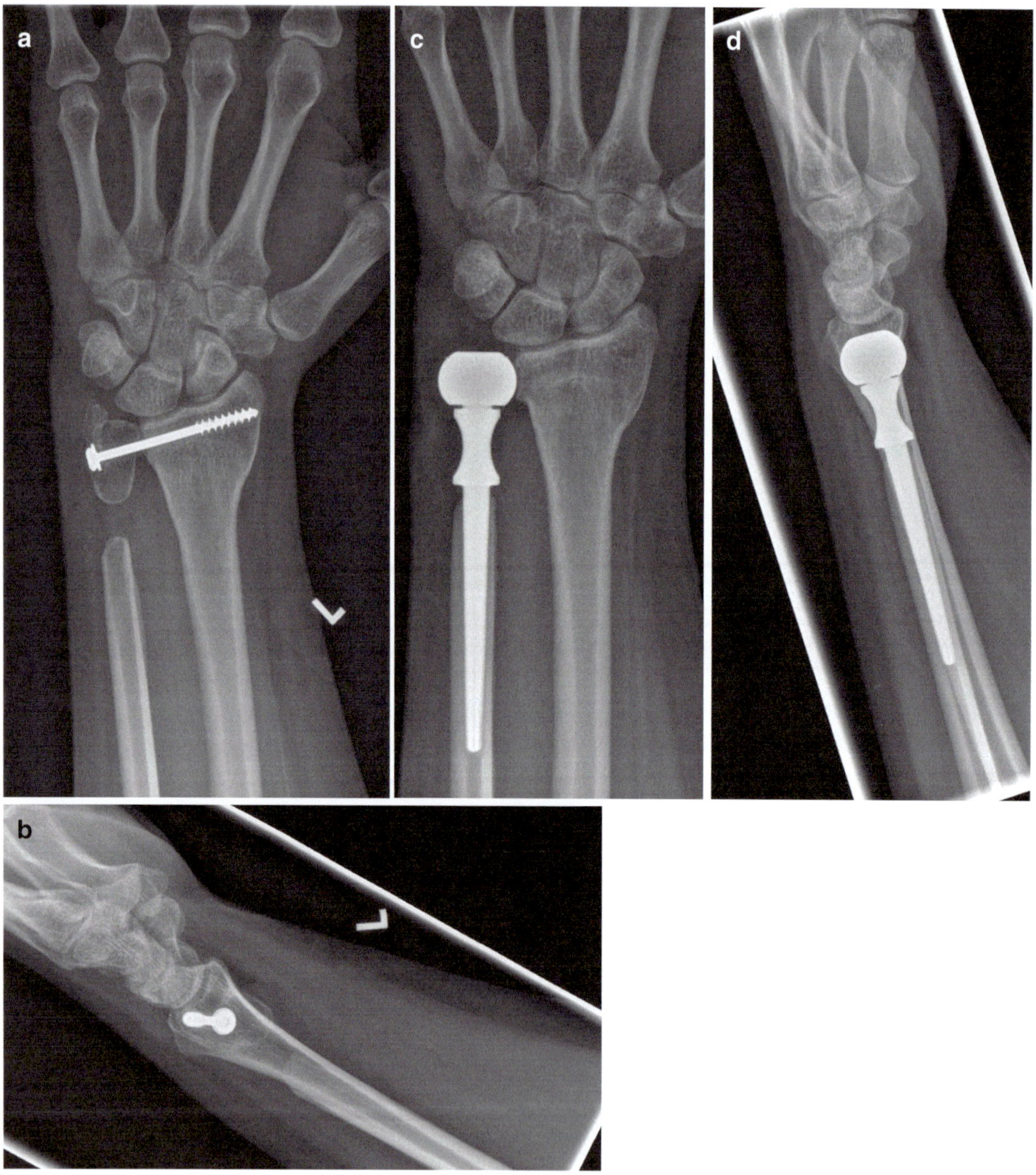

Fig. 8.14 Postoperative images of a Sauve-Kapandji procedure, revised to a Herbert distal ulna prosthesis. Remodeling of the ulnar border of the distal radial metaphysis can be seen in response to abutment of the unstable ulnar stump. The Herbert distal ulna prosthesis is modular, consisting of a press-fit titanium stem, variable neck lengths to allow for differing levels of ulna resection, and a ceramic head which replicates the anatomy of the native distal ulna. It relies on ECU function for DRUJ stability as the TFCC attachments are excised. AP (**a**) and lateral (**b**) view of Sauve-Kapanji procedure. AP (**c**) and lateral (**d**) of Herbert distal ulna replacement

where the radius and ulna are fused in the mid-diaphysis.

Arthroplasties can be divided into ulnar head replacements or DRUJ total arthroplasty.

Ulnar head replacement designs are either a monoblock or modular design, usually consisting of a metal stem and either metal, ceramic, or pyrocarbon articulation. The modular design allows for an extended neck, which can be useful when revising a Sauve-Kapandji procedure, where the osteotomy site is often too proximal for a standard prosthesis (Fig. 8.15).

DRUJ total arthroplasties can again be subdivided into two categories, constrained and semiconstrained. They are considered in patients who have erosion of the sigmoid notch, either at presentation or following distal ulna replacement. Semiconstrained prostheses (Fig. 8.16) have the theoretical advantage of allowing the normal gliding and rolling action of the DRUJ, whereas constrained prostheses permit rotation only. There is, however, only short-term follow-up of small numbers for these prostheses and as yet no conclusions as to which is superior in the long term.

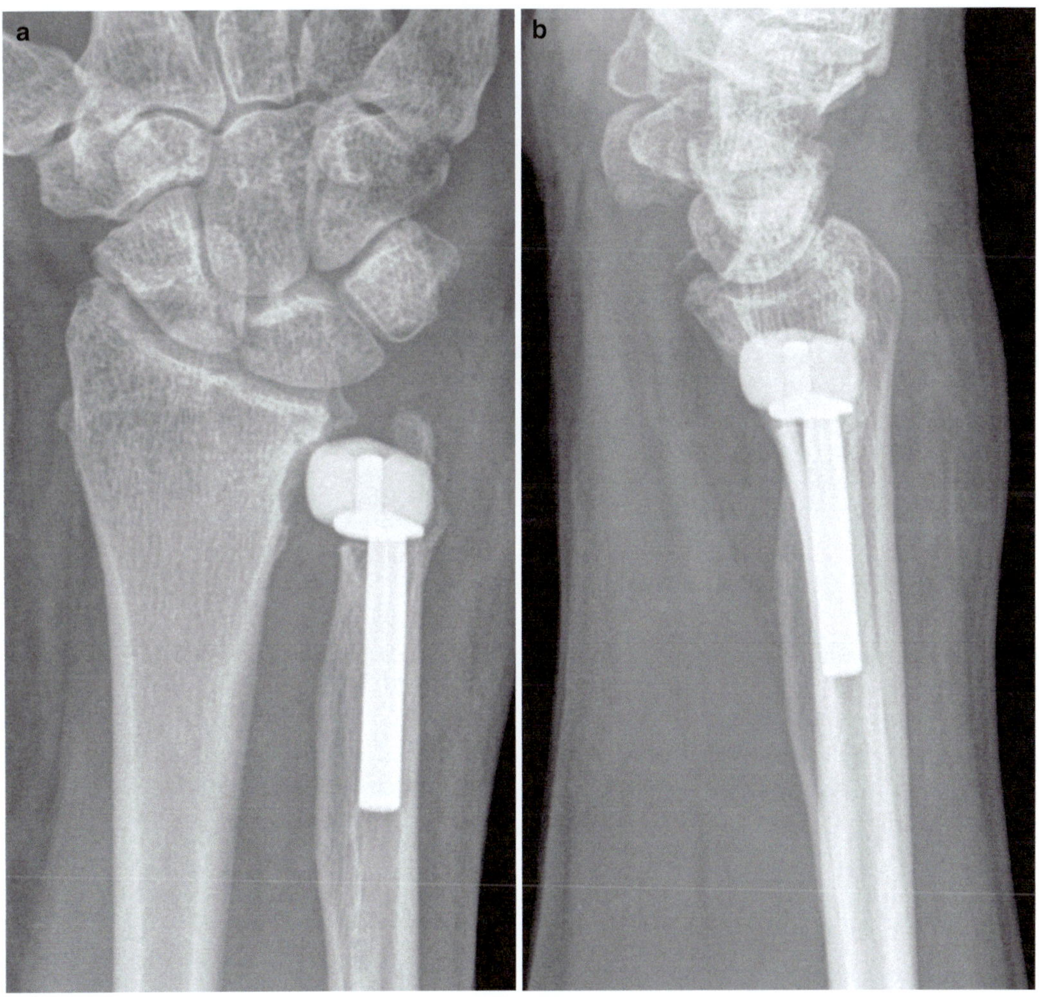

Fig. 8.15 Eclypse ulnar head replacement. This is a modular prosthesis. With a titanium press fit (uncemented) stem and pyrocarbon head. It is designed to replicate the ulnar head. Mobility between the cylindrical peg and the pyrocarbon spacer allows some rotation and proximo-distal translation, and it can be inserted without detaching the normal soft tissue stabilizers of the DRUJ, thus maintaining the normal dynamics of the joint. AP (**a**) and lateral (**b**) view

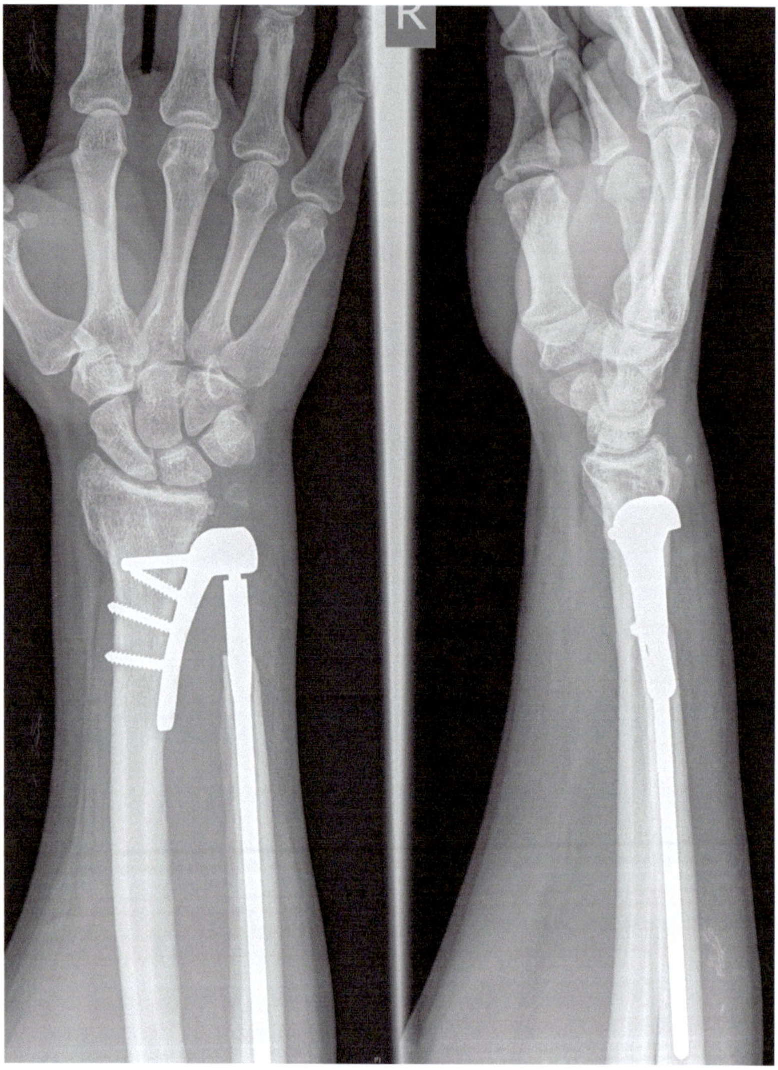

Fig. 8.16 The Scheker (Aptis), semiconstrained total distal radioulnar joint prosthesis. This is used for arthritis of the distal radioulnar joint with instability or following distal ulna resection with stump instability. The constrained design means that stability is maintained even in the absence of the normal soft tissue constraints. Replacement of the sigmoid notch overcomes the problem of notch erosion, and the Scheker can be used as a revision prosthesis. A cobalt-chrome plate is attached to the distal radial metaphysis using a peg and screw fixation. A socket protrudes from this. A cobalt-chrome peg is inserted into the ulnar shaft. This has a highly polished stem distally, onto which is inserted a polyethylene ball. This ball articulates with the cobalt-chrome socket on the radial plate

In summary, arthroplasty for the joints in the hand and wrist is in its infancy when compared to the advances that have been made in larger joints. The prostheses tend to have only short-term follow-up, and a consensus on the best designs has yet to be reached.

References

1. Swanson AB. Silicone rubber implants for replacement of destroyed joints in the hand. Surg Clin North Am. 1968;48:1113–27.
2. Linscheid RL, Beckenbaugh RD. Arthroplasty of the metacarpophalangeal joint. In: Morrey BF, editor. Joint replacement arthroplasty. New York: Churchill Livingstone; 2003.
3. Nunez VA, Citron ND. Short term results of Ascension pyrolytic carbon metacarpophalangeal joint replacement arthroplasty for osteoarthritis. Chir Main. 2005;24:161–4.
4. Parker WL, Rizzo M, Moran SL, et al. Preliminary results of nonconstrained pyrolytic carbon arthroplasty for metacarpophalangeal arthritis. J Hand Surg Am. 2007;32:1496–505.
5. Simpson-White RW, Chojnowski AJ. Pyrocarbon metacarpophalangeal joint replacement in primary osteoarthritis. J Hand Surg Eur. 2014;39(6):575–81.

6. Namdari S, Weiss A-PC. Anatomically neutral silicone small joint arthroplasty for osteoarthritis. J Hand Surg Am. 2009;34A:292–300.
7. Reissner L, Schindele S, Henlser S, Marks M, Herren DB. Ten year follow-up of pyrocarbon implants for proximal interphalangeal joint replacement. J Hand Surg Eur. 2014;39E(6):582–6.
8. Davis TC, Brady O, Dias JJ. Excision of the trapezium for osteoarthritis of the trapeziometacarpal joint: a study of the benefit of ligament reconstruction or tendon interposition. J Hand Surg Am. 2004;29:1069–77.
9. Huang K, Hollevoet N, Giddins G. Thumb carpometacarpal joint total arthroplasty: a systematic review. J Hand Surg Eur. 2015;40(4):338–50.
10. Krukhaug Y, Lie SS, Havelin LI, Furnes O, Hove LM, Hallan G. The results of 479 thumb carpometacarpal joint replacements reported in the Norwegian Arthroplasty Register. J Hand Surg Eur. 2014;39E(8):819–25.
11. Siddiqui A, Onwordi L, Packer G. Thumb CMCJ prosthetic arthroplasty using ARPE: a review of 241 cases. Presented at BSSH meeting, 18th October 2013.
12. Adams BD. Wrist arthroplasty: partial and total. Hand Clin. 2013;29:79–89.
13. Yeoh D, Tourret L. Total wrist arthroplasty: a systematic review of the evidence from the last five years. J Hand Surg. 2015;40E(5):458–68.

Radionuclide Imaging of Skeletal Implants

9

Vetri Sudar Jayaprakasam and Patrick Fielding

Radionuclides are atomic species that are inherently unstable and decay emitting energy in the form of ionising radiation. Nuclear medicine or radionuclide imaging studies use a variety of radionuclides, usually bound to a further molecule to form a radiopharmaceutical. The radionuclide acts as the marker that allows localisation and formation of an image with a camera/scanner system, whilst the radiopharmaceutical (with the carrier molecule) gives the tracer specificity.

Two distinct types of radionuclides are used in clinical practice: those that decay by single-photon emission and those that decay by positron emission. Single-photon-emitting radionuclides and radiopharmaceuticals derived from them are routinely detected with gamma cameras, and this form of imaging is available in most hospitals. Scans of this type include isotope bone scans, labelled white cell scans, gallium scans and labelled colloid scans. These form the first line of radionuclide imaging for most patients with suspected complications of skeletal implants.

There has been a recent interest in the use of positron emission tomography (PET)-based tracers in imaging complications of prosthetic joints. Tracers decaying by positron emission have included 18-F fluorodeoxyglucose (FDG), the uptake of which reflects metabolic activity, and sodium fluoride (NaF), the uptake of which reflects bone turnover. Whilst PET imaging does have an emerging literature, most centres will routinely use single-photon-emitting radionuclides as the first nuclear medicine investigation of choice, and the majority of this chapter is devoted to discussion of these.

All forms of nuclear medicine investigations use ionising radiation, and the approximate doses received for each investigation are given in each section. As a comparison, the UK average background radiation exposure is around 2.5 millisieverts (mSv) per year.

V. S. Jayaprakasam · P. Fielding (✉)
University Hospital of Wales, Cardiff, UK
e-mail: vetri.jayaprakasam@wales.nhs.uk; Patrick.Fielding@wales.nhs.uk

S. Agarwal, G. J. Bansal (eds.), *Radiology of Orthopedic Implants*,
https://doi.org/10.1007/978-3-319-76009-4_9

Imaging Technology

Single-photon-emitting radionuclides are imaged with a gamma camera. Usually planar images are acquired initially. Planar images demonstrate the distribution of tracer from a particular viewpoint with respect to the patient. Standard views would include anterior and posterior images. It is also possible to obtain tomographic images of the distribution of single-photon-emitting tracers. This process is known as single-photon emission (computed) tomography (SPECT or PET imaging). These may be combined with CT images with a variety of resolutions. The examinations performed in this way and the hybrid images produced are known as SPECT/CT images. It is important to note that SPECT and SPECT/CT are not scans or investigations as of themselves but are only a refinement of existing investigations to clarify the exact distribution of a single-photon-emitting tracer.

PET imaging is only ever acquired as tomographic (3D) images. It is always combined with cross-sectional imaging, usually with CT or occasionally MRI. PET images have intrinsically higher spatial resolution than SPECT images due to differences in hardware and instrumentation. The CT component of a PET/CT examination will also tend to be of a higher resolution than those in SPECT/CT examinations.

Isotope Bone Scans and Skeletal Implants

Isotope bone scans use bisphosphonate derivatives to assess bone turnover. Skeletal uptake is proportional to osteoblastic activity and to blood flow. Scans for assessment of the problematic skeletal implant are usually performed as three-phase studies (Fig. 9.1). For these, the patient is positioned on the gamma camera table, and the initial images are obtained in the first 60 s following tracer injection. These are labelled as “flow” images. “Blood pool” images are obtained between 2 and 5 min. Subsequently, delayed images are obtained between 2 and 4 h. Early-phase images reflect perfusion and vascularity, whereas delayed images reflect osteoblastic activity. The scans allow evaluation of the local anatomy, in addition to the joint under investigation (Fig. 9.2).

Administered activities are typically of the order of 600 MBq intravenously, which yields a radiation dose of 3 mSv.

It is hypothesised that in the case of periprosthetic infection that there will be increased uptake on all three phases, whereas in aseptic loosening, there is no hyperaemia on the early phases but increased uptake on delayed imaging (Fig. 9.3). Table 9.1 shows typical described patterns in the uncomplicated prosthesis, in aseptic loosening and in periprosthetic infection.

In a study [1] at a single institution, 75 patients who had undergone total knee replacements and presented with pain were studied. The mean interval between surgery and re-presentation was 3 years. The patients underwent two-phase bone scans and were assigned as normal if uptake was within normal limits on both phases, as infected if there was abnormal uptake on both phases and as aseptic loosening if increased uptake was seen on the delayed phase images only. Although this approach was unreliable at distinguishing infection from aseptic loosening, of 43 patients in whom the bone scan was felt to be normal, 41 were felt to be indeed normal on prolonged follow-up with two patients being eventually diagnosed with aseptic loosening and none with infection. This early study underlines a key principle in relation to isotope bone scans in the painful prosthetic joint—if an isotope bone scan is

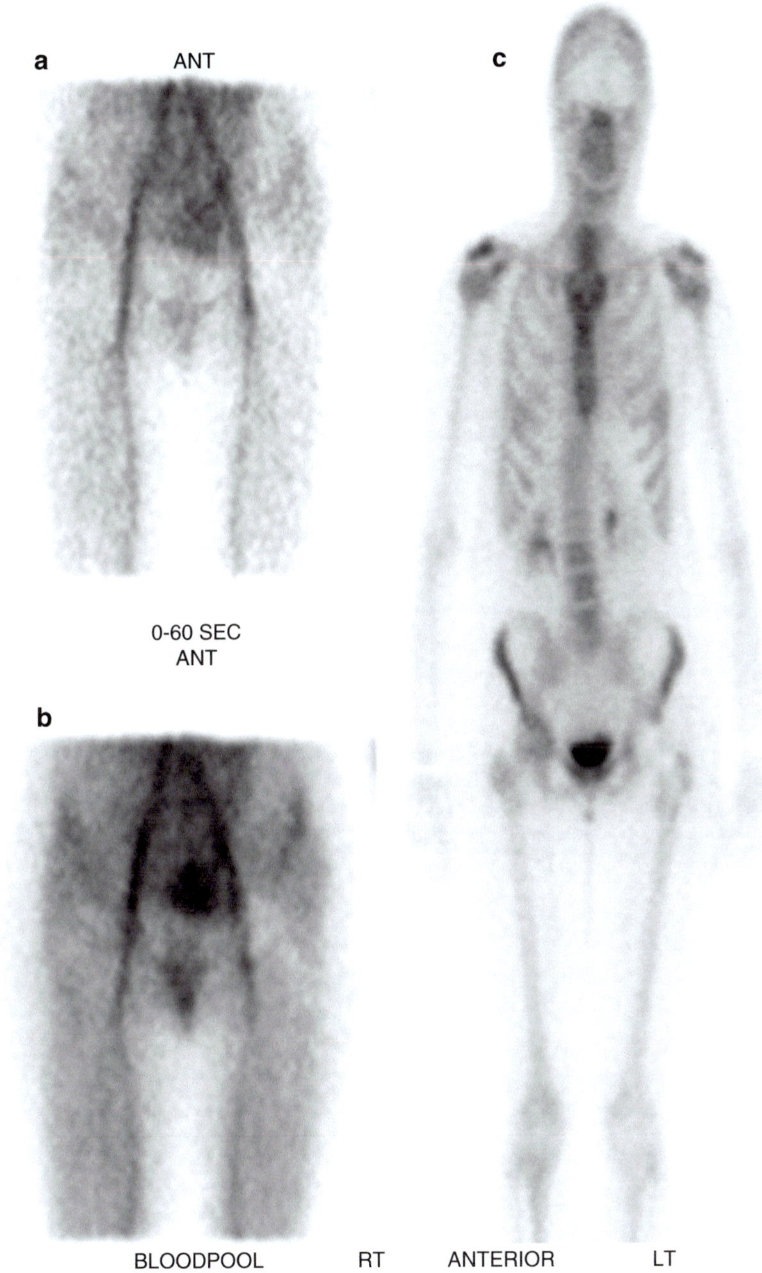

Fig. 9.1 A 64-year-old female patient who underwent a left uncemented THR 15 months prior to this scan. She presented with left-sided groin pain. Plain films and inflammatory markers were unremarkable. Images from isotope bone scan following 500 MBq of Tc 99m HDP. Images shown are anterior views only although posterior images are usually also acquired. (**a**) is the anterior perfusion or flow image (first 60 s, notice prominent vessels), (**b**) shows blood pool images acquired between 2 and 5 min and reflects capillary blood flow and (**c**) shows delayed images obtained at 3 h following tracer injection. The scan was felt to be normal, and the patient remains well after 2 years of clinical follow-up

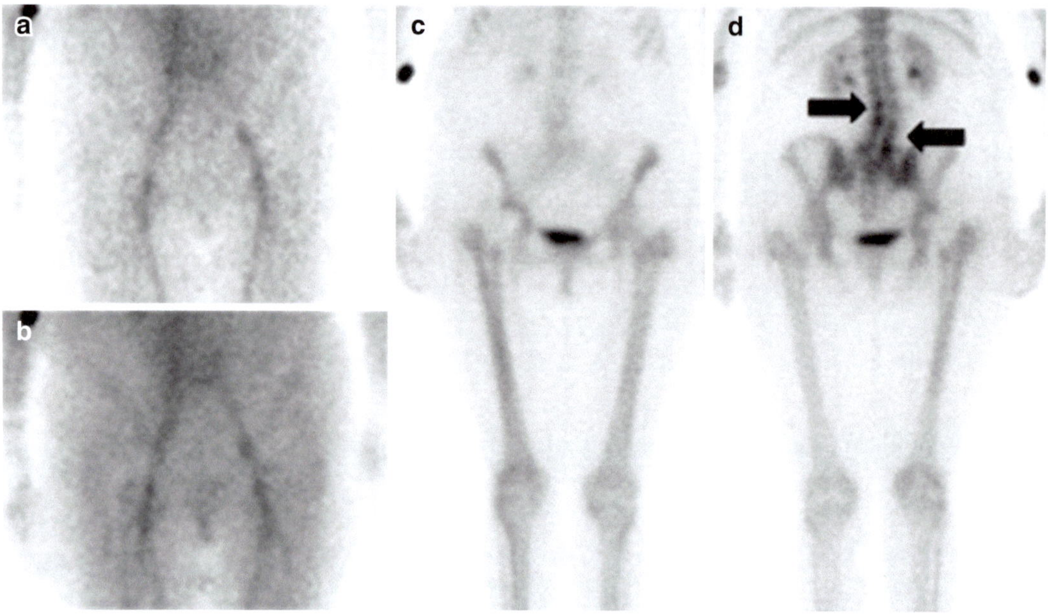

Fig. 9.2 A 71-year-old patient who underwent a revision right total hip replacement 6 months prior to the scan. He had been experiencing right sided hip pain radiating down the right leg. Three-phase studies following 500 MBq of Tc 99m HDP. (**a**, **b**) are anterior flow and blood pool images which are within normal limits. (**c**) is anterior and (**d**) is posterior delayed images. Despite the early stage following surgery, tracer uptake around the hip prosthesis is within normal limits. There is however a lumbar scoliosis with degenerative pattern uptake of tracer (arrows) in association with this. This may have been the cause for ongoing pain. When performing isotope imaging for assessment of prosthetic joints, it is important to include a wider anatomical area on the delayed phase images. Typically for hip and knee prostheses, a field of view from the lumbar spine to below the knees is recommended

entirely normal then a significant prosthetic complication is unlikely (Figs. 9.4, 9.5, 9.6, 9.7, 9.8, 9.9, 9.10, 9.11, 9.12, 9.13, 9.14, 9.15, 9.16 and 9.17).

As isotope bone scans demonstrate bone turnover, it can be expected that scans performed immediately (in the first few days or weeks) following a skeletal implant will show intense abnormal tracer uptake around the prosthesis. A degree of increased tracer uptake is to be expected for some time after implantation. As a general guide, some increased uptake is to be expected in the first year in an uncomplicated hip replacement and some increased tracer uptake is to be expected for up to 2 years in knee replacements [2].

Several early studies have focussed on the pattern of abnormal uptake in the differentiation of loosening and infection. It has been suggested that in aseptic loosening, the uptake will be focal, but uptake may be either diffuse or focal in the case of infection. If uptake is diffuse, then infection should certainly be considered [3].

In another series [4] of 71 patients, with painful hip and knee prostheses, all of whom eventually underwent revision surgery; the relative merits of the erythrocyte sedimentation rate (ESR), joint aspiration and a three-phase bone scan were evaluated. All patients underwent three-phase bone scintigraphy, measurement of ESR, and 70 patients also underwent joint aspiration. Bone scans were interpreted as positive for infection if they revealed uptake around the prosthesis on all three phases in the absence of any other explanation. The final consensus of the state of the joint was derived from the surgical appear-

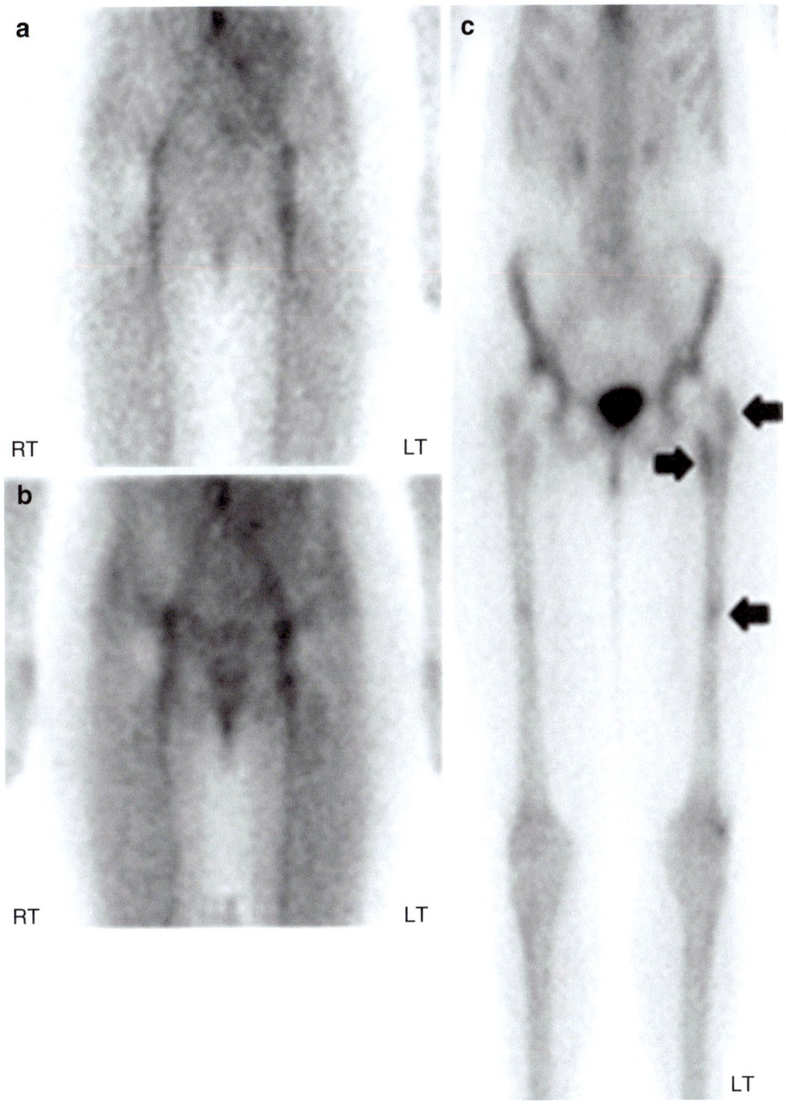

Fig. 9.3 A 59-year-old male patient, 3 years following left total hip replacement and 5 years following right total hip replacement. The patient presented with left-sided hip pain and was asymptomatic on the right side. Images following 500 MBq of Tc 99m HDP. Only the anterior images are shown. The early perfusion and blood pool images are normal (**a**, **b**). Delayed images (**c**) show focal increased tracer uptake in relation to the tip and both trochanteric regions (arrows). This pattern of abnormality is classically associated with aseptic loosening—which is normal early phase imaging and focal uptake on delayed phase imaging

Table 9.1 Typical patterns in 3 phase bone scintigraphy in joint prostheses

Phase	Uncomplicated	Aseptic loosening	Infection
Early and blood pool	Normal	Normal	Increased
Delayed	Normal	Increased focal pattern	Increased diffuse pattern

ances and the presence or absence of appropriate microbiology. Of the nine joints felt to be definitely infected, only three showed the classical appearances on three-phase bone scans. In this study the sensitivity and specificity of three-phase bone scans combined with radiographs were 38% and 41%, respectively. It appears therefore that whilst a totally normal three-phase bone scan is reassuring, as a diagnostic tool on its own, isotope bone scans are unable to distinguish between infection and aseptic loosening as the cause for a painful prosthesis.

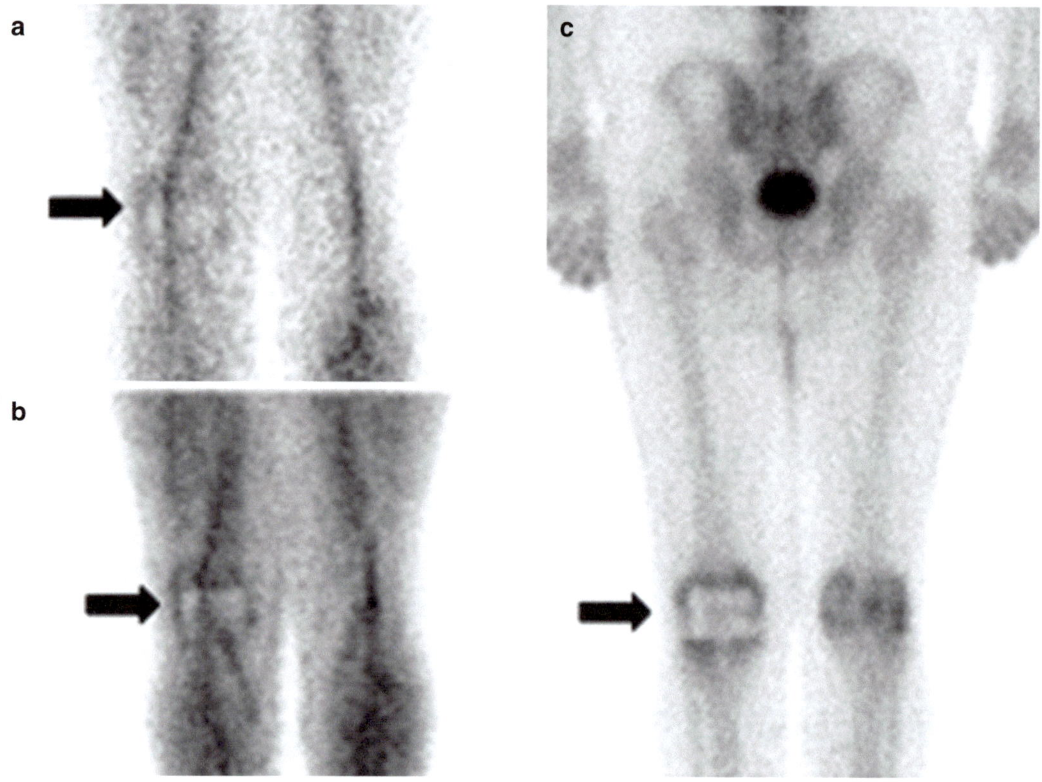

Fig. 9.4 A 52-year-old man had undergone a left knee replacement 4 years previously. He complained of pain, inflammatory markers and plain films were equivocal. Three-phase isotope bone scan. The early perfusion and blood pool images show diffuse increased tracer uptake around both components of the prosthesis (**a**, **b**). This persists on the delayed images (**c**). Only posterior images are shown. There should not be any increased uptake at this stage following prosthetic implantation. The diffuse uptake on all three phases is the pattern most classically associated with infection, although this is not an absolutely accurate predictor. In this case subsequent labelled white cell imaging suggested prosthetic infection, and this was subsequently confirmed at surgery

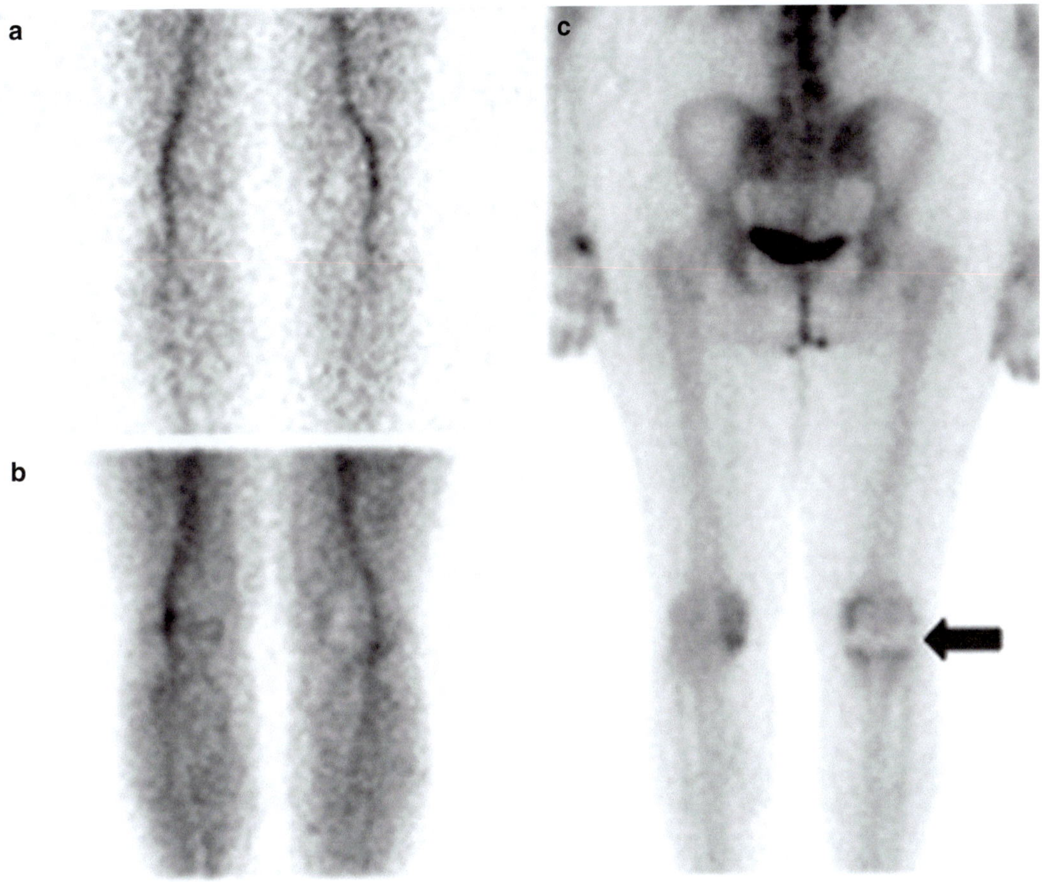

Fig. 9.5 A 59-year-old female patient who had undergone a right total knee replacement 3 years ago and patellar resurfacing 1 year previously. There was ongoing pain. The clinical impression was of aseptic loosening. A three-phase bone scan was undertaken, and the images shown are posterior views. There is no significant abnormality on the perfusion or blood pool imaging (**a**, **b**). Delayed images (**c**) show focal increased tracer uptake in relation to the tibial and femoral components. The scintigraphic pattern is compatible with aseptic loosening

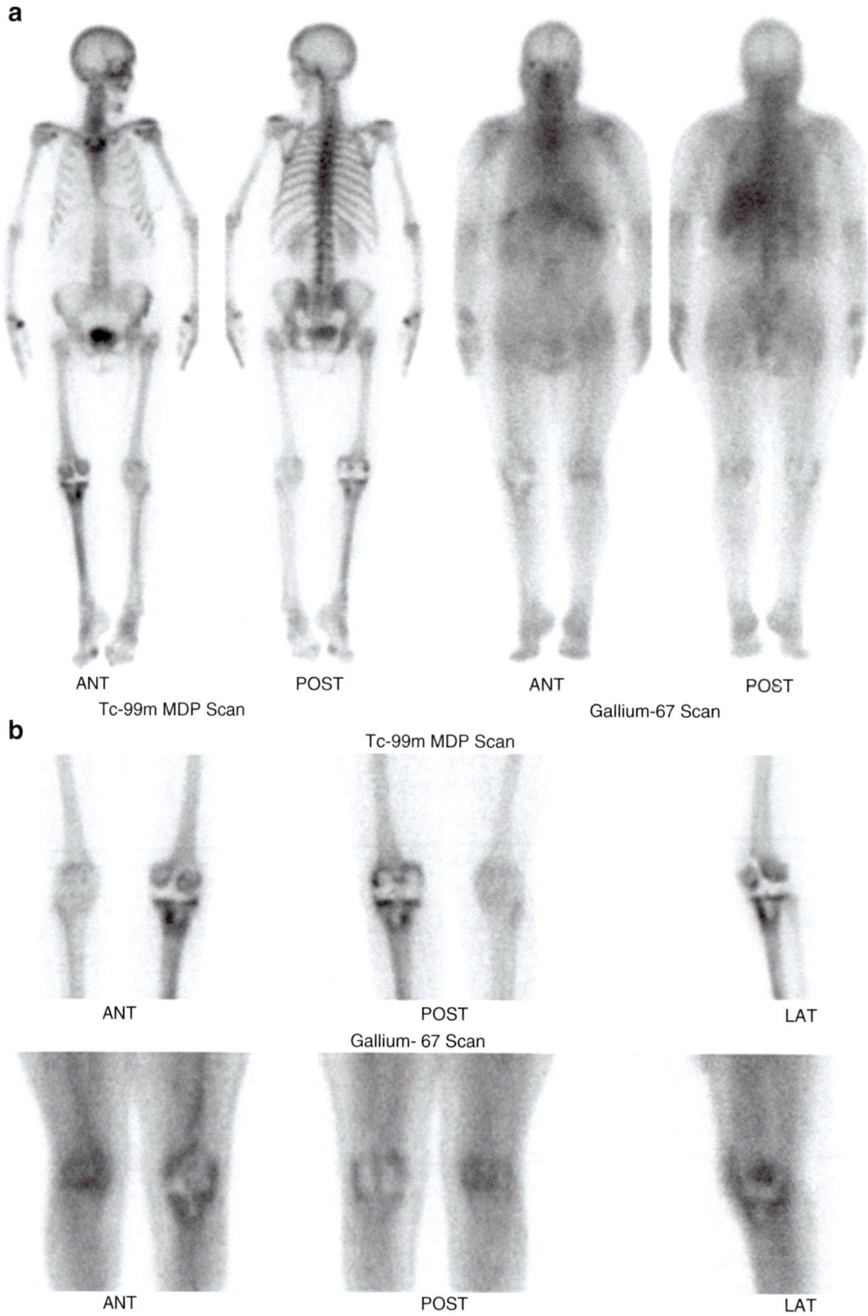

Fig. 9.6 A 73-year-old female underwent left knee total arthroplasty 10 months ago. Presented with pain on the left knee. Clinical examination showed slight oedema, and the left knee was warm to touch. A whole body Tc-99m MDP scan followed by whole body gallium-67 scintigraphy was performed. (**a**) shows the whole body anterior and posterior views of the Tc-99m MDP scan and gallium-67 imaging. (**b**) shows the static anterior, posterior and left lateral knee views of the Tc-99m MDP bone scan (top row) and gallium-67 imaging (bottom row). The Tc-99m MDP bone scan shows increased uptake in relation to the tibial component of the prosthesis. Mild increased uptake is also seen within the femoral component. The gallium-67 scan (both static and whole body views) shows relatively normal uptake in relation to the left knee. Prosthetic infection was ruled out

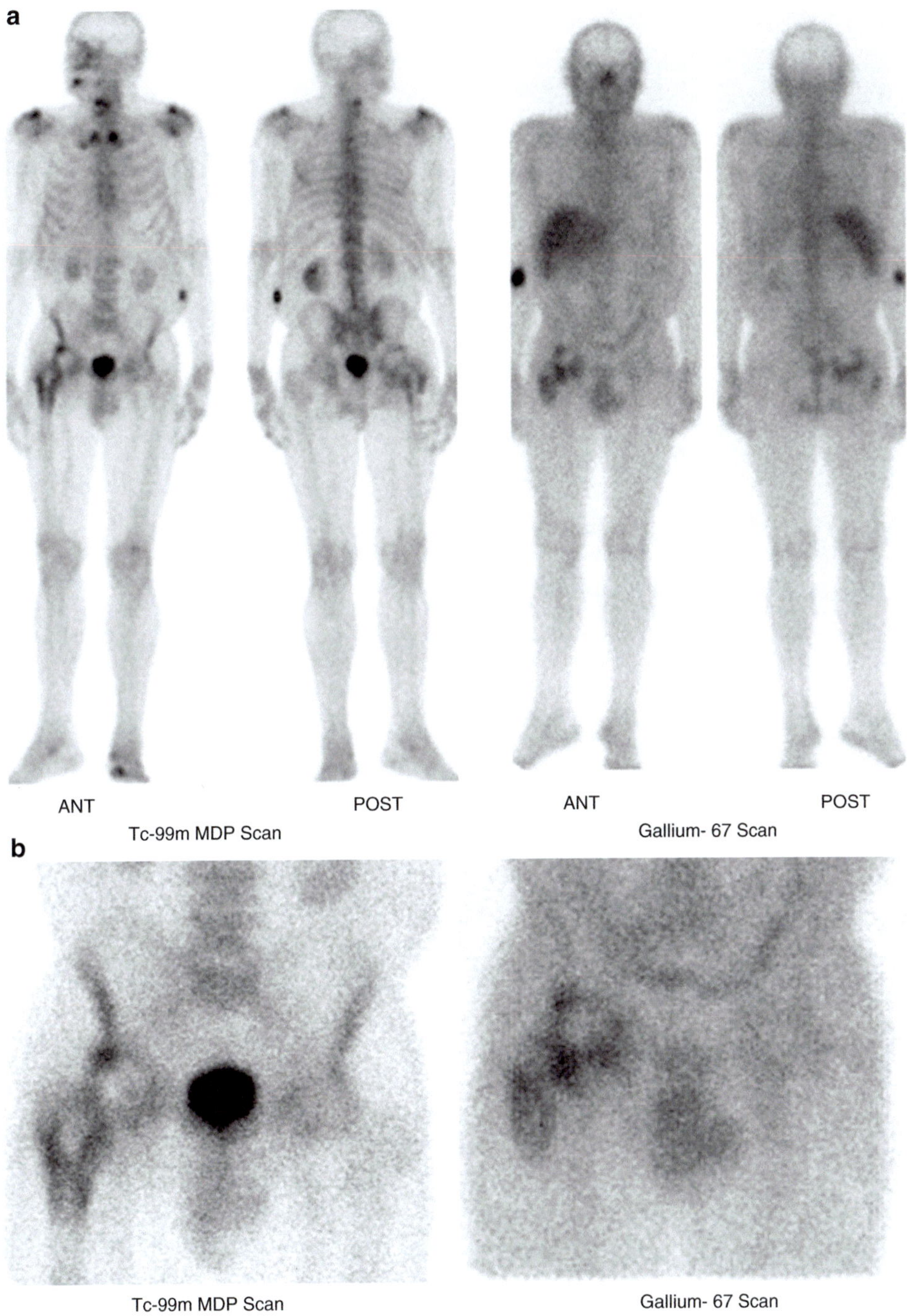

Fig. 9.7 Whole body images (**a**) and static anterior pelvic views (**b**) of Tc-99m MDP bone scan and gallium-67 imaging in a patient who had undergone right total hip arthroplasty a few years ago and presented with right hip pain. The Tc-99m bone scan shows increased tracer uptake, particularly in relation to the femoral component of the prosthesis. The gallium-67 images also show increased tracer accumulation in relation to the prosthesis. This was proven to be an infected prosthesis. Note the normal physiological distribution of gallium-67 within the liver and soft tissues

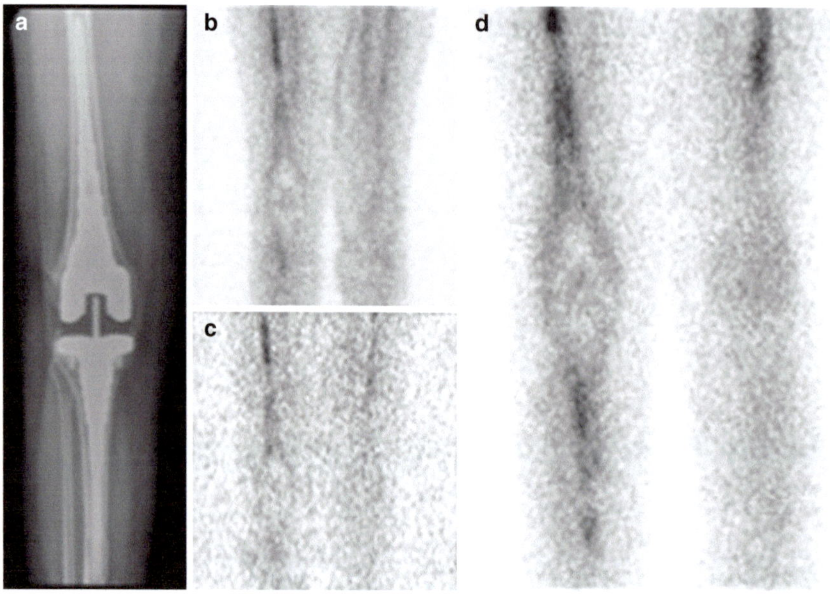

Fig. 9.8 A 79-year-old female underwent a revision right knee replacement 1 year previously. Clinical presentation was pain at the level of the joint line, and inflammatory markers were equivocal. X rays (**a**) were felt to be unremarkable. A labelled white cell scan was performed with 200 MBq of leukocytes labelled with HMPAO. Images at 4 h (**b**) and 24 h (**c**) showed low-grade increased tracer uptake around the tibial and femoral stems. In order to evaluate further, colloid scintigraphy was undertaken with 300 MBq of colloid. Images were obtained at 2 h (**d**). Only the anterior views are shown. The colloid scan shows at least as marked tracer uptake as the white cell scan; hence the low-grade white cell accumulation is taken to be related to marrow redistribution rather than periprosthetic infection

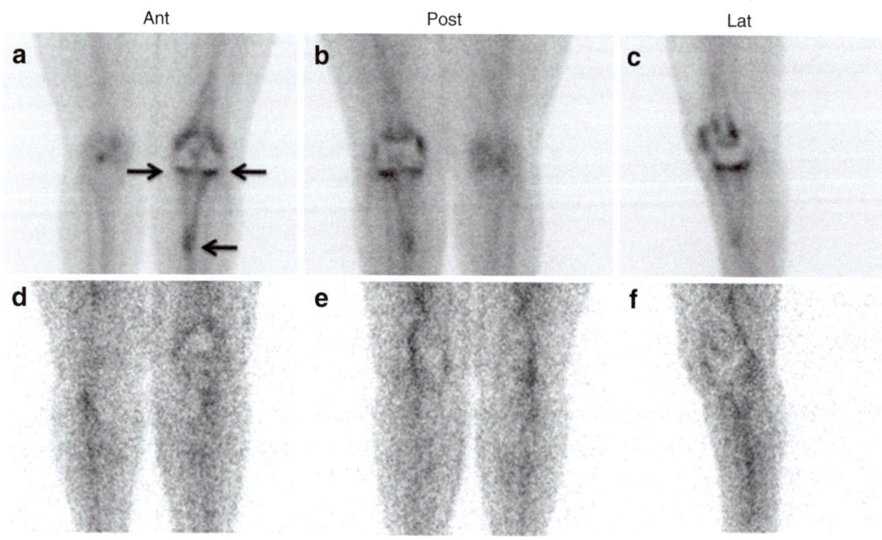

Fig. 9.9 An 84-year-old lady presented with continued pain around the left knee 11 months post left revision total knee arthroplasty for nickel allergy. Tc-99m bone scan followed by Tc-99m-labelled leukocyte scan was performed. Delayed static anterior, posterior and left lateral Tc-99m MDP bone scan views (**a–c**) of the left knee show increased tracer uptake in relation to the tibial component of the left knee prosthesis, particularly at the plateau and the tip of the prosthesis (arrows). Some increased uptake is also seen in relation to the femoral component. At 4 h anterior, posterior and left lateral views of Tc-99m-labelled WBC scan (**d–f**) show normal white cell distribution. Patient was managed conservatively. Pain subsided over the next 6 months, and the patient remained symptom-free on 2-year follow-up

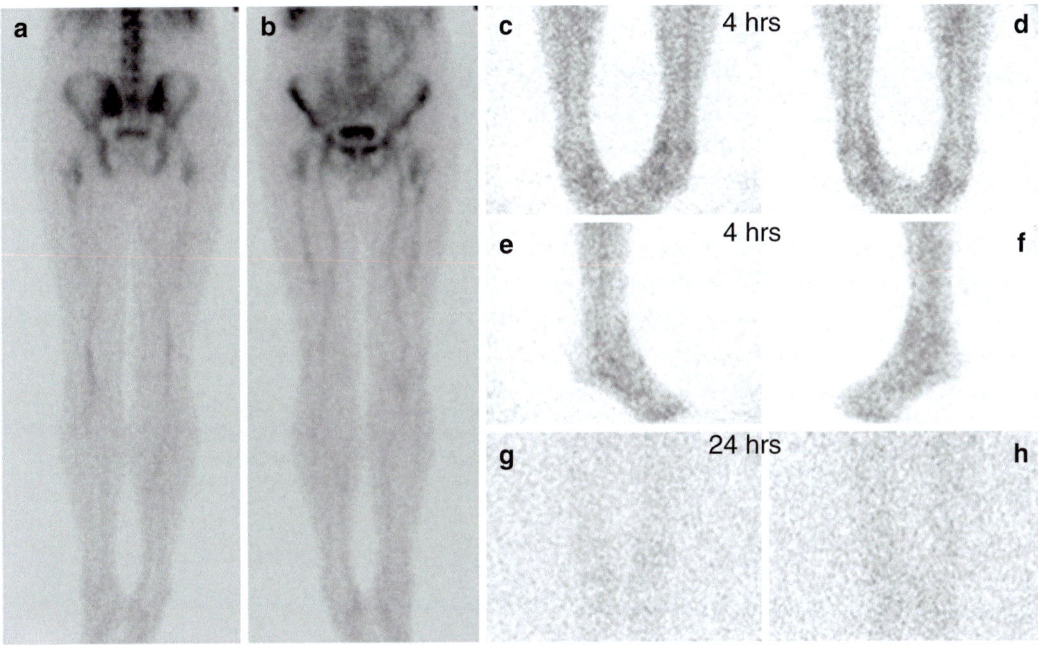

Fig. 9.10 Tc-99m-labelled leukocyte scan in a 70-year-old male presenting with pain along the anterior aspect of the right ankle 5 months following right ankle replacement. The 4 h planar anterior and posterior images from pelvis to the ankles (**a**, **b**), anterior (**c**), posterior (**d**) and lateral views (**e**, **f**) and 24-h anterior (**g**) and posterior (**h**) of the ankles show a normal pattern uptake. No evidence of infection. Note the normal uptake within the lower limb vessels

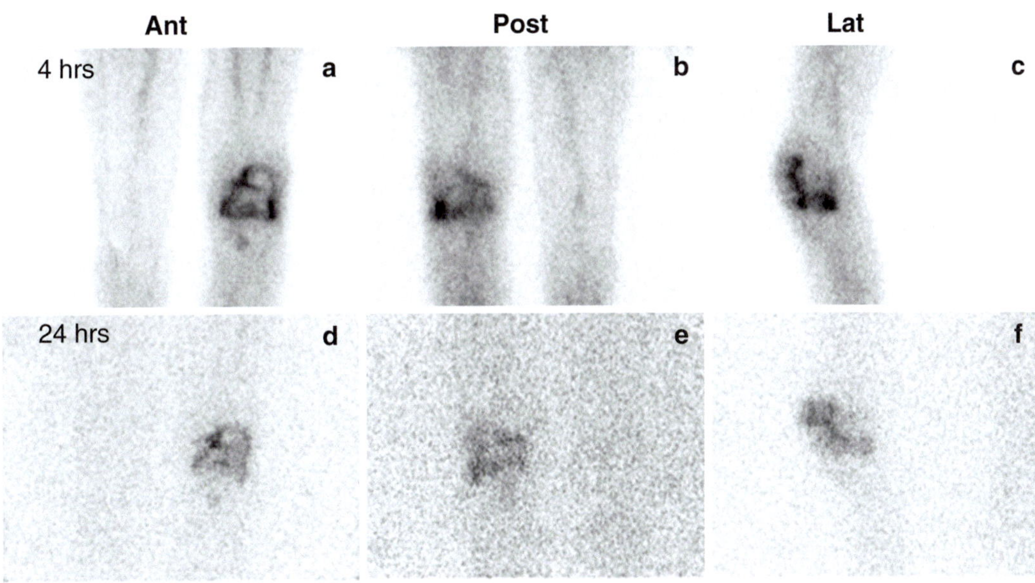

Fig. 9.11 Tc-99m-labelled leukocyte scan in a 80-year-old male presenting with continued pain 8 months following total knee arthroplasty. The 4 h anterior (**a**), posterior (**b**) and lateral views (**c**) of the knees shows intense tracer uptake within the femoral component, which persists at 24 h (**d**–**f**). Small focus of uptake is also seen within the tibial component. Appearances are consistent with infection. Patient underwent revision left total knee replacement with infection proven on intraoperative cultures

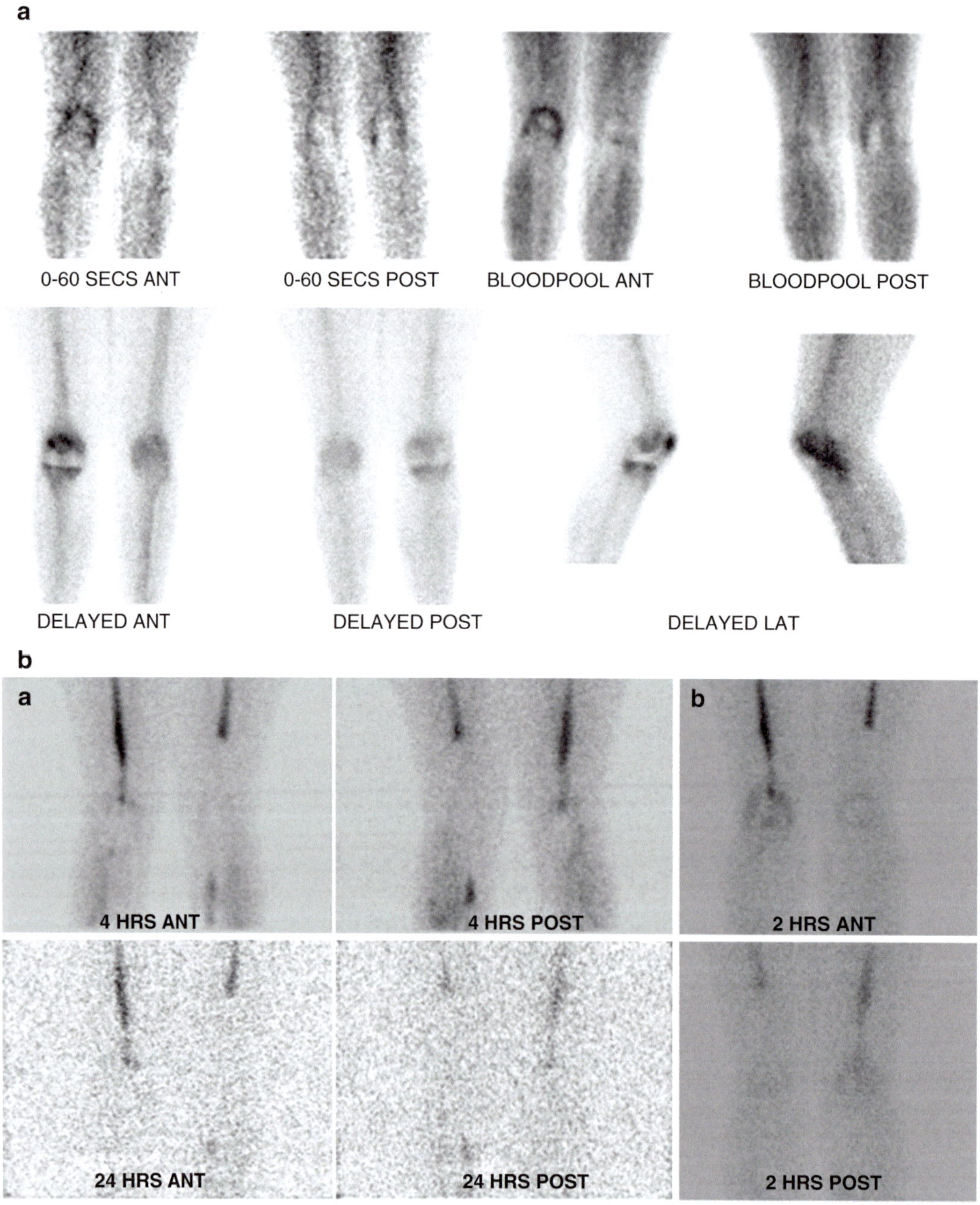

Fig. 9.12 Three-phase Tc-99m MDP bone scan (**a**) and a combined WBC marrow scan (**b**) in a 54-year-old female who had undergone right knee replacement 3 years ago. Patient complained of swelling and pain around the right knee. On the early (0–60 s anterior and posterior) and blood pool images, there is hyperaemia of the knee, particularly around the femoral component. Delayed anterior, posterior and lateral images show increased activity surrounding the femoral component and underneath the tibial component. Four- and 24-h Tc-99m-labelled leukocyte scan {**b**(**a**)} shows tracer activity extending asymmetrically along the femoral shaft up to the femoral component. This pattern of uptake matches with the Tc-99m colloid scan {**b**(**b**)} performed a week later. Appearances are consistent with aseptic loosening. In view of ongoing symptoms, a revision of the right total knee replacement was undertaken

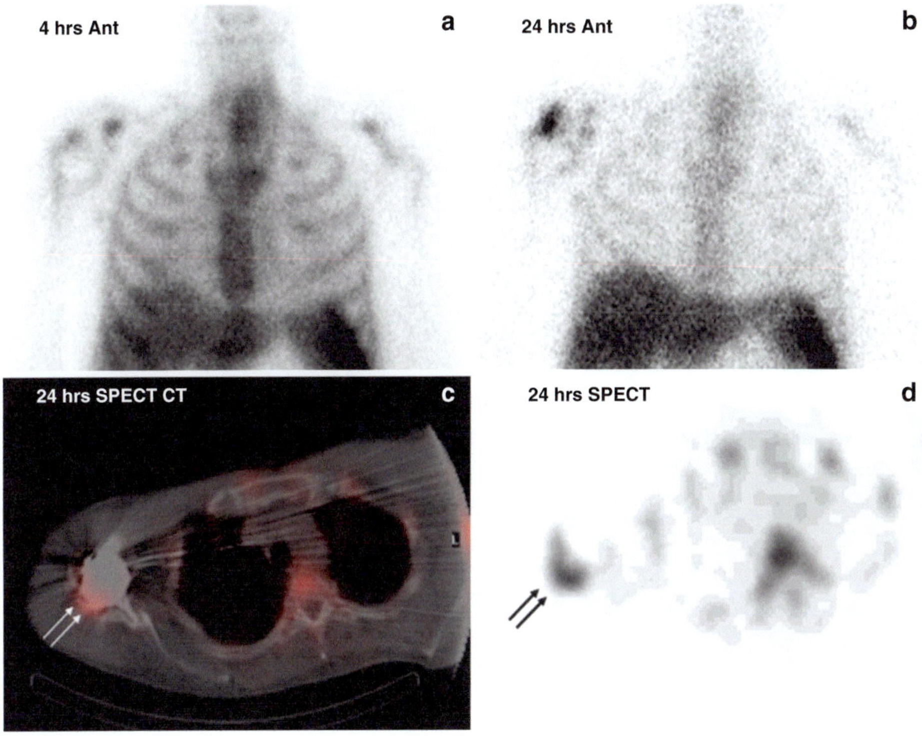

Fig. 9.13 Tc-99m-labelled leukocyte scan in a 67-year-old male. Right shoulder replacement was performed 1 year previously. Clinical presentation was right shoulder pain with raised inflammatory markers. Four-hour (**a**) and 24-h (**b**) anterior views show abnormal uptake in relation to the right shoulder. A SPECT CT (**c**, **d**) performed at 24 h shows the activity was located along the posterolateral aspect (arrows) of the humeral component of the prosthesis, consistent with infection. The patient underwent two-stage revision of the right shoulder replacement

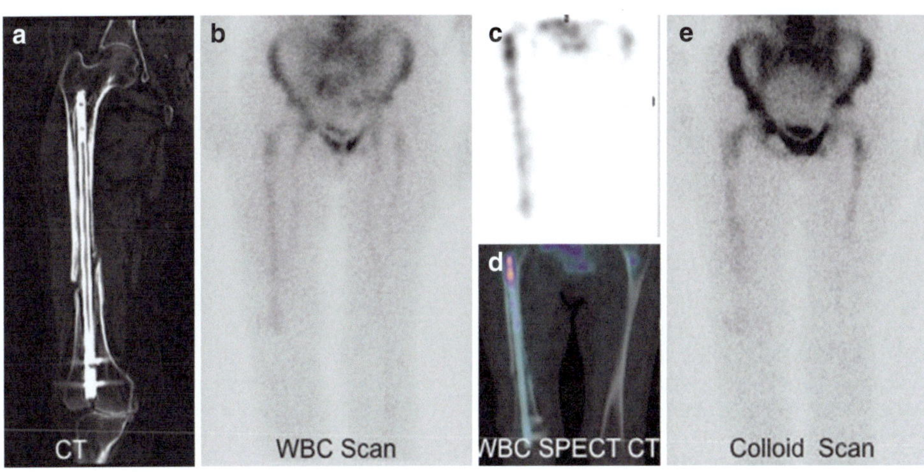

Fig. 9.14 A 75-year-old female underwent retrograde nailing for femoral shaft fracture 12 years previously. She presented with constant pain around the fracture site. Coronal CT image (**a**) shows non-union of the fracture of the shaft of the right femur. Planar 4-hour (**b**) and SPECT CT (**c**, **d**) Tc-99m-labelled leukocyte imaging shows moderate grade uptake along the entire length of the femoral shaft. The SPECT CT confirms that the uptake is around the prosthesis. A Tc-99m colloid scan (**e**) performed a week later shows congruent uptake along the length of the femoral shaft. There was no scintigraphic evidence of infection

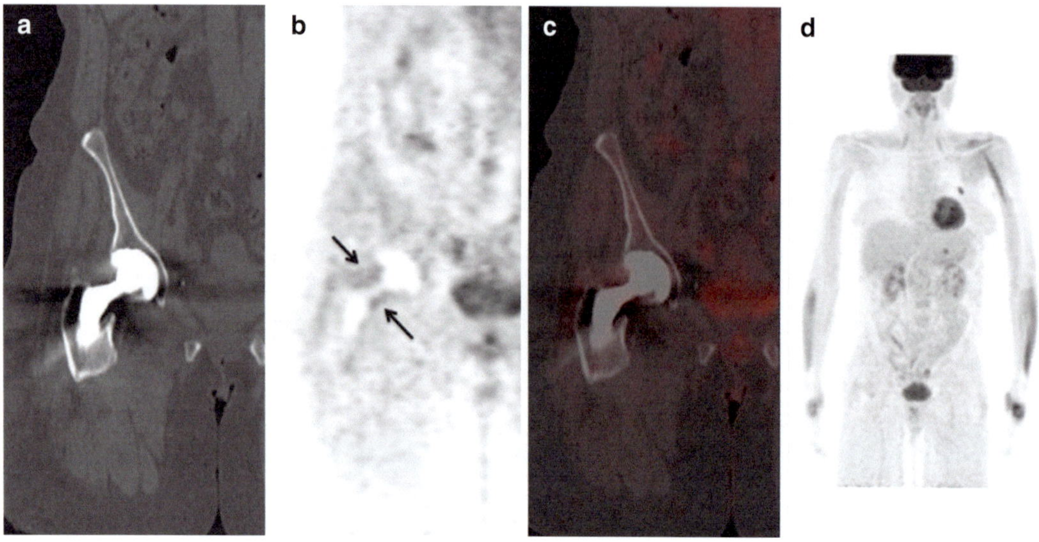

Fig. 9.15 An 18F-FDG PET CT in a 65-year-old female with right femoral retrograde intramedullary nail. Coronal CT images (**a**) show the metalwork in the right femur. Coronal PET (**b**) and coronal fused PET CT (**c**) images show normal FDG uptake in relation to the implant. Note the mild increased uptake adjacent to the prosthetic neck along the prosthesis-soft tissue interface (arrows) which is considered within normal limits. Whole body maximum intensity projection (MIP) images (**d**) show physiological uptake within the brain, myocardium, liver and muscles. 18F-FDG is excreted via kidneys (unlike normal glucose) and is accumulated in the bladder

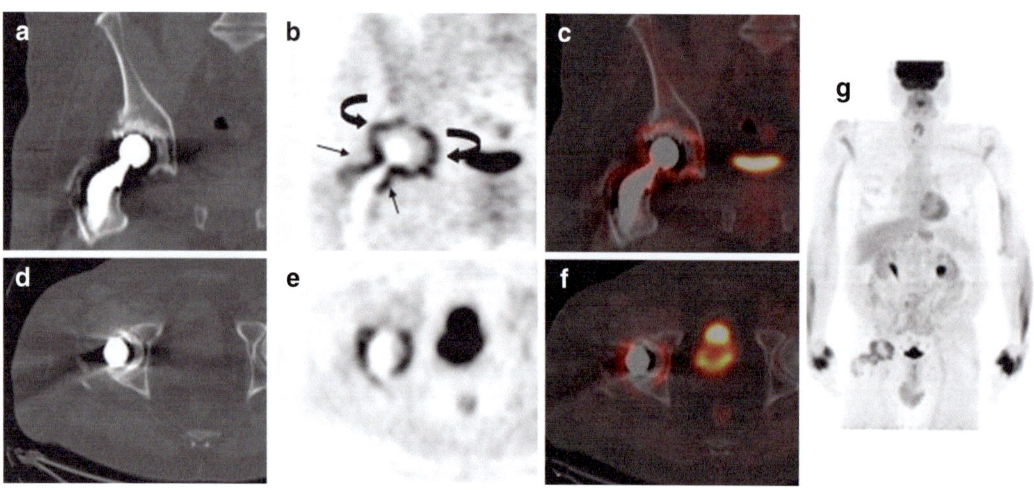

Fig. 9.16 An 18F-FDG PET CT in a 70-year-old male with asymptomatic right hip prosthesis. Coronal (**a**) and axial (**d**) CT images show right hip prosthesis. Coronal (**b**) and axial (**e**) PET and coronal (**c**) and axial (**f**) fused PET CT images show intense uptake around the neck of the femoral prosthesis (straight arrows) and between the prosthesis-bone interface in relation to the acetabular component (curved arrows). Maximum intensity projection (MIP) images (**g**) show uptake within the head and neck of the femoral prosthesis. No abnormal tracer uptake is seen in relation to the prosthesis within the femoral shaft. The site of uptake (prosthesis-bone interface) is considered more significant than the intensity (SUVmax) of the uptake. Uptake limited to the femoral head portion of the prosthesis is suggestive of aseptic loosening. Patient remained symptom-free at 1-year follow-up

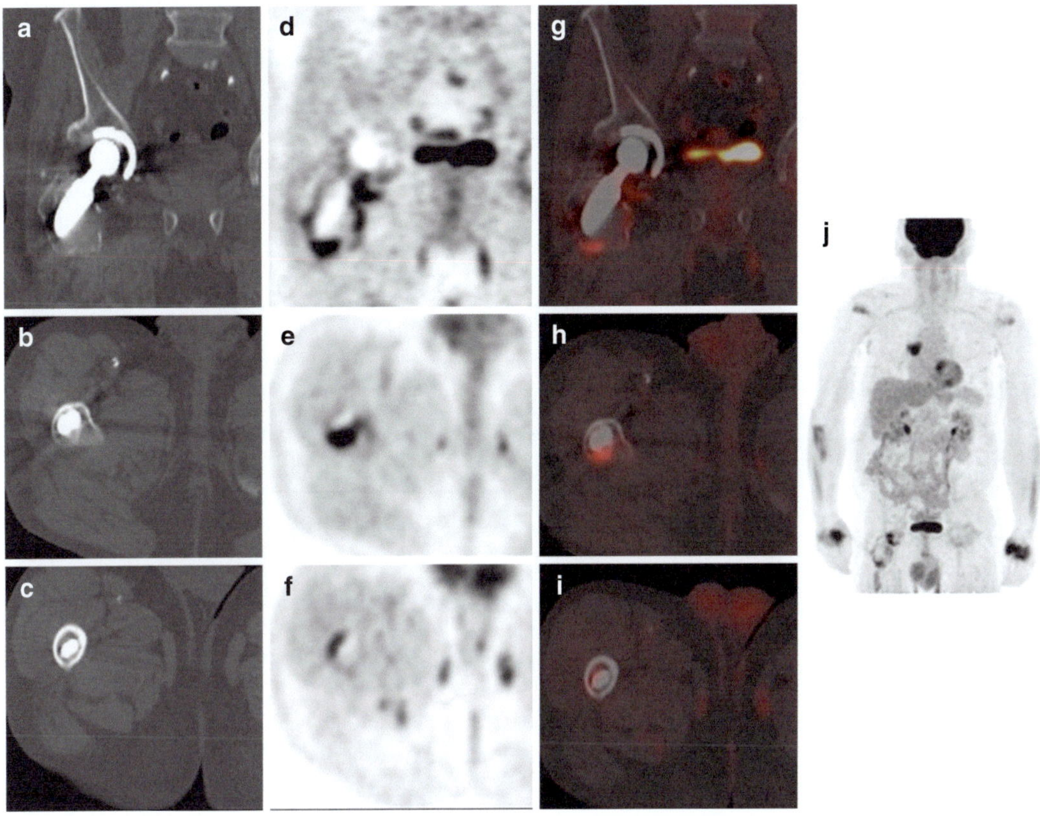

Fig. 9.17 A 71-year-old male patient underwent 18F-FDG PET CT for an unrelated indication. Coronal (**a**) and axial (**b**, **c**) CT images show right hip prosthesis. Coronal (**d**) and axial (**e**, **f**) PET and coronal (**g**) and axial (**h**, **i**) fused PET CT images show intense uptake along the bone-prosthesis interface of the femoral component of the prosthesis. There is also intense uptake in relation to the neck of the prosthesis. Appearances are suggestive of infection. Maximum intensity projection (MIP) image (**j**) shows uptake in relation to the right hip prosthesis. Note intense uptake in relation to the right lung cancer for which the patient was initially referred

Gallium/Bone Scintigraphy

Gallium-67 has been used for many years in nuclear medicine as a non-specific tracer for infection, inflammation and malignancy. As isotope bone scans alone have been found to be insufficient to discriminate between aseptic loosening and infection, a combination of gallium scintigraphy and bone scintigraphy has been suggested as a means for the distinction between prosthetic infection and aseptic prosthetic complications.

Gallium-67 has a long half-life of 3.26 days. It is administered intravenously as the citrate salt and binds non-specifically to neutrophil and bacterial cell membranes. Images are typically obtained at 24 and 48 h following injection and are acquired with a medium-energy collimator over a period of around 30 min. Administered activities are usually in the region of 150 MBq, and this yields a fairly high radiation dose of around 15 mSv.

In a typical approach, the patient undergoes gallium and isotope bone scans sequentially. The combined scan is ascribed as positive if there is "spatial incongruence" between the uptakes of the two tracers. Using a final consensus of surgery, microbiology or 2-year clinical follow-up, a sensitivity of 66% and specificity of 81% have been reported for this approach [5].

Other authors have however found imaging with labelled leukocytes to be superior to gallium/bone imaging. In a review [6] of 57 consecutive patients with a mixture of suspected prosthetic infections and native osteomyelitis, the sensitivity of leukocyte scanning was estimated to be 100% for acute infections, whereas combined gallium scanning showed the typical pattern of incongruent uptake in only 28% of patients thought to have infection.

Gallium imaging has the disadvantages of higher radiation doses, poorer image quality and the fact that images have to be acquired over several days. For these reasons, combined with the fact that the results from labelled leukocyte imaging is at least as good as gallium imaging has led most centres to use labelled leukocytes in preference to gallium imaging.

Labelled Leukocyte and Colloid Scintigraphy

A normal isotope bone scan has a good negative predictive value. In other words, with a normal three-phase bone scan, the chances of a significant periprosthetic complication are very low. However, isotope bone scans alone cannot reliably distinguish between infection and aseptic loosening.

This limitation has led to development of leukocyte-labelled radionuclide studies, and this, combined with marrow studies, is still considered the most accurate [7] and most widely available test for the evaluation of possible prosthetic infection.

Radiolabelled leukocytes have been used in detection of infection and inflammation since the 1970s [8, 9]. Initially the leukocytes were labelled with In-111 oxine non-selectively. But over the years, Tc-99m hexamethylene-propylene amine oxime (HMPAO) has gradually replaced In-111 oxine as the radionuclide of choice for labelling leukocytes because of low cost, general availability and favourable imaging characteristics [10]. The long half-life of In-111 oxine (67 h) compared to the Tc-99m (6 h) may be useful under certain circumstances. Another advantage of using In-111 is in combined WBC and marrow imaging when the images can be acquired simultaneous or immediately after the WBC scans. However the less favourable photon energy, long waiting times (up to 30 h) and low-resolution images make it a less desirable radioisotope in clinical practice [11, 12].

The presence of an orthopaedic implant causes variations in normal marrow distribution [13]. For this reason labelled leukocyte accumulation can occur in uninfected musculoskeletal pathologies and result in reduced sensitivity and specificity [14, 15]. The basis for the combined WBC/marrow imaging is that the WBC accumulates in both normal marrow and infection, whereas the colloid accumulates only in normal marrow and not in infection.

Radiopharmaceutical Preparation

Commercial Tc-99m HMPAO kits have been available since the late 1990s. However, the labelling of the white blood cells (WBC) is still cumbersome. The kit is reconstituted with a freshly eluted Tc-99m pertechnetate, which forms a hydrophilic Tc-99m HMPAO complex in aqueous solution [16]. As this complex is unstable in aqueous solution, it should be prepared immediately before use [17].

Around 20–50 mL of the patient's blood is drawn into a syringe containing an acid-citrate-dextrose (ACD) anticoagulant solution. Mixed leukocytes are separated by centrifugation and sedimentation. If purified granulocytes are required, gradient centrifugation is required. For most clinical practices, mixed leukocyte is used for labelling with Tc-99m HMPAO and is considered to perform satisfactorily [18].

The procedure for labelling In-111 oxine radioisotope with mixed leukocytes is similar to labelling with Tc-HMPAO [19]. However the radioisotope has to be ordered in advance in contrast to Tc-99m, which is readily available from the portable generators. The labelling efficiency and the in vivo stability of In-111 oxine are better than the Tc-HMPAO.

Special precautions need to be taken by the operator when handling blood and blood products. As the labelled blood is reinjected into the patient, strict aseptic conditions should be followed during labelling, and for practical purposes, commonly only one patient is labelled at a time.

The most commonly used tracers for marrow imaging are Tc-99m sulphur colloid and nanocolloid. Sulphur colloid particles range in size from 100 to 1000 nm, and about 5% of the particle gets distributed within the marrow. The nanocolloid particles measure less than 80 nm in size, and about 10% gets distributed in the marrow. There is however considerable background blood pool and urinary tract activity with nanocolloid [20]. The sulphur colloid is more commonly used in the USA, whereas the nanocolloid is commonly used in Europe [21].

For adults, the usual administered dose is 180–375 MBq of Tc-99m HMPAO-labelled WBC with an effective dose of 2 mSv. Around 10–20 MBq is administered for In-111 oxine-labelled WBC imaging. This gives an effective dose of around 12 mSv in total. The bone marrow imaging is performed by injecting 370 MBq of freshly prepared Tc-99m colloid (effective dose of around 4 mSv).

Image Acquisition

It is generally agreed that for musculoskeletal infections, Tc-HMPAO WBC imaging should be performed at two time points. The first imaging is 3–4 h after labelled leukocyte injection, and the second is a late imaging at 16–24 h. Early imaging at 30 min–1 h is optional for bone marrow uptake but is generally omitted [22]. Planar anterior and posterior whole body or of the involved site along with contralateral site for comparison are acquired at both these time points using a large field of view gamma camera with a low-energy, high-resolution collimator [23].

For In-111 WBC scan, planar images are acquired at 1–4 and/or at 16–30 h following tracer injection using a large field of view gamma camera fitted with medium-energy collimator. Delayed images should be obtained if the early images are negative [24].

The addition of single-photon emission computed tomography with computer tomography (SPECT/CT) has shown to improve identification, localisation, accuracy and reader confidence [25, 26]. In particular, SPECT/CT can help in differentiating skeletal uptake from soft tissue uptake [27]. SPECT/CT can be performed at late (4 h) or delayed (20–24 h) time point and is usually guided by the uptake on the planar imaging. The presence of a metallic implant with consequent beam-hardening artefact on CT does not appear to reduce the diagnostic accuracy of the scan, and evaluation of the non-attenuation-corrected images help in further assessment under these circumstances [28].

Colloid marrow images are acquired 30 min after tracer injection using a large field of view gamma camera. This can be performed at the time of injecting In-111 oxine-labelled WBC or immediately after completion of WBC scan. However, if Tc-HMPAO labelling is used, the WBC and marrow scan should be performed 48–72 h apart [29]. The advantage of performing WBC scans first is that if it is negative or normal, the marrow scan can be omitted.

Normal Distribution

Normal uptake of the Tc-HMPAO-labelled leukocytes is seen within the spleen, liver, bone marrow, kidneys, bowel, bladder and blood vessels. Renal and bladder activity appears within 15–30 min of the tracer injection, and the patients should be advised to void before the acquisition and over the course of 24 h following tracer injection to reduce the radiation dose to the bladder. Physiological bowel activity may be seen at 4 h, usually within the right iliac fossa and increases over time [23, 30]. Normal lung uptake is seen on the early images which gradually decreases over time and by 4 h becomes similar to background uptake [31].

Normal biodistribution of the In-111-labelled WBC is restricted to the liver, spleen and bone marrow. No bowel or bladder activity is present.

Pathological Uptake

In clinical practice, the planar images are visually analysed initially. The study is considered "negative" if no uptake is seen in relation to the prosthesis on either the 4 or 24 h images. A "positive" study is characterised by at least one focus of tracer uptake seen at the region of interest. The uptake typically increases over time from the 4 h images to the 24 h images.

Based on bacteriology and/or follow-up, Esper et al. found the sensitivity and specificity of the Tc-HMPAO WBC scan to be around 83% and 100%, respectively [32]. Erba et al. demonstrated a sensitivity of 88% and 100% for visual analysis of hip and knee prosthesis with radiolabelled WBC scan and a specificity of 82% and 62%, respectively [22]. Similar results were found in other studies using Tc-HMPAO-labelled leukocytes scan [33, 34].

In-111-labelled WBC scan showed a sensitivity and specificity of 77% and 86% in a study performed by Scher et al. [35]. Other studies using In-111 WBC scans have reported sensitivity of 83–100% and a specificity of 45–73% [36–38].

Bar-Shalom et al. [39] showed that addition of SPECT/CT improved diagnosis, localisation and assessment of the extent of disease in 48% of patients undergoing gallium-67 and WBC scan. SPECT/CT offered a significant contribution to final diagnosis in 35.7% of patients undergoing WBC scans in a study performed by Filippi et al. [27] SPECT/CT scans are not useful when the planar imaging is negative.

For a scintigraphic diagnosis of periprosthetic infection, uptake of white cells should be seen in areas in which there is no colloid uptake (spatial incongruence) or uptake of labelled white cells should be much more intense than the uptake of colloid. Seabold et al. [40] performed Tc-99m albumin colloid study on 34 patients with abnormal WBC scan. The marrow imaging improved specificity from 59% to 92%. The combined accuracy of WBC/marrow imaging is around 90%.

Imaging Using Labelled Antigranulocyte Antibodies

As an alternative to scintigraphy with labelled leukocytes, several studies have evaluated the role of technetium-labelled murine Fab fragments directed against NCA-90, a cell membrane protein found on granulocytes. The only commercially available version of this is sulesomab (LeukoScan™), labelled with technetium [41]. Typically an activity of around 900 MBq is administered yielding a dose of around 7.7 mSv. These have the advantage of a single injection without the need to remove and label blood products.

In patients with possible infection of either hip or knee prostheses, a sensitivity, specificity and positive predictive value of up to 100% for the diagnosis of prosthetic infection have been reported when used in combination with colloid imaging [42]. Another study [43], involving 78 consecutive patients with knee prosthesis, recommended dual time imaging at 4 h (early) and 24 h (delayed) to avoid false-positive results and to increase specificity.

The data on LeukoScan™ is however limited to a few trials and centres. Other drawbacks are that it is expensive and the use of mouse antibodies can trigger an allergic reaction. Therefore many departments continue to prefer labelled white cells in view of the much greater volume of data for accuracy.

Positron Emission Tomography/Computed Tomography (PET/CT)

In the recent years, PET/CT has been increasingly used in the evaluation of the prosthetic joint infections. The commonly used radiotracer is 18F-fluorodeoxyglucose (FDG), which is an analogue of glucose. The principle behind using this tracer is that there is increased glucose consumption by the infected tissues when compared with the normal tissues, leading to increased accumulation of the tracer at the site of infection.

Around 300–400 MBq of 18F-FDG is injected intravenously, and the images are obtained at 60–90 min. Usually the CT images are obtained without any intravenous contrast. The high resolution and high target to background uptake of tracers make it a favourable imaging modality. However, it is still not widely available and remains a relatively expensive modality.

In a preliminary study [44], FDG PET was performed in 23 patients with 28 prostheses referred for suspected prosthetic infection or loosening. The evaluation criteria for synovitis were when the uptake was seen solely within the synovial structures surrounding the prosthesis. When the uptake was seen at the bone prosthesis interface, it was considered either infection (if the uptake was intense) or aseptic loosening (if the uptake was intermediate). FDG PET correctly identified four prosthesis as infected, four prosthesis as loosening, 13 prosthesis with synovitis and three as unsuspected for loosening or infection. One case was false negative for loosening.

Another study compared FDG PET to combined In-111-labelled leukocyte/Tc-99m sulphur colloid imaging in 88 prostheses [45]. FDG PET was found to more sensitive in hip prosthesis evaluation (P = 0.0625). On its own, the FDG PET showed a sensitivity of 82% and specificity of 93% for detection of hip prosthesis infection and sensitivity of 95% and specificity of 88% for knee prosthesis infection.

The advantage of using FDG PET/CT is easy availability of the tracer and relatively straightforward technique. There is no need for handling blood products, scanning is completed in one visit, and the images are of higher quality. However the volume of literature is relatively limited, and more research is required before FDG PET/CT can be considered as a replacement for WBC/marrow imaging for detection of skeletal implant infections.

Imaging of Spinal Implants

In spinal surgical implants, isotope bone scans may be helpful for the identification of areas of increased biomechanical stress. In this circumstance SPECT/CT may be very helpful in the precise localisation of any abnormal uptake, particularly with reference to the anatomy of the metalwork. As there is normally a substantial amount of haematopoietic marrow in the vertebral bodies, labelled white cells will normally accumulate here. In cases of infection, there may be associated avascular necrosis and loss of the normal marrow, and areas of vertebral osteomyelitis related to spinal metalwork may show increased or decreased activity. For these reasons, in suspected spinal periprosthetic infection, imaging with labelled white cell scans is not routinely recommended.

References

1. Rushton N, Coakley AJ, Tudor J, Wraight EP. The value of technetium and gallium scanning in assessing pain after total hip replacement. J Bone Joint Surg Br. 1982;64(3):313–8.
2. Smith SL, Wastie ML, Forster I. Radionuclide bone scintigraphy in the detection of significant complications after total knee joint replacement. Clin Radiol. 2001;56(3):221–4.
3. Levitsky KA, Hozack WJ, Balderston RA, Rothman RH, Gluckman SJ, Maslack MM, et al. Evaluation of the painful prosthetic joint. Relative value of bone scan, sedimentation rate, and joint aspiration. J Arthroplasty. 1991;6(3):237–44.
4. Gemmel F, Van den Wyngaert H, Love C, Welling MM, Gemmel P, Palestro CJ. Prosthetic joint infections: radionuclide state-of-the-art imaging. Eur J Nucl Med Mol Imaging. 2012;39(5):892–909.
5. Merkel KD, Brown ML, Fitzgerald RH. Sequential technetium-99m HMDP-gallium-67 citrate imaging for the evaluation of infection in the painful prosthesis. J Nucl Med. 1986;27(9):1413–7.
6. Schauwecker DS, Park HM, Mock BH, Burt RW, Kernick CB, Ruoff AC, et al. Evaluation of complicating osteomyelitis with Tc-99m MDP, In-111 granulocytes, and Ga-67 citrate. J Nucl Med. 1984;25(8):849–53.
7. Palestro CJ, Swyer AJ, Kim CK, Goldsmith SJ. Infected knee prosthesis: diagnosis with In-111 leukocyte, Tc-99m sulfur colloid, and Tc-99m MDP imaging. Radiology. 1991;179(3):645–8.
8. McAfee JG, Thakur ML. Survey of radioactive agents for in vitro labeling of phagocytic leukocytes. I. Soluble agents. J Nucl Med. 1976;17(6):480–7.
9. McAfee JG, Thakur ML. Survey of radioactive agents for in vitro labeling of phagocytic leukocytes. II. Particles. J Nucl Med. 1976;17(6):488–92.
10. Peters AM, Danpure HJ, Osman S, Hawker RJ, Henderson BL, Hodgson HJ, et al. Clinical experience with 99mTc-hexamethylpropylene-amineoxime for labelling leucocytes and imaging inflammation. Lancet. 1986;2(8513):946–9.
11. Palestro CJ, Love C, Bhargava KK. Labeled leukocyte imaging: current status and future directions. Q J Nucl Med Mol Imaging. 2009;53(1):105–23.
12. Palestro CJ, Torres MA. Radionuclide imaging of nonosseous infection. Q J Nucl Med. 1999;43(1):46–60.
13. Bosetti M, Cannas M. The effect of bioactive glasses on bone marrow stromal cells differentiation. Biomaterials. 2005;26(18):3873–9.

14. Palestro CJ, Mehta HH, Patel M, Freeman SJ, Harrington WN, Tomas MB, et al. Marrow versus infection in the Charcot joint: indium-111 leukocyte and technetium-99m sulfur colloid scintigraphy. J Nucl Med. 1998;39(2):346–50.
15. Palestro CJ, Roumanas P, Swyer AJ, Kim CK, Goldsmith SJ. Diagnosis of musculoskeletal infection using combined In-111 labeled leukocyte and Tc-99m SC marrow imaging. Clin Nucl Med. 1992;17(4):269–73.
16. de Vries EF, Roca M, Jamar F, Israel O, Signore A. Guidelines for the labelling of leucocytes with (99m)Tc-HMPAO. Inflammation/Infection Taskgroup of the European Association of Nuclear Medicine. Eur J Nucl Med Mol Imaging. 2010;37(4):842–8.
17. Hammersley PA, Nkohkwo AT. Studies on white blood cell labelling: (99)Tc(m)-HMPAO preferentially labels granulocytes. Nucl Med Commun. 2001;22(9):981–6.
18. Peters AM. The utility of [99mTc]HMPAO-leukocytes for imaging infection. Semin Nucl Med. 1994;24(2):110–27.
19. Roca M, de Vries EF, Jamar F, Israel O, Signore A. Guidelines for the labelling of leucocytes with (111)In-oxine. Inflammation/Infection Taskgroup of the European Association of Nuclear Medicine. Eur J Nucl Med Mol Imaging. 2010;37(4):835–41.
20. Agool A, Glaudemans AW, Boersma HH, Dierckx RA, Vellenga E, Slart RH. Radionuclide imaging of bone marrow disorders. Eur J Nucl Med Mol Imaging. 2011;38(1):166–78.
21. Wilhelm AJ, Mijnhout GS, Franssen EJ. Radiopharmaceuticals in sentinel lymph-node detection—an overview. Eur J Nucl Med. 1999;26(4 Suppl):S36–42.
22. Erba PA, Glaudemans AW, Veltman NC, Sollini M, Pacilio M, Galli F, et al. Image acquisition and interpretation criteria for 99mTc-HMPAO-labelled white blood cell scintigraphy: results of a multicentre study. Eur J Nucl Med Mol Imaging. 2014;41(4):615–23.
23. Palestro CJ, ML. Brown, Forstrom LA, Bennett S. Greenspan, McAfee JG, Royal HD, et al. Society of nuclear medicine procedure guideline for 99mTc-exametazime (HMPAO)-labeled leukocyte scintigraphy for suspected infection/inflammation, version 3.0. Society of nuclear medicine procedure guidelines; 2004.
24. Palestro CJ, Brown ML, Forstrom LA, McAfee JG, Royal HD, Schauwecker DS, et al. Society of nuclear medicine procedure guideline for 111In-leukocyte scintigraphy for suspected infection/inflammation, version 3.0. Society of nuclear medicine procedure guidelines; 2004.
25. Kim HO, Na SJ, Oh SJ, Jung BS, Lee SH, Chang JS, et al. Usefulness of adding SPECT/CT to 99mTc-hexamethylpropylene amine oxime (HMPAO)-labeled leukocyte imaging for diagnosing prosthetic joint infections. J Comput Assist Tomogr. 2014;38(2):313–9.
26. Djekidel M, Brown RK, Piert M. Benefits of hybrid SPECT/CT for (111)In-oxine- and Tc-99m-hexamethylpropylene amine oxime-labeled leukocyte imaging. Clin Nucl Med. 2011;36(7):e50–6.
27. Filippi L, Schillaci O. Usefulness of hybrid SPECT/CT in 99mTc-HMPAO-labeled leukocyte scintigraphy for bone and joint infections. J Nucl Med. 2006;47(12):1908–13.
28. Hulme KW, Kappadath SC. Implications of CT noise and artifacts for quantitative 99mTc SPECT/CT imaging. Med Phys. 2014;41(4):042502.
29. Palestro CJ, Love C, Tronco GG, Tomas MB, Rini JN. Combined labeled leukocyte and technetium 99m sulfur colloid bone marrow imaging for diagnosing musculoskeletal infection. Radiographics. 2006;26(3):859–70.
30. Love C, Palestro CJ. Radionuclide imaging of inflammation and infection in the acute care setting. Semin Nucl Med. 2013;43(2):102–13.
31. Love C, Opoku-Agyemang P, Tomas MB, Pugliese PV, Bhargava KK, Palestro CJ. Pulmonary activity on labeled leukocyte images: physiologic, pathologic, and imaging correlation. Radiographics. 2002;22(6):1385–93.
32. el Esper I, Dacquet V, Paillard J, Bascoulergue G, Tahon MM, Fonroget J. 99Tcm-HMPAO-labelled leucocyte scintigraphy in suspected chronic osteomyelitis related to an orthopaedic device: clinical usefulness. Nucl Med Commun. 1992;13(11):799–805.
33. Devillers A, Moisan A, Jean S, Arvieux C, Bourguet P. Technetium-99m hexamethylpropylene amine oxime leucocyte scintigraphy for the diagnosis of bone and joint infections: a retrospective study in 116 patients. Eur J Nucl Med. 1995;22(4):302–7.
34. Pelosi E, Baiocco C, Pennone M, Migliaretti G, Varetto T, Maiello A, et al. 99mTc-HMPAO-leukocyte scintigraphy in patients with symptomatic total hip or knee arthroplasty: improved diagnostic accuracy by means of semiquantitative evaluation. J Nucl Med. 2004;45(3):438–44.
35. Scher DM, Pak K, Lonner JH, Finkel JE, Zuckerman JD, Di Cesare PE. The predictive value of indium-111 leukocyte scans in the diagnosis of infected total hip, knee, or resection arthroplasties. J Arthroplast. 2000;15(3):295–300.
36. Wukich DK, Abreu SH, Callaghan JJ, Van Nostrand D, Savory CG, Eggli DF, et al. Diagnosis of infection by preoperative scintigraphy with indium-labeled white blood cells. J Bone Joint Surg Am. 1987;69(9):1353–60.
37. Rand JA, Brown ML. The value of indium 111 leukocyte scanning in the evaluation of painful or infected total knee arthroplasties. Clin Orthop Relat Res. 1990;259:179–82.
38. Magnuson JE, Brown ML, Hauser MF, Berquist TH, Fitzgerald RH, Klee GG. In-111-labeled leukocyte scintigraphy in suspected orthopedic prosthesis infection: comparison with other imaging modalities. Radiology. 1988;168(1):235–9.

39. Bar-Shalom R, Yefremov N, Guralnik L, Keidar Z, Engel A, Nitecki S, et al. SPECT/CT using 67Ga and 111In-labeled leukocyte scintigraphy for diagnosis of infection. J Nucl Med. 2006;47(4):587–94.
40. Seabold JE, Nepola JV, Marsh JL, Hawes DR, Justin EP, Ponto JA, et al. Postoperative bone marrow alterations: potential pitfalls in the diagnosis of osteomyelitis with In-111-labeled leukocyte scintigraphy. Radiology. 1991;180(3):741–7.
41. Becker W, Palestro CJ, Winship J, Feld T, Pinsky CM, Wolf F, et al. Rapid imaging of infections with a monoclonal antibody fragment (LeukoScan). Clin Orthop Relat Res. 1996;(329):263–72.
42. Sousa R, Massada M, Pereira A, Fontes F, Amorim I, Oliveira A. Diagnostic accuracy of combined 99mTc-sulesomab and 99mTc-nanocolloid bone marrow imaging in detecting prosthetic joint infection. Nucl Med Commun. 2011;32(9):834–9.
43. Rubello D, Rampin L, Banti E, Massaro A, Cittadin S, Cattelan AM, et al. Diagnosis of infected total knee arthroplasty with anti-granulocyte scintigraphy: the importance of a dual-time acquisition protocol. Nucl Med Commun. 2008;29(4):331–5.
44. Manthey N, Reinhard P, Moog F, Knesewitsch P, Hahn K, Tatsch K. The use of [18 F]fluorodeoxyglucose positron emission tomography to differentiate between synovitis, loosening and infection of hip and knee prostheses. Nucl Med Commun. 2002;23(7):645–53.
45. Basu S, Kwee TC, Saboury B, Garino JP, Nelson CL, Zhuang H, et al. FDG PET for diagnosing infection in hip and knee prostheses: prospective study in 221 prostheses and subgroup comparison with combined (111)In-labeled leukocyte/(99m)Tc-sulfur colloid bone marrow imaging in 88 prostheses. Clin Nucl Med. 2014;39(7):609–15.

Index

S. Agarwal, G. J. Bansal (eds.), *Radiology of Orthopedic Implants*,
https://doi.org/10.1007/978-3-319-76009-4

MIX
Papier aus verantwortungsvollen Quellen
Paper from responsible sources
FSC® C105338

If you have any concerns about our products,
you can contact us on
ProductSafety@springernature.com

In case Publisher is established outside the EU,
the EU authorized representative is:
Springer Nature Customer Service Center GmbH
Europaplatz 3, 69115 Heidelberg, Germany

Printed by Libri Plureos GmbH
in Hamburg, Germany